UNDERSTANDING THE DANGERS OF CESAREAN BIRTH

Recent Titles in
The Praeger Series on Contemporary Health and Living

UNDERSTANDING THE DANGERS OF CESAREAN BIRTH

Making Informed Decisions

NICETTE JUKELEVICS

Foreword by
Charles Mahan, M.D.

The Praeger Series on Contemporary Health and Living
Julie Silver, M.D., Series Editor

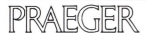

Westport, Connecticut
London

Library of Congress Cataloging-in-Publication Data

Jukelevics, Nicette, 1948–
   Understanding the dangers of cesarean birth : making informed decisions / Nicette Jukelevics ;
foreword by Charles Mahan.
      p.   cm. – (The Praeger series on contemporary health and living, ISSN 1932–8079)
   Includes bibliographical references and index.
   ISBN-13: 978–0–275–99906–3 (alk. paper)
   1. Cesarean section.   2. Mothers—Health and hygiene.   3. Self-care, Health.   I. Title.
   RG761.J85   2008
   618.8′6–dc22   2008020492

British Library Cataloguing in Publication Data is available.

Library of Congress Catalog Card Number: 2008020492
ISBN: 978–0–275–99906–3
ISSN: 1932–8079

First published in 2008

Praeger Publishers, 88 Post Road West, Westport, CT 06881
An imprint of Greenwood Publishing Group, Inc.
www.praeger.com

Printed in the United States of America

The paper used in this book complies with the
Permanent Paper Standard issued by the National
Information Standards Organization (Z39.48–1984).

10 9 8 7 6 5 4 3 2 1

This book is for general information only. No book can ever substitute for the judgment of a
medical professional. If you have worries or concerns, contact your doctor.

In memory of my mother, Grace,

and

for my husband Tibor, my daughter, Lisa, and my son, Eric. I am grateful for your love, support, and encouragement, and especially for your personal contributions to this book.

CONTENTS

SERIES FOREWORD

Over the past hundred years, there have been incredible medical break-throughs that have prevented or cured illness in billions of people and helped many more improve their health while living with chronic conditions. A few of the most important twentieth-century discoveries include antibiotics, organ transplants, and vaccines. The twenty-first century has already heralded important new treatments including such things as a vaccine to prevent human papillomavirus from infecting and potentially leading to cervical cancer in women. Polio is on the verge of being eradicated worldwide, making it only the second infectious disease behind smallpox to ever be erased as a human health threat.

In this series, experts from many disciplines share with readers important and updated medical knowledge. All aspects of health are considered including subjects that are disease-specific and preventive medical care. Disseminating this information will help individuals to improve their health as well as researchers to determine where there are gaps in our current knowledge and policy-makers to assess the most pressing needs in health care.

Series Editor Julie Silver, M.D.
Assistant Professor
Harvard Medical School
Department of Physical Medicine and Rehabilitation

FOREWORD

I have been practicing obstetrics and gynecology either from a patient care or public health perspective for over 40 years and have never seen our once-proud specialty in the dire straits that it is now in America. The author of this book carefully and effectively presents the social and scientific evidence that, in one very serious intervention in birth, cesarean section, things have rapidly spun out of control—from the occasionally necessary surgical procedure to one that actually outnumbers vaginal birth in some of our hospitals.

How has this accelerating increase in delivery by major abdominal surgery, which now accounts for over 30 percent of all births, benefited our country in terms of birth outcomes since the turn of this century? Not much is the answer. Our infant mortality rates, dropping nicely the last 20 years, have stalled and are flat, leaving the United States thirty-second of all developed countries by this important measure. (Infant mortality is considered the best overall measure of how a country cares for the health of all of its citizens.)

Our premature birthrates, stable for over 70 years (while other countries lowered theirs satisfactorily), have started to rise rapidly this century. This has been especially true of late preterm births, from 35 to 37 completed weeks. This group represents the main reason preterm births are increasing, and as this book points out, many of these children have permanent development problems and learning disabilities since they were born before their brains were mature. Our studies in Florida are showing that as much as two-thirds of our increase in late preterm births is associated with the increasing use of cesareans, often without a trial of labor.

Perhaps most alarming is the increase in maternal deaths in the past 5 years. Many of these are postcesarean and due to infection, uncontrolled bleeding, and blood clots that travel to the lungs. This is the first trend upward in mothers dying during or after birth that we have seen for over 100 years in the United States.

So the cesarean rate goes up, and our nation's birth outcomes get worse; is there anything good to be said for this major abdominal operation? Well, on the financial side of the issue, scheduled cesareans save time for the hospital and doctor, and time is money. The uncynical answer is that around 15 percent of people giving birth really need a cesarean that can be lifesaving for some mothers and babies. But when we go over that number, we venture far into the realm of unnecessary surgery, as we did years ago with hysterectomies, and this becomes a public health problem. And as this book reveals, birth by cesarean can have a serious psychological impact on mothers and their ability to care for their newborn the way they would like to.

In this book expectant mothers, birth activists, and maternity care professionals will find mother-centered, comprehensive, evidence-based information and extensive resources to help avoid a medically unnecessary cesarean section. Mothers will also find that they have many choices about how they want to give birth and where and with whom they can have a satisfying birth and reduce their odds for a cesarean. Health professionals will better understand how routine medical interventions and birth practices complicate labor and increase health risks for mothers and babies and how changes can be made to facilitate labor and birth. If a mother is going to have a cesarean birth she will find excellent suggestions to help her make informed decisions about the surgical procedure, anesthesia, postpartum recovery, and enhancing her opportunity for mother–infant attachment and breastfeeding.

From my perspective, I would like to present some ideas as to how we can turn this around and rescue normal birth from unnecessary technological interventions. Some of these actions may seem quite radical to some, but harsh times call for innovative thinking and tough moves. After all, where has our polite acquiescing to the medical-industrial establishment gotten us? Lots of scars on lots of bellies and some of the worst mother and child health outcomes in the world! Read this book. Learn from the author's research on cesarean section, her many years of experience in prenatal and childbirth education. Then come back again to consider these proposals for making change on a national level.

ACTION STEPS

Change Care Providers and Set Standards

As the evidence in this book shows, midwives should be the primary care givers for all healthy pregnant women in the United States. Over the next 10 years, general OB-GYN residency training programs should be phased out and only a critical number of maternal-fetal medicine physician specialists trained to provide backup to midwives for high-risk pregnancies.

The national Medicare program that pays hospitals to train residents can shift those payments to train midwives. Medicare should also fund efficient distance education programs such as the Frontier School of Nursing's CNEP program housed in Kentucky, which produces more midwives and nurse practitioners each year than any program in the country. Since the newest generation of obstetricians has announced it doesn't want to work nights and week-ends, more no-labor cesareans should be expected. A pleasant and rewarding lifestyle could be had with practice groups of two maternal-fetal medicine doctors, six midwives, and six doulas—plus better outcomes and fewer cesareans.

Speaking of doulas (women professionally trained to provide emotional and physical support in labor), every pregnant woman should have one before, during, and after birth. You will read about the health benefits of doula care in this book. Doulas can be recruited from low-income communities and trained using Welfare-to-Work monies. Insurance companies should be mandated to pay for doula services. State laws and regulations need to change, so that midwives can practice independently without formal ties to doctors.

National and state practice standards should be set for when, where, and why a cesarean can be performed and when it cannot. The standards would be linked to payment with yearly audits and payback penalties if they were not followed. Doctors often argue that this is "cookbook medicine" and inter-feres with the "art" of medicine, whatever that is, but the fact of life is that medicine is the only major industry in the United States where reimbursement for services is not linked to adherence to a set of scientific evidence–based standards. Regulation is a scary word for some, but it is seriously needed in U.S. health care today. It would actually help protect doctors and midwives from malpractice suits—as long as they followed the standards.

Payer Reform

All payers, public and private, should be expected to pay according to the performance and outcome standards discussed above. If insurers are not conforming to good practice, such as not paying for VBACs, meet with your state government insurance commissioners to help bring them in to line. Lobby your state Medicaid program directors via your favorite local legislator to change how they pay for birth services. One idea: $2,000 for a VBAC; $1,800 for a vaginal birth; and $1,000 for a cesarean.

Legal Maneuvers

To restore the important option of VBAC around the country, train friendly doctors and nurses to become expert witnesses in legal liability cases to help out doctors or midwives who have been sued for not doing a cesarean. This would build goodwill toward normal birth advocates in the practice community.

Boycott doctors and hospitals that won't provide VBACs, and direct patients to ones that do. If this fails, work with friendly legislators to get state regulators of hospitals and the Medicaid program to drop them off the Medicaid payment list, if they don't comply. Since Medicaid pays for about half the births in most states, this could have a big impact. Get birth advocates placed on local hospital boards and on advisory boards for the state agencies mentioned earlier.

In some states, nurse practice acts are hostile to midwife and nurse prac-titioner practice: work to get these changed. If hospitals won't let midwives on staff or insurers refuse to pay for midwife, doula, birth center, or home birth care, ask a friendly lawyer to threaten to report them to the Federal Trade Commission for restraint of trade. The National Quality Forum (NQF), a volunteer consensus standard-setting organization and leading government advisory body, has endorsed quality measures which include perinatal care, including from the last trimester of pregnancy through hospital discharge for both mothers and newborns. The NQF's endorsed measures include care provided by clinicians, hospitals, and freestanding birth centers. The Coalition for Improving Maternity Services and other advocacy groups should encourage entities that set maternity care quality measures, health plans, hospitals, health professional groups, payers of maternity and newborn care and health systems to use the NQF evidence-based quality measures. This will ensure that mothers and babies get the care that they deserve.

If all of the above fail, or in spite of it nothing changes, involve the trial lawyers. Ask to make brief presentations to trial lawyer association meetings about the damage to mothers and especially babies due to elective induction of labor and elective cesarean with no medical indication. They'll catch on quickly and, hopefully with a few high profile lawsuits aimed at poor infant outcomes due to unnecessary cesareans, so will the doctors and hospitals.

POLITICS—NOT AS USUAL

The first 8 years of this new century have not been kind to those of us interested in better health for Americans. After 15 years, health and health care have once again risen to the top of the nation's concerns. Opportunity for positive change abounds. If we want change, we each need to be much more politically active than we have been. We need to be in the politicians' faces and minds as much and as effectively as the insurance lobbyists are. We need to support more women to run for office and nurture them to support normal birth. A few good friends in Congress or the state legislature can make a world of difference.

When people are running for office, whether county commission, state legislature, Congress, or President, childbirth advocacy groups should send them lists of questions about what they will do to support your issues and publish their responses in the local newspaper and newsletters or on the Web. Also, after they are in office, ask your local paper to publish the votes on all issues and how each representative voted.

Petition your governor to establish a statewide cabinet in the governor's office, specifically devoted to women's and children's issues.

Have your people in Congress actively support the currently developing National Children's Study which will follow children into adulthood so we can better learn the long-term consequences of unnecessary interventions at the time of birth. Most importantly, vote each time and support good candidates with money and/or work. And our biggest need is more midwives, doulas, and advocates for normal birth to run for office.

EDUCATING THE UNEDUCATED—AMERICANS

I think it's safe to say that the average American woman hasn't a clue about what she ought to expect to have a normal pregnancy, birth, and baby. Heck, most labor and delivery nurses don't know that definitive studies 20 years ago showed that the most ubiquitous technology in their delivery units—the electronic fetal monitor—doesn't give useful information. Most obstetricians don't know that late preterm babies have brains that are not fully developed.

This is why new and unique efforts need to be made to reach the public with good information. The Coalition for Improving Maternity Services (CIMS) G.A.C. (Grassroots Advocacy Committee) movement is one such exciting idea. You will read about several other national efforts to promote accurate and transparent information on cesareans in this book. We need to do assertiveness training for our best advocates, so they can argue their case for normal birth toe-to-toe with interventionist doctors and nurses. We need to find new ways to spark interest in childbirth education classes where attendance has been declining rapidly this century. We need to recruit famous people who have enjoyed normal births to speak to the public for us to counteract the damage done by the popular culture. Great examples are Cindy Crawford and Ricky Lake, both of whom appear in excellent new childbirth films.

New York's law requiring hospitals to publish birth data is an excellent model, but consumers also need detailed information about the practice habits and outcomes of every doctor and midwife in their communities. A yearly questionnaire should be sent to each practitioner with a list of questions about his or her practice that we would all like to know, and the answers would be published online or in print. If they declined to answer, that would be noted—and then there would be a good chance they'd answer next time! The CIMS Birth Survey (www.thebirthsurvey.com) and proprietary groups like Angie's List are taking steps in this direction.

Another highly effective modality we have used in the past in Florida is using a self-test. People love them. The Healthy Baby Test was a one-page tear-off sheet placed in laundromats, buses, and churches, and if a person took the test and had a high score, she was directed to call the March of Dimes, local health department, or her health care provider. We couldn't restock them fast enough.

STORMING THE MEDIA

Stop letting *The Today Show* (for example) have an "expert doctor" tell its audience that cesarean on maternal request is "probably OK" with no opposing view. Call and write the network when news shows or soap operas portray the wrong information.

Monitor government publications and Web sites, and if they give inaccurate or biased information, write the appropriate agency to protest, with a copy to your senator and congressperson.

If you like to write, send guest editorial or community columnist pieces to your local paper, summarizing some of the more alarming information in this book. Or send a book review of this and other pregnancy-related books to the paper and be harshly critical of the ones (and there are many) with inaccurate, and sometimes dangerous, information.

Regularly read the obstetric and midwifery journals. When less than scientifically rigorous articles are published or the media reports uncritically on faulty study conclusions comment on them in professional publications, Web sites, blogs, and the popular press.

There have been many fine articles published recently that back up the concerns exposed in this book and it would be great if the CIMS, Childbirth Connection, Lamaze International, the International Childbirth Education Association, and similar organizations would publish press releases the day positive articles appear. Using the media to your advantage does not have to be expensive. It just takes a little time, thought, ingenuity, and a rapid response.

INFORMED CONSENT THAT REALLY INFORMS

Hardly any patient, man or woman, rich or poor, could tell you what was on that outpatient procedure or hospital consent form they just signed. So when the rare mother does die from a pulmonary embolus after her cesarean, it is a double shock to the family because, as they are likely to say, "Nobody told us she might be more likely to die after that operation compared to normal birth!" The way we currently manage so-called informed consent is generally useless as information (especially in court) and very effectively hides the danger of medical procedures from patients.

In my opinion this is the area where use of the information in this book could help take the biggest step to reform. Use it to develop true informed consent forms that contain all pertinent factual information about the pros and cons of the procedure and give it to expectant mothers to study and absorb and query at the right times, not on admission to the hospital.

This book and all of the recent research that Childbirth Connection has done on birth interventions provide all the scientific evidence one needs to build a comprehensive set of consent forms. There should be separate forms for labor induction, epidural, VBAC, cesarean, repeat cesarean, forceps, vacuum extraction, and vaginal birth. The possible benefits of the procedure should be covered, but the hidden dangers should be highlighted. Also all women, after reading the chapter on the impact of cesareans on the baby, should get a copy of the new March of Dimes "Brain Card."

When should women get these consent forms? They should get a complete set of forms at their preconception visit—an individual form covering one of the areas at each prenatal visit starting with the cesarean form. And if they are having a normal vaginal birth but have to have an unexpected emergency cesarean then the VBAC and repeat cesarean forms to help think about the future should also be sent home to them.

As an OB-GYN resident I was taught a valuable way to present informed consent in my opinion. The doctor or midwife sits down with the woman at a prenatal visit to cover, say, the epidural consent at this visit. They underline key positive and negative effects of the procedure, send the form home for the patient to discuss with family and friends, and ask her to return with the form and any questions she may have. The discussion is noted in the chart, and in each of the consent forms it is noted what the woman thinks she might prefer at that time—agreeing that she can always change her mind. This is not only true informed consent but also a great teaching opportunity which is what prenatal care is supposed to be all about but has drifted away from recently.

THE LAST HARANGUE

If you just read this book, shelve it, and go about your business—surprise—change will not occur. We are the richest country in the history of the world, and we are seriously endangering our future by letting healthy birth be stolen from us. This is immediately becoming apparent with the poor outcomes of late preterm babies.

We have been passive, complacent, apathetic, and lacking concern for our neighbors' and our country's children, even our own. If those of us who fervently believe in healthy births don't develop a new activism, a new assertiveness, a new meanness toward the technocrats who are ruining our birth experiences and outcomes, things will keep on getting worse this century.

Childbirth advocates are nice people—probably too nice to effect real change. Are we going to stay nice or shed that image and get fierce for a cause that is so important for the future of our families and our country? As the famous line in the old movie goes, "I'm mad as hell, and I'm not taking it any more." Are we mad enough to stop doing business as usual and get out and change things for mothers and babies? I sure hope so. I'm with you.

Charles Mahan, M.D., F.A.C.O.G.
Dean and Proffesor Emeritus
University of South Florida Colleges
of Public Health & Medicine

PREFACE

Every childbearing woman is a giver of life and should be honored and respected no matter how her child is born. Birth can be a creative, transformative, and an empowering experience. It can also be traumatic, disempowering, and oppressive. A cesarean is a potentially lifesaving procedure, but increasingly, we are learning that performing these operations above a certain level does not increase health outcomes for mothers or their infants. In fact, high numbers of cesareans put healthy mothers and their babies at risk. The infant mortality rate is rising in the United States despite our highest cesarean rate ever, 31.1 percent in 2006. More babies are being born preterm and not surviving. More mothers having cesareans are experiencing serious complications in subsequent pregnancies. The Centers for Disease Control has linked these outcomes with increasing inductions, and the rising number of cesareans, many of them performed without labor for "no indicated risk." That is, no medical diagnosis was recorded in the birth records.

Many outdated birth practices are still being implemented illogically in hospital births, most leading to complications that eventually lead to a cesarean section. Current national obstetric policies are encouraging women to have a cesarean even when no medical indication exists. They are also limiting women's options and leaving them no choice but to have routine repeat operations, the majority of which could be avoided. These policies are divisive and violate human rights. Concern about the health impact of rising cesareans is worldwide. Countries like Britain and Brazil are already implementing policies to reduce cesareans on a national scale.

In my 30 years in maternal-child health as a perinatal and childbirth educator, I have seen childbirth become more technologically intensive and more restrictive of women's choices. Women becoming more and more fearful of giving birth and less and less aware of their options. I decided to write this book because I firmly believe that many childbearing women, their families, along with an increasing number of maternity-care professionals are disturbed and concerned about the unprecedented number of healthy women who are giving birth unnecessarily by major abdominal surgery. Many, I believe, are doing so without knowledge of the risks associated with the operation and its impact on their early parenting experience. The words themselves, cesarean section, c-section, section, cesarean birth, c-birth, and cesarean delivery, are value laden and invoke powerful feelings and responses from mothers themselves.

My many years in maternal-child health began as a part-time interest. A way to stay home and raise my daughter during the day and maintain my professional training and interest in teaching a few hours at night. Retraining to be a childbirth educator seemed to make perfect sense. When my son was born, almost 5 years later, it served me well. Classes were taught at night or on weekends. Over the years I felt honored and privileged to be a part of such an important and hopeful time in parents' lives. I shared a small part of their joy and excitement as they came to learn about a healthy pregnancy in their first trimester, and as they prepared for childbirth, learned about newborn baby care, and in their first year when new mothers would come with their infants to "Mommy & Me" classes. I was also privileged to provide labor support to several mothers who attended my VBAC (vaginal birth after cesarean) classes. I was asked by a few mothers to go in with them into the operating room for a cesarean birth. I kept in touch with them in the first weeks after they gave birth.

No matter their age, culture, race, religion, or profession, I learned that all parents had the same hopes and dreams for themselves and their family. They all wanted what was best for their children. I also learned that if given accurate information and encouraged to participate in their own care, mothers would eventually make their own best decisions—decisions that made sense and felt right for them given their own personal history, values, and life circumstances. Mothers taught me that each woman and pregnancy is unique. What may be empowering to one, say laboring and giving birth without any drugs, may be extremely frightening and distressing to another. For some mothers, a cesarean may be the safest way, medically or psychologically, to give birth. For others a cesarean may be experienced as a form of institutional violence.

As time passed we began to include information about electronic fetal monitoring in childbirth classes, that is, how fetal heart rate is recorded second by second. We taught fathers how to read the fetal monitor strips. The technology was always fascinating and reassuring. As things changed we added information about ultrasound screenings: stress tests; nonstress tests; amniocentesis; inductions; cervical ripening agents; use of IV lines; amniotomy (breaking the bag of waters); epidurals for labor; folley catheters (to empty the bladder); forceps and vacuum extractors. As more and more women were giving birth by cesarean section we added information about the procedure, options for anesthesia, and postoperative recovery. What began as lessons on innovations and practices that promised to keep mothers' labors short and pain-free and babies safe from brain damage or death became, over the years, lessons in how to avoid these very same procedures.

Many maternity care professionals were disturbed by the studies that began to be published about the harms associated with the routine use of these birth practices. They did not reflect evidence-based care. In the words of the authors of *A Guide to Effective Care in Pregnancy and Childbirth*, the "gold standard" for evidence-based maternity care, "Evidence-based care has been defined as the [conscientious, judicious, and explicit use of current best evidence in making decisions about the care of individual patients]."

Used routinely for healthy women, these practices complicated labor, made it more painful, increased risks for infection, hyperstimulated contractions, increased the incidence of fetal distress (nonreassuring fetal heart rate), and consequently, cesareans. The interventions compromised the health of newborns and made it more difficult to breastfeed. Mothers were having a more difficult time caring for their infants. They spent less and less time in the hospital recovering from their birth. Mothers who had a cesarean were being discharged too soon considering they were still also full-fledged surgical patients. In the first few days at home many new parents found it difficult to deal alone with newborn jaundice, dehydration, and feeding difficulties with the baby. Mothers who were still healing from an episiotomy, an instrumental delivery, or the side effects of major abdominal surgery, were blaming themselves for not being better mothers.

As we continued to learn about the complications associated with these interventions, some of us felt compelled to teach parents about informed consent, informed refusal, and patient rights. Some of us who also taught hospital-based classes were reprimanded. Occasionally a physician would call my department head at a hospital I was working for and complain that patients who attended a specific childbirth class on a specific night had learned that electronic monitoring increased the risk for cesareans, an amniotomy raised the odds for infection and fetal distress, an epidural may lead to an instrumental delivery, or that VBAC (vaginal birth after a prior cesarean) was safe. Whenever I was called in, my response would always be the same, "Yes, I said all those things and here are the studies to back it up."

Occasionally, when I was asked to support a mother laboring for a VBAC, I saw firsthand how labor was managed. I learned that the decision to go ahead with a cesarean could be based on factors that have nothing to do with the health status of the mother or her unborn child. Occasionally a physician on call who had to monitor patients at two separate hospitals a few miles from each other would decide after a few trips back and forth that labor was "slow," or "was not going anywhere." Or it was 3 AM, and the physician had been on call since 7 AM the previous morning, and just performed an emergency cesarean on a mother who came in with dangerously high blood pressure. Since he had to wake up the assisting surgeon in the middle of the night to come to the hospital and since the operating team was already assembled, the physician worried that he might have to do this again in a couple of hours if complications developed with the mother laboring for a VBAC. I have great respect for the many nurses who used creative ways to avoid a cesarean they felt was not needed, since both the mother and her baby were not in any danger.

In all my years of hospital-based and community-based teaching, I can say that individually maternity care professionals are dedicated, work hard, and feel they are doing their best to serve the women and families they care for. Somehow, forces beyond any one individual's control seemed to be pushing for more interventions, faster labors, more documentation to avoid malpractice suits, and less time with patients.

Years ago I chose to have two unmedicated births with my husband at my side. My caregivers were supportive and I received excellent care. I know that is not the right choice for all women. When with my first pregnancy I asked my doctor about a referral to a childbirth preparation class because I wanted to avoid medication, he supported my choice, but with the referral he said, "O.K. you want to have a natural childbirth, but you don't want your child to grow up to be an elevator operator, do you?" Those words meant little to me at the time but were never forgotten. Years later I understood that my obstetrician wanted the best for me but firmly believed that babies can suffer from brain damage or death if he couldn't intervene in labor some way.

I hope that childbearing women and their families may find some value in this book: learn about their options and make more choices about how they want to give birth. I have tried to base my book on the best current evidence, confident that women are capable and have the right to make their own best decisions. My hope is also to make a small difference with the health professionals who dedicate their lives to caring for childbearing women and their families; to gain some knowledge, and perhaps find the inspiration and courage to help make the changes many believe are long overdue.

Acknowledgments

Thousands of expectant parents and many maternity care professionals have crossed my path in these last three decades, and they have enriched my understanding and appreciation of childbirth and family. I have learned much. I have volunteered with and have been inspired by many strong and dedicated women. Women whose love for mothers and babies, whose trust and confidence in the value and power of a good birth, despite the obstacles, has never waivered.

I am grateful for the contributions of so many people who so generously gave of their time, shared their resources, their expertise, and wisdom, all of which has greatly enriched this book. All have offered their assistance without having first read the manuscript and therefore they may not agree with my perspective on the current state of childbirth in this country.

I am deeply grateful to Sarah J. Buckley, MD; Richard Nelson, MD; Susan Jenkins, JD; Ina May Gaskin, CPM; Marsden Wagner, MD, MS; Penny Simkin, PT; Larry Leeman, MD, MPH; Ginger Breedlove, PhD, CNM; J. Zhang, PhD, MD; Douglas Brooks, MD; Rebecca Jacobs, Fay Menacker, DrPH, CPNP, Peggy O'Mara, Katherine Campbell Phillips, MPH; and the U.S. Agency for Healthcare Research and Quality, Healthcare Cost and Utilization Project. Also to Shana dela Cruz and Martens & Kiefer, thank you for your illustrations, which have made this book come alive. To Dr. Matthew A. Clark, my deep appreciation for formatting my first jumbled draft into a meaningful and professional manuscript and reviewing the accuracy of the surgical procedure.

To Childbirth Connection, and the CIMS Expert Work Group (EWG), my gratitude for their research and contribution to the literature on issues that significantly impact childbearing women and their families. They have filled in a huge gap in the birth literature. I continue to be inspired by the CIMS Leadership, past and present, by their vision and tireless dedication to improving maternity care.

Dr. Michele Lauria, thank you for your careful and insightful review of the chapters on cesarean section and VBAC. To Mary Zwart, Duteh Midwife,

Robbie Davis-Floyd, Mayri Sagady Leslie, CNM, Idadarragh, CPM, and Maureen Corry, MPH, I thank you for taking the time to edit and comment on the chapter on midwives. Special thanks to Linda Herrick, RN CD (DONA), Ellie Shea, RN CD (DONA), Ginger Breedlove, CNM, PhD, and Dr. Douglas Brooks for their contribution to the chapter on doulas. To Carol Sakala, PhD, and Ruth Wilf, CNM, PhD, I am deeply grateful for your support and faith in the value of this project.

To Ruth Ancheta, thank you for your generosity in allowing me to reproduce your drawings. Many more women will now stand up for themselves and refuse to lie down to give birth. For my editor, Debbie Carvalko at Praeger, many thanks for your guidance and patience as I worked my way through this new process of book publishing. I'm especially thankful to Diony Young who suggested I send my controversial book proposal to Praeger Publishers.

To Judy, Diane, and my sister J, my heartfelt appreciation for your love, support, and encouragement throughout this long and challenging journey. For my daughter, Lisa, who literally midwifed me through this arduous but ultimately satisfying journey, thank you for not letting me quit several times along the way and reminding me that young women like you "need this book."

And to Dr. Charles Mahan, who did not know me, but agreed to write the Forword based on my overview and outline of the book, I owe you a debt of gratitude: for validating this work, for having the integrity and courage to speak up, and inspiring women and health professionals to create a new activism to give birth back to women where it duly belongs.

ABBREVIATIONS

AABC	American Association of Birth Centers
AAFP	American Association of Family Physicians
ABM	Academy of Breastfeeding Medicine
ACNM	American College of Nurse-Midwives
ACOG	American College of Obstetricians and Gynecologists
AFAR	Alliance Francophone pour l'Accouchement Respecté
AHRQ	Agency for Healthcare Research and Quality
AMA	American Medical Association
APHA	American Public Health Association
AWHONN	the Association of Women's Health, Obstetrics, and Neonatal Nursing
BFHI	Baby-Friendly Hospital Initiative
CDC	Centers for Disease Control
CDMR	cesarean delivery on maternal request
CfM	Citizens for Midwifery
CIMS	Coalition for Improving Maternity Services
CM	certified midwife
CNM	certified nurse midwife
CPM	certified professional midwife
CSE	combined spinal-epidural

DIC	disseminated intravascular coagulation
DONA	Doulas of North America
DVT	deep vein thrombosis
EFM	electronic fetal monitoring
ECV	external cephalic version
FBS	fetal blood sampling
FDA	Federal Drug Administration
FIGO	the International Federation of Gynecology and Obstetrics
GAC	Grassroots Advocacy Committee
HIPPA	Health Insurance Portability and Accountability Act of 1996 (U.S.)
HIV	human immunodeficiency virus
ICAN	International Cesarean Awareness Network
ICEA	International Childbirth Education Association
IOM	Institute of Medicine
IV	intravenous fluids
LOA	left occiput anterior
LTM II	Listening to Mothers II Survey
MANA	Midwives Alliance of North America
MCA	Maternity Center Association
MCWP	Maternity Care Working Party
MFCI	Mother-Friendly Childbirth Initiative
MRSA	methicillin-resistant staphylococcus aurous
NARM	North American Registry of Midwives
NCCA	National Commission on Certifying Agencies
NEC	necrotizing enterocolitis
NICE	National Institute for Clinical Excellence
NICHD	National Institute of Child Health and Development
NCQA	National committee for Quality Assurance

NICU	neonatal intensive care unit
NIH	National Institutes of Health
NIR	no indicated risk
NNEPQIN	Northern New England Perinatal Quality Improvement Network
NQF	National Quality Forum
OB-GYN	obstetrician/gynecologist, obstetrics/gynology
OP	occiput posterior
PCA	patient controlled analgesia
PLICO	Physicians Liability Insurance Company
PROM	premature rupture of the membranes
PTSD	Posttraumatic Stress Disorder
RDS	respiratory distress syndrome
REDUCE	Research and Education to Reduce Unnecessary Cesareans
ROA	right occiput anterior
SOGC	Society of Obstetricians and Gynecologists of Canada
TOLAC	trial of labor after a cesarean
VBAC	vaginal birth after a prior cesarean
WHO	World Health Organization

INTRODUCTION

The American health care delivery system is in need of fundamental change. Many patients, doctors, nurses, and health care leaders are concerned that the care delivered is not, essentially, the care we should receive... The frustration levels of both patients and clinicians have probably never been higher. Yet the problems remain. Health care today harms too frequently and routinely fails to deliver its potential benefits. Americans should be able to count on receiving care that meets their needs and is based on the best scientific knowledge. Yet there is strong evidence that this frequently is not the case.[1]

Despite unprecedented access to medical research findings and the rapid development of medical technology, the quality of care in the United States leaves much to be desired. How appropriate, safe, effective, and economically sound is that care, are issues that have only recently begun to be explored and examined. In 1996, the Institute of Medicine (IOM) launched an intensive and comprehensive effort to evaluate and improve the quality of health care that Americans receive. The Institute defined the quality of care as "the degree to which health services for individuals and populations increase the likelihood of desired health outcomes and are consistent with current professional knowledge."[2] In more general terms, medical care, drugs, tests, and procedures should recommended, prescribed, or performed by health care professionals if they are likely to increase the odds for improved health outcomes and are based on sound scientific knowledge. The Institute of Medicine identified pregnancy and childbirth-appropriate prenatal and intrapartum care, as one of twenty priority areas for health care improvement.[3]

Cesarean section is the most common major surgical procedure performed in the United States. More than 1.3 million in 2006. The majority of the operations do not increase the odds for improved health outcomes and many of the indications for which they are performed are not based on sound scientific knowledge. Rather, the high rate of cesarean deliveries puts both women and babies at increased short-term and long-term health risks. In 2006 the U.S.

cesarean rate was 31.1 percent the highest ever recorded and a 50 percent increase since 1996.[4] Medical experts, including the U.S. National Health Service, maintain that at least one-third to one-half of these operations can safely be avoided.[5, 6]

According to the Medical Leadership Council, an association of over 2,500 U.S. hospitals, the operations are often performed based on outdated medical assumptions, lack of clear clinical guidelines, fear of liability, and economic advantages that are often measured in time rather than dollars. The lack of accountability for physicians' or hospitals' cesarean rate also contributes to the high number of cesarean births.[7] The routine use of medical interventions including elective inductions of labor and electronic fetal monitoring are contributing to the rising number of cesareans. There would be fewer cesareans if more women with a breech were offered the option of an external version, a safe method of turning a breech to a vertex (head down) presentation, and more women given the choice of laboring after a prior cesarean delivery.[8]

Cesareans are also increasing for low-risk, full-term women giving birth for the first time. If they become pregnant again, they are highly likely to have a repeat operation. In 2003, 23.6 percent of low-risk women gave birth by cesarean. The term "low risk" is defined as at least 37 completed weeks of gestation with a singleton pregnancy and a vertex (head-down) presentation. These are healthy women least likely to need a cesarean. Almost 90 percent of low-risk women with a prior cesarean birth had a repeat operation[9] despite evidence that 75 percent of low-risk women with one prior cesarean can labor and have a safe VBAC (vaginal birth after cesarean). Women with no medical indications are having planned cesareans. The Centers for Disease Control (CDC) estimate that up to 7 percent of women have a primary cesarean (first cesarean) with no indicated risk.[10] Increasing cesareans are not exclusive to the United States. "Modern" American obstetrics has been imported by many other countries where cesarean rates have reached alarming rates, especially for women of higher economic status in countries with a public health service. High cesarean rates can be found in countries worldwide: in Latin America,[11] the Republic of Korea,[12] Thailand,[13] Britain,[14] Puerto Rico,[15] and Italy.[16]

More than two decades ago the World Health Organization found no improved health outcomes for countries with a higher than 15 percent cesarean rate. Countries with a less than 15 percent cesarean rate had equal or better maternal and infant health outcomes.[17] The WHO recommendation was based on research, debate, and eventual consensus between members of a multidisciplinary international team who examined the perinatal services of twenty-three European member states as well as those of Canada, Australia, and China. Respected researchers state that "the optimal rate is not known, but little improvement in outcome appears to occur when rates rise above a minimum level."[18]

Toward the end of the 1970s, when the U.S. cesarean rate was 16 percent, the benefits of a surgical delivery no longer seemed to outweigh the risks. Dr. Mortimer Rosen (who chaired the National Institute of Child Health and Human Development Consensus Panel on Cesarean Childbirth in 1979) wrote,

"We were delivering more and more babies by cesarean, but about the same percentage of them died and about the same percentage were born with brain damage or other problems."[19] More than a decade ago a national survey of U.S. hospital cesarean rates by the Public Citizen's Health Research Group found that many Level III hospitals (those with a neonatal intensive care unit), the ones most likely to serve a higher risk population had lower overall cesarean rates than those without. Hospitals affiliated with a medical school (large teaching hospitals), many also with neonatal intensive care units (NICUs) had lower primary and total cesarean rates and much higher VBAC rates compared to community and private institutions.[20] Healthy mothers were having more cesareans.

In 1995, as part of the Institute for Healthcare Improvement's Breakthrough Series, health care organizations from the United States and Canada worked together to safely reduce their cesarean section rates, while maintaining maternal and infant outcomes. By instituting evidence-based measures, making changes in hospital policy, and reducing the use of routine medical procedures associated with a higher risk for cesarean, several institutions were able to reduce their cesarean rate to 15 percent or less without compromising maternal or infant health.[21] In 1998, the Institute of Medicine's National Roundtable on Health Care Quality concluded that there was an "urgent need to improve health care quality" in the United States. The report pointed to the overuse, underuse, and misuse of medical procedures and services. "Overuse occurs when a health care service is provided under circumstances in which its potential for harm exceeds the possible benefit."[22] Cesarean section is a prime example of the overuse of a major surgical procedure. Cesarean sections do not prevent pelvic floor disorders later in life,[23] do not reduce the risk of cerebral palsy,[24] do not necessarily improve outcomes for a second twin,[25] overall are not as safe as vaginal birth,[26] are not safer than vaginal birth after a cesarean[27] and do not necessarily improve outcomes for macrosomic "big" babies.[28]

Cesarean section puts healthy women and their infants at risk for complications. Although cesarean section is safer than ever before, it is still a major abdominal surgery and exposes women to surgical complications and risks from anesthesia, which they would not otherwise experience. A woman who has one cesarean will always be at risk for a uterine rupture (when a uterine scar separates or gives way) in a subsequent pregnancy, whether she labors for a VBAC or has an elective repeat cesarean delivery. Cumulative cesareans significantly increase the risk for placental problems, hemorrhage, and a hysterectomy. In a subsequent pregnancy women are more likely to give birth to a low-birth or preterm baby, or a baby with a malformation or central nervous system injury. Compared to a vaginal birth maternal mortality is at least twice as high with a cesarean delivery.[29]

Birth by cesarean also affects psychosocial outcomes. A review of several studies (meta-analysis) found that compared to mothers who delivered vaginally, cesarean mothers expressed less immediate and long-term satisfaction with their births, took longer to interact with their infants, had less positive reactions to them after birth, and interacted less with them at home.[30] With a cesarean birth mothers are more likely to experience depression, negative early reaction to their infant, and poorer psychological health. Personal accounts from women who have had a cesarean, as well as emerging research, suggest that despite a healthy baby and a timely physical recovery, some women experience cesarean birth as a traumatic event.[31]

According to the March of Dimes, a leading nonprofit research organization dedicated to preventing birth defects, premature birth, and infant mortality, the rising numbers of scheduled cesareans and medically induced labors may be contributing to the growing number of babies who are born late preterm, between 34 and 36 weeks gestation. Nearly half a million babies are born too soon each year and late preterm babies now account for 70 percent of all premature births. They are the fastest growing subgroup of premature babies. Preterm babies are more likely to need care from a special care nursery (NICU), and are more likely to be rehospitalized after discharge.[32]

Breastfeeding is a time-sensitive relationship that is established more easily if there is skin-to-skin contact between the mother and her baby within the first 30 minutes of birth. Cesarean surgery and complications from the operation can interfere with the initiation of breastfeeding. Breastfeeding provides health advantages that last many years after the infant is weaned.[33, 34]

Many Cesarean Sections Can Safely Be Avoided

In the last three decades researchers have found that a variety of non-medical factors affected the cesarean rate. The number of operations seemed to be associated with: the physician's style of practice; private health insurance; certain regions of the country; type of hospital (private, community, or university affiliated); staff scheduling; physician-on-call patterns; nursing style; day of the week; and the culture of the hospital. In the 1960s the cesarean rate in the United States was 6.6 percent. By the end of the 1970s it had increased to 15.2 percent. Despite the National Institutes of Health's investigation into increasing cesareans and recommendations that thousands of operations could safely be avoided, more and more women each year gave birth by cesarean, until 1988, when the rate reached 24.7 percent and VBACs began to be encouraged. Since the majority of cesareans were repeat operations, as more and more women with a prior cesarean labored and gave birth vaginally, the rate slowly began to drop. Cesarean rates decreased between 1989 and 1996, when it began an uphill trend again. In 1999 the American College of Obstetricians and Gynecologists issued controversial and financially prohibitive VBAC guidelines, which discouraged hospitals from providing care to women who wanted a VBAC. These guidelines virtually illiminated that option for women across the country. In 2006 less than 10 percent of women with a prior cesarean had a VBAC. Currently cesareans are increasing across the board for all women, all ages, all weight gain categories, all races, all economic classes, all health conditions, and in all regions of the country. Researchers have found little evidence that the rise in cesareans is due to increasing medical risk factors.[35]

Figure I.1
Rates for Total Cesarean Section, Primary Cesarean Section and Vaginal Birth after Cesarean Section (VBAC), United States, 1989–2006

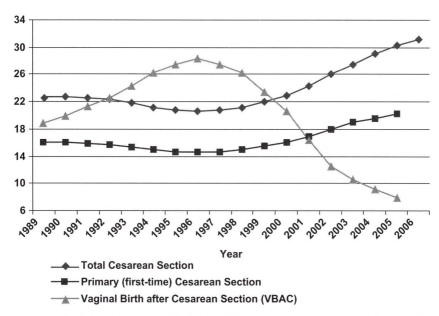

Source: U.S. National Center for Health Statistics. (For comparability, 2004 and 2005 primary cesarean section and VBAC rates are limited to thirty-seven jurisdictions with unrevised birth certificates, encompassing 69 percent of 2005 births; 2006 total cesarean section rate is preliminary.) © 2008 Childbirth Connection. Used with permission.

The majority of cesareans have, historically, been performed for four medical indications: routine repeat operations, non-progressive labor (dystocia), non-reassuring fetal heart tones (fetal distress), and breech. For each of these indications many cesareans can be avoided by changing birth practices without compromising maternal and infant health. If one agrees with the Institute of Medicine's definition of quality of care as "the degree to which health services for individuals and populations increase the likelihood of desired health outcomes and are consistent with current professional knowledge," then it can be said that overall childbearing women deserve a much higher quality of care.

PART I

BACKGROUND

1

FREE FALL

Free fall: Encarta English Dictionary (North American edition)

1. Descent with unopened parachute. A descent through the air with an unopened parachute as the first part of a parachute jump.
2. Rapid decline. A sudden rapid, and uncontrollable decline or descent in a particular system.

In the United States, policies that ultimately dictate provision of maternity care are drafted and issued not by government public health agencies but, in effect, by a private membership association with no federal oversight and no accountability to the public. Those policies issued by the American College of Obstetricians and Gynecologists (ACOG) are, by default, adopted by clinicians and hospitals—often without critical examination. In turn they come to be regarded as the standard of care by which medical issues are determined in litigation. Without further scrutiny, these privately issued policy statements become the basis upon which reimbursement for maternity care services is approved or disapproved—standards by which malpractice insurance companies evaluate their coverage determinations and claim-setting practices. Above all, these policies affect women's lives, health, and well-being. They also affect the health and well-being of their infants and families.

In the words of one of its past presidents, the American College of Obstetricians and Gynecologists is the "world's richest, largest, and most influential organization devoted to women's health."[1] And yet, only 23 percent of all obstetric practice recommendations issued by the organization are category Level A; that is, based on good and consistent scientific evidence, according to criteria established by the U.S. Preventive Health Services Task Force. (Task Force criteria range from Level A to Level E.) One-third of all recommendations include no Level A sources at all. The national maternity care policies in countries like Britain are evidence-based and drafted and approved with the input of dozens of stakeholders (multidisciplinary professional associations, consumer advocacy groups, hospitals, and others). Yet, overall, less than two physicians were involved in the drafting of each of the fifty-five obstetrics and gynecology practice bulletins current in 2006. Around the world, those who craft health policies and practice guidelines look to the Cochrane Database of Systematic Reviews, considered the "gold standard" for scientific evidence on health care issues. But only 1 percent of the 3,953 references cited in all of ACOG's practice bulletins are citations from the Cochrane Database. The ACOG drafts maternity care policies in part to minimize the probability of malpractice claims against their members.[2] Those policies do not optimize the health of childbearing women and their infants.

Medical associations have been reporting that increasing malpractice suits and exorbitant premiums have impacted their ability to provide quality care to their patients. Ironically, and perhaps reflecting a conflict of interest, medical malpractice insurance companies owned and operated by physicians currently provide coverage for more than 60 percent of all physicians in private practice.[3] A deep-seated belief by both physicians and consumers that has been identified for the increasing cesarean rate is the threat of litigation. Apparently consumers have been filing an unprecedented number of malpractice claims that have reaped havoc in their physicians' lives and pockets. But at least one survey of 658 members of the Central Association of Obstetricians and Gynecologists found that cumulatively physicians had been in practice 17,136 years. Each surveyed member had one claim for every 11 years of practice and a trial every 69 years. The authors of the study published in the American Journal of Obstetrics and Gynecology concluded that professional liability claims are uncommon.[4]

A report on medical malpractice payout trends between 1991 and 2004 by the watch dog group Public Citizen's Congress Watch concluded that there was no evidence that the steep rise in some doctors' insurance rates was due to lawsuits and patients seeking legal compensation.[5]

Similarly, a report by the Harvard School of Public Health found that in Pennsylvania the liability "crisis" was not responsible for the mass exodus of OB/GYNs and family physicians. Physicians had been leaving the state at the same rate before the liability "crisis."[6]

Decades ago, scientific evidence proved beyond any doubt that the routine use of electronic fetal monitors (EFM) do not improve health outcomes but increase the number of cesareans. Malpractice attorneys are however still advertising to potential litigants that EFM can identify babies at risk for fetal hypoxia (inadequate oxygen in body tissues), so that physicians can timely intervene and prevent neurological damage or death. "The sooner the clinician intervenes, the higher the probability of avoiding irreversible brain damage," states one legal firm's Web site.[7]

At well-respected and nationally recognized teaching hospitals it is not unusual to have ten to twenty anesthesiologists on the staff administering epidural analgesia for labor, each practicing independently according to her or his preferred technique, with some whose patients have low and others whose patients have high cesarean rates.[8]

At a time when the Centers for Disease Control[9] and the National Institutes of Child Health and Development Maternal-Fetal Medicine Unit[10] have published evidence associating increasing cesarean rates with severe maternal complications, late preterm births, and infant mortality, the policies, press releases, and ethics statements issued by ACOG are leaning toward more cesarean sections—more scheduled cesareans for no medical indication and more routine repeat cesareans. Maternal mortality for planned cesareans in healthy women is at least twice that for normal birth.[11] In 2006 the cesarean rate was 31.1 percent—twice the rate recommended by the U.S. National Health Service. One in three women gave birth by cesarean section, a record high. ACOG leaders are championing women's right to "choose" a cesarean section, a major abdominal surgery, when no medical indication warrants it. Yet the ACOG's policies on vaginal birth after a prior cesarean (VBAC) deny women the right to avoid a routine repeat cesarean. Contrary to the current national fears, planning a VBAC is safe. This option is not denied within certain safety guidelines to women in any other industrialized nation. Since 1999, when this anti-VBAC policy was crafted, more than 300 hospitals have decided not to provide medical care for women who want to plan a VBAC.[12] In 2005 more than 90 percent of women with a prior cesarean birth had a repeat operation. What is even more egregious is that no one has yet challenged these violations of human rights.

THE NATIONAL BILL FOR CESAREANS

The United States spends more money on health care than any other developed country in the world. In 2003 the average charge for a vaginal delivery without complications was $6,200 compared to $11,500 for a cesarean section without complications and $15,500 with complications.[13]

In 2005 there were 4.1 million births in the United States, out of which 99 percent took place in a hospital. The national pregnancy and delivery hospital charge in 2005 was $44 billion. Cesareans accounted for 31 percent of all maternal discharges. The national bill for newborn care was $35 billion. Pregnancy and delivery and newborn care were the second and third most expensive conditions treated in U.S. hospitals and the two most expensive conditions billed to Medicaid and private insurance. These two conditions were also the second and fourth most expensive conditions billed to the uninsured. Charges for pregnancy/delivery and newborn care grew 75 percent and 78 percent respectively between 1997 and 2005. Inpatient hospital charges do not include individual physician fees, outpatient emergency care, or outpatient care.[14] More than 40 percent of all births nationwide are covered by Medicaid.[15]

Babies born by scheduled cesarean section are more likely to be born preterm, have low birth weight, and suffer from respiratory distress syndrome.

In 2005 the conditions with the longest hospital stays for all U.S. hospitalized patients regardless of age were related to infants—respiratory distress syndrome, premature birth, and low birth weight. The average stay for infants with respiratory distress syndrome was 25.7 days at an average cost of $114,200 per stay. In 2005 about 16,000 babies were diagnosed with respiratory distress syndrome, double the rate in 1997.[16]

For families who have a medical savings account, the out-of-pocket cost of a cesarean delivery can reach $9,000. For a preterm baby who may need to spend several days in neonatal intensive care the personal cost can run as high as $21,000.[17]

HEALTH COSTS FROM NOT MAXIMIZING MIDWIFERY CARE

Evidence shows that professional midwifery care in or out of hospital settings results in better maternal and infant outcomes compared with physicians caring for similar populations. Low-risk women cared for by midwives have fewer complications in labor and birth. With midwives patients have less epidurals, fewer cesareans, and more VBACs. Babies are less likely to be born preterm or with low birth weight and less likely to suffer from fetal distress and birth trauma. They are also less likely to require resuscitation or special care in a neonatal intensive care unit (NICU). With midwifery care more mothers initiate and continue breastfeeding, a significant health advantage for both infants and mothers.[18] Despite these health outcomes, in the last few years several hospital-based midwifery services have been shut down for financial reasons—many from hospitals associated with a university medical or midwifery school.

Midwives perform fewer billable procedures like routine electronic fetal monitoring, use of IVs, epidurals, episiotomies, forceps, and vacuum deliveries. Their patients are less likely to need a cesarean section. They are also less likely to bill for treatment of newborn complications and additional hospital days in special care units. Evidence shows that home birth in North America and birth in freestanding birth centers, the majority of which are attended by midwives, are safe for low-risk women and they reduce rates of complications and cesarean sections. Medical associations, however, have in many states actively lobbied to restrict midwifery care, home births, and birth in birth centers, effectively limiting women's choices and consequently burdening families with higher hospital-based costs for labor, delivery, and newborn care. Giving birth in a birth center costs an average of $1,600.[19]

CURRENT HEALTH STATUS OF CHILDBEARING WOMEN AND BABIES

So what is the current health status of U.S. childbearing women and their infants? Compared to maternal and infant health in other countries what does a cesarean rate of 31 percent and an annual price tag of $75 billion for maternity and newborn care a year achieve?

High cesarean rates have not improved the health of mothers. The overall maternal mortality rate in the United States has been increasing and is now 11 per 100,000 live births, more than three times higher than the national health target for the year 2010. The rate is one of the highest among industrialized nations. Maternal mortality among black women is almost four times higher than among non-Hispanic white women. The U.S. Healthy People target is to lower maternal mortality rates to 3.3 per 100,000 live births.[20]

A United Nations working group placed the United States forty-first among 171 countries for the risk of death from complications of pregnancy and childbirth over a woman's reproductive lifetime. One in 4,800 women in the United States is likely to die from pregnancy-related causes compared to one in 9,600 in Kuwait, one in 13,300 in Australia, one in 17,800 in Denmark, and one in 47,600 in Ireland. For every woman who dies, several thousands suffer disability. One in five U.S. women experiences major complications during pregnancy and one in four will have serious complications during and after delivery. More than 40 percent of women experience some kind of maternal morbidity—an illness or injury directly related to pregnancy and childbirth. Pre-eclampsia (toxemia or pregnancy-induced hypertension and presence of protein in the urine) is the most common complication of pregnant women in the United States.[21]

The United States has more neonatologists and neonatal intensive care beds per person than Australia, Canada, and the United Kingdom but has higher rates of low birth weight infants.[22] The United States ranks thirty-second in the industrialized world for newborn mortality. Fewer newborns die in Lithuania, Denmark, Slovenia, Ireland, Greece, Portugal, Israel, Iceland, the Czech Republic, and Japan than in the United States.[23] The number of healthy women who give birth for the first time by cesarean for nonmedical reasons (no indicated risk) has been increasing these last few years. The rate was 20.6 percent in 2004. Neonatal mortality is almost two times higher for babies born by planned cesarean to healthy women.[24]

RECORD HIGH CESAREANS RUN CONTRARY TO NATIONAL HEALTH OBJECTIVES TO IMPROVE MATERNAL AND INFANT HEALTH

Performing a cesarean section on one out of three women runs contrary to the U.S. Healthy People 2010 goals. Healthy People 2010 is a comprehensive set of disease prevention and health promotion objectives for the country. The objectives were created by scientists both inside and outside of government and identify a wide range of public health priorities and specific, measurable targets. The Healthy People Consortium is an alliance of more than 350 national organizations, and 250 state, public health, and environmental agencies have made a commitment to support the goals of Healthy People, the nation's health agenda. Healthy People has set specific targets for maternal, infant, and child health. Among them is to reduce martenal mortality rates to 3.3

per 100,000, reduce cesareans among low-risk women to 15.5 percent and increase VBACs to 63 percent by the year 2010.[25] High cesarean rates also challenge the Healthy People 2010 goals to increase the proportion of mothers who breastfeed their babies.

Increasing breastfeeding rates is a major goal of the CDC Program to Prevent Obesity and Other Chronic Diseases. It is also a public health goal of the American Academy of Pediatrics. The CDC has identified cesarean section as a risk factor for the initiation and continuity of breastfeeding. Cesarean section impacts the newborn's ability to breastfeed. Medications and procedures administered to mothers during birth affect the infants' behavior which in turn affects the newborn's ability to be breastfeed. Understandably, mothers who are just beginning to recover from major abdominal surgery have difficulty providing for their newborn's needs in the way they would like to.

CESAREAN DELIVERY AND THE CHALLENGE FOR THE MEDIA

In today's warp speed distribution of news and events and the existence of thousands of Web sites that report on women's health care, the media inadvertently plays a significant role in reporting on the "normality" of cesarean section. It often reports on maternity care issues based not on independent investigation and personal communications with individuals, but on press releases written and distributed by the medical societies themselves. These press releases can only report good news or "news" the society wants to create. The issues are clearly laid out, expert quotes from society members are included, and conclusions are clearly defined. Three cogent examples of the issues reported on are "maternal request" cesareans (mothers driving up the cesarean rate), the belief that cesareans can protect women from damage to their pelvic floor (incontinence), and the belief that repeat cesarean sections are as safe as normal birth and safer than laboring after a prior cesarean birth.

When the press casually reports on celebrities who give birth by cesarean, the public perceives the surgical procedure as commonplace and even desirable. Media reports about cesarean and VBAC have a tendency to directly impact consumer beliefs on the issues and consequently patterns of maternity care. While the media is not expected to have the knowledge to weed out medical studies of less than excellent quality, health care journalists should take the time to learn as much as they can about evidence-based maternity care and how current patterns of care run contrary to the quality of care childbearing women should be receiving. The Association for Health Care Journalists has taken the lead in educating journalists about evidence-based care and has published excellent reports and resources on health care quality and specific health issues. However, to date maternity care has not yet been a focus of their attention.[26]

THE NEED FOR INFORMED MATERNITY CARE CONSUMERS

There is a lack of awareness among the general public about what constitutes quality of health care in general, especially quality maternity care. The U.S. Agency for Healthcare Research and Quality (AHRQ) found that it's "difficult to draw broad conclusions about the performance of the nation's health care system in caring for mothers and children because of the gaps in our knowledge about the quality of care for these populations."[27]

When the need arises to make a decision about a health care plan, a care provider, birth practices, or a birthing facility women have few guidelines to follow and no easy access to the information. In fact any entity today can establish itself as a source of quality care measures, set a number of arbitrary quality measures, and give awards to institutions, provider groups, or health plans based on those arbitrary chosen measures. This current state of affairs has made these measures meaningless and almost incomprehensible to consumers. Except for the states of New York and Massachusetts, where reporting of maternity practices is mandated by law, hospital cesarean rates, induction rates, and other birth practices that increase the risk for cesareans are not easily available to the public. Women have no easy way of knowing if comparable hospitals in their own community have a 15 percent or 50 percent cesarean rate unless they make a special effort to obtain that information from their state health departments.

Women have few standards by which to choose quality coverage for maternity care. The National Committee for Quality Assurance (NCQA) is a private, not-for-profit organization that sets standards for quality of care and service for health plans. In its 2005 report on the state of health care quality the NCQA found that "consumers do not yet have access to the kind of objective information they need to make informed decisions about their care... They need to know which practices, hospitals and health plans have systems in place to improve quality and safety and which ones make themselves publicly accountable, and they need to know how to find their way to high performance providers."

The NCQA accreditation is nationally recognized as a seal of approval. Their health plan report cards are used by U.S. Fortune 500 employers, federal and state governments, as well as consumers. Currently, key measures of quality for maternity care only include prenatal and postpartum care. The NCQA 2007 State of Health Care Quality Report Cards include no benchmarks for intrapartum care (labor and birth).[28]

Hospital ranking has little to do with the inpatient quality of maternity care women receive.

Maternity care professionals and childbearing women may soon have transparent evidence-based measures that they can use to evaluate the quality of childbirth and newborn care against national benchmarks. The National Quality Forum (NQF), a consensus body of private and public groups with interest in maternity care advises the federal government on key issues to improve the nation's quality of health. The NQF Voluntary Consensus Standards for Perinatal Care Streering Committee has endorsed specific measures known to improve perinatal care from the last trimester through hospital discharge, benchmarks never before considered on a national level. The measures will go through the multi-stakeholder's endorsement process before final approval in the fall of 2008. Among others, the committee encourages all maternity care stakeholders to focus on the following measures to improve the health of mothers and babies:

- The number of elective cesareans performed before 39 weeks.
- The number of cesareans performed on low-risk women.
- The number of women undergoing a cesarean who have received prophylactic antibiotics.
- The rate of OB-related anesthesia complications.
- The rate of deep vein thrombosis (blood clot in the leg) and pulmonary embolism, a side effect of cesarean section.
- The number of preterm infants (24–32 weeks with intact membranes) who receive steroids to reduce their risk of respiratory distress syndrome, other complications, and death.
- The number of newborns who have a bilirubin screening before discharge to prevent potential brain damage or death.
- The number of newborns who are fed only breast milk before discharge.[29]

A national survey of women's childbearing experiences in 2005, Listening to Mothers II conducted for Childbirth Connection in New York by Harris Interactive, found that women were poorly informed about the risks of cesarean section despite their belief that they ought to be told about the risks associated with the procedure.[30]

Besides the Healthy People 2010 goals, which are recommendations rather than national health policies, there is no comprehensive national effort to reduce the number of cesarean deliveries in the United States. Childbearing families need access to accurate and comprehensive information about birth practices and cesarean delivery and its impact on maternal and infant health.

ESPECIALLY FOR MOTHERS

National guidelines for maternity care in the United States have not yet been fully updated to reflect the best scientific evidence. Many maternity care practices are outdated and can cause women and babies unnecessary harm and can complicate labor to the extent that many women end up with a cesarean section that could have been avoided. Fear of malpractice can be so strong as to prevent practitioners and hospitals from providing the high quality care that mothers and babies deserve. Take the time to find out which care practices are effective and beneficial and which ones are questionable or can potentially cause harm. Learn about what you should expect from your care providers, hospitals, and health plans. Ask questions about options that may be available to you.

Resources

A Guide to Effective Care in Pregnancy and Childbirth can be obtained in full by visiting http://www.childbirthconnection.org/article.asp?ClickedLink=329&ck=10218&area=27 (last accessed May 23, 2008).

Agency for Healthcare Quality and Research, Consumers and Patients, http://www.ahrq.gov/consumer/ (last accessed May 23, 2008).

Center for Medical Consumers, http://medicalconsumers.org/pages/center.html, (last accessed May 23, 2008).

Cochrane Plain Language Reviews, Pregnancy and Childbirth at http://www.cochrane.org/reviews/en/topics/87_reviews.html (last accessed May 23, 2008).

2

NONDISCLOSURE: THE MISSING INFORMATION FOR MAKING INFORMED DECISIONS

Every woman should have the opportunity to receive accurate and up-to-date information about the benefits and risks of all procedures, drugs, and tests suggested for use during pregnancy, birth, and the postpartum period, with the rights to informed consent and informed refusal.[1]

In 2001 the U.S. Institute of Medicine released a landmark report that examined the state of the nation's health care industry. The report found that the industry "floundered in its ability to provide safe, high-quality care consistently to all Americans." The Institute of Medicine operates under the National Academies of Sciences and is an adviser to the federal government on issues regarding medical care, research, and education. In its report, *Crossing the Quality Chasm*, the Institute included ten specific recommendations to make the health care system more responsive to patients' needs. One key recommendation was to provide evidence-based information to the public to allow them to make informed decisions about all aspects of their health care that ultimately affects their lives. Instead of professionals controlling care, the Institute advised the patient should be the source of control. Instead of care providers making decisions based on their own personal training and experience, it recommended decisions be made by the patient, based on evidence-based information. Instead of the current "culture of secrecy" it urged that "transparency" was essential.[2] An earlier study on health care quality had found that in the United States "more information was available on the quality of airlines, restaurants, cars, and VCRs than on the quality of health care."[3]

With regard to maternity care, women's access to evidence-based information is even more critical, since less than one quarter of the current recommendations issued in obstetrics practice bulletins published by the American College of Obstetricians and Gynecologists (ACOG) are based on sound and consistent scientific evidence.[4]

Access to or denial of accurate and unbiased health care information ultimately affects women's lives. Participating in making health care decisions is important because clinical decisions also involve personal value judgments. Women may value the risks and benefits of major surgery such as a cesarean section differently then their care providers, family, or friends. Since women's decisions regarding childbirth also impact the health of their infant, the information should include the impact on infant health and well-being. Accurate and comprehensive information can also provide a more realistic expectation of the benefits and harms of cesarean delivery.[5]

As noted by the Institute of Medicine, however, currently "control over decisions, access, and information is typically in the hands of caregivers and is ceded to patients only when caregivers choose to do so." Although there has been a growing effort by care providers and institutions to make the transition from an authoritarian model of care to a model that provides more transparency and encourages shared decision-making, the Institute found the efforts were "far from complete."[6] The International Federation of Gynecology and Obstetrics (FIGO) states: "Assuring accuracy of information is an obligation of the profession as assuring patient trust is the foundation of the therapeutic physician/patient relationship."[7]

WHAT DO WOMEN KNOW ABOUT CESAREANS?

On the whole, in the United States, medical societies and hospital associations have been slow to respond with regard to providing evidence-based comprehensive information on maternity care practices that impact women's lives. Although cesarean section is the single most common operation performed in U.S. hospitals (1.3 million surgeries in 2006), the women who have the surgery can find it difficult to access accurate, comprehensive, and nonbiased information. At least 12 million expectant mothers of a best-selling book on pregnancy and birth have read, "Even though it is technically considered major surgery, a cesarean carries relatively minor risks-closer to those of a tonsillectomy than of a gallbladder operation, for instance-that can generally be treated easily."[8] A cesarean is a highly invasive procedure and unlike gallbladder surgery cannot be performed laparoscopically (minimally invasive surgery) to reduce the risks of complications and infections.

Many women are not adequately prepared for what to expect from the operation. They are not familiar with the risks associated with the surgery and do not have enough information to help them choose among the safest physicians and hospitals if the surgery is planned in advance. They may not have enough information to help them decide whether or not they should go ahead with the operation at all. Health care has been identified as a high-risk industry, like aviation, by the Institute of Medicine, one that is a decade or more behind many others in ensuring basic safety.[9]

The *Listening to Mothers II* Survey (LTM II) found that 81 percent of the women felt they ought to know all the side effects and complications of cesarean delivery before making a decision about the procedure. But surprisingly, survey results showed that of the women who had a cesarean, between 42 percent and 46 percent were "not sure" how best to answer four key questions about risks associated with the surgery. Up to one-third of the mothers answered at least one question incorrectly. And only 10 percent of the mothers who had a first cesarean said that they were involved in making the decision. More than half of the mothers who had a repeat operation indicated that their care provider made that decision for them before labor.[10]

In the last few years there has been an increasing trend from leading U.S. obstetricians favoring elective cesarean for no medical reason, championing patient autonomy and honoring a woman's right to make an informed decision about cesarean delivery.[11, 12]

Some, in defiance of the U.S. National Health Service Healthy People 2010 objectives to reduce cesarean rates, have argued that, "It's time to target a new cesarean delivery rate . . . a total cesarean section rate in the range of 30 percent is appropriate and clinically justified."[13] Other leaders in obstetrics have stated the "Healthy People goal is based on worldwide data that came out of the 1970s and early 1980s, and it just doesn't fit with modern medicine."[14]

Some physicians who view childbirth as similar to "rolling a bowling ball through the vagina" recommend a planned cesarean section to prevent lifelong damage to the pelvic floor,[15] a recommendation that is questionable given current evidence. In debates with professional colleagues some physicians have argued, "If patients can choose to have . . . rhinoplasty [cosmetic surgery on the nose], a breast enlargement and reduction, abdominoplasty [tummy tuck], and liposuction . . . why can't the same patient choose to have a primary elective cesarean section?"[16] In national news magazines a prominent obstetrician has stated that "many physicians are willing to perform an elective C-section once the mother understands the risks and benefits."[17]

A woman's right to accept or refuse any medical procedure, drug, or treatment is clearly established in medical ethics and the law. But, it appears that women are not fully informed about the risks associated with a cesarean. And they may not be making an *informed decision* when they consent to the surgery. In 2006, 1.3 million women gave birth by cesarean section. What did they know about the risks of the operation for themselves and their baby?

To Make an Informed Decision Women Need Accurate, Comprehensive, and Nonbiased Information

In the United States, the Health Insurance Portability and Accountability Act of 1996 (HIPAA) makes it a federal requirement for caregivers to provide accurate information to patients. HIPAA ensures the rights and responsibility of all citizens to participate fully in all decisions related to their health care.[18]

The U.S. Consumer Bill of Rights and Responsibilities mandates health care professionals to provide their patients with easily understood information and the opportunity to decide among all treatment options consistent with the informed consent process, including the option of no treatment at all.

Health care professionals are required by law to discuss all risks, benefits, and consequences to treatment or nontreatment and give their patients the opportunity to refuse treatment and to express preferences about future treatment decisions.[19]

Women are empowered when they are included in the decision-making process. Their participation increases caregiver accountability and can improve health outcomes. Good quality health information is important to women if they are going to be actively involved in making decisions about maternity care. But, comprehensive information on cesarean delivery varies widely and evidence-based information may be hard to come by from medical association patient education pamphlets and even from some federal government health information Web sites, both of which women are likely to trust as reliable and authoritative sources of information.

What Is the Quality of Authoritative Sources of Information?

More than three out of four U.S. women are turning to the Internet for information on pregnancy and birth[20] to share their stories and experiences, and to seek support for their specific conditions. The quality of the information found in some authoritative sources of information on childbirth on the Internet is mixed. Sometimes they are excellent, accurate, and comprehensive. At other times incomplete, biased, and don't take into consideration women's personal values and preferences. With regard to information on cesareans, the reasons for needing a cesarean are often listed. The procedure is more or less described, what happens when, but the full range of risks and alternatives to the surgery are not. Information is sometimes outdated, excluded, or misrepresented. Some resources omit all complications related to the surgery. Often no additional sources for further information are mentioned. Childbirth is often presented as being extremely dangerous and cesareans as extremely safe. Consumers view medical association pamphlets and government health information Web sites as authoritative and trustworthy and may have no way to evaluate the quality of that information.

Information about Cesarean and VBAC

One on-line leaflet from the American College of Surgeons states, "A cesarean section is performed only after an obstetrician has carefully weighed the factors involved in a woman's pregnancy and has decided that performing a cesarean section is necessary." The only reference to the risks associated with the operation is this phrase, "in most instances, it is not considered a dangerous or risky procedure."[21]

A patient publication from the American College of Obstetricians and Gynecologists states, "There are many reasons why a cesarean birth may be used to deliver your baby. It may be the best approach for both you and your baby. A cesarean delivery may be planned in advance when certain conditions are known. In some cases, if problems arise, the decision is made during labor." Here again, the doctor is the one making the decisions. No discussion is encouraged. The woman has no voice. Her right to refuse interventions is not stated. The pamphlet continues, "Sometimes the doctor can start or speed up labor with medication if labor is moving slowly ... Because of this, doctors may watch for several hours before deciding a cesarean birth is needed."[22] No statement suggests to the mother that induction can increase the risk for an irregular fetal heart rate, intrapartum fever, shoulder dystocia, instrumental delivery, and cesarean section.[23]

Women are given no other alternative methods to facilitate labor—such as freedom of movement, positioning, and having continuous emotional support in labor—factors proven to lower the odds for a cesarean. This pamphlet lists short-term complications related to the surgery but does not mention any long-term effects or added risks in a future pregnancy; uterine rupture, placenta previa, a repeat operation, miscarriage, or preterm birth. Similarly, the ACOG patient education pamphlet on VBAC does not include these same avoidable risks when women plan a VBAC.

In the on-line journal of the American Medical Association, *Patient Page, Cesarean Delivery,* there is an obvious bias for routine repeat cesarean section rather than for VBAC. Only one sentence is devoted to previous cesarean birth. It states, "The doctor may discuss with the mother that having delivered one baby by cesarean might mean it would be best to have other babies delivered by cesarean." This educational pamphlet includes one sentence on the risks of cesarean: "Cesarean delivery is major surgery, but sometimes it is the safest way to deliver a baby."[24]

Searching for comprehensive, unbiased information about cesareans and VBAC from federal government Web sites can sometimes be frustrating and confusing. While some links are excellent sources of evidence-based, patient centered information, others are not. A few obviously favor cesarean section as the safest method of childbirth. An interactive tutorial on cesarean delivery posted on the National Library of Medicine, MedlinePlus, states, "Long labor is very exhausting and risky for the mother and baby. The doctor may try other solutions to dilate the cervix, but if these fail, a C-section might be the recommended option." Here again, there is no mention of any other nonsurgical alternatives to helping labor progress. The only solution presented is a surgical one. In the same tutorial one also reads, "Sometimes forceps are used to help the baby go faster ... Using forceps is very safe and helps prevent possible complications if the delivery is not going fast enough."[25, 26]

Informing women that forceps are very safe is a highly inaccurate statement. Use of forceps with an episiotomy causes serious long-term injury to the muscles of the pelvic floor, including sexual function, and future problems with incontinence.[27] Forceps can cause bruising, intracranial pressure, and facial nerve damage that can affect the newborn's ability to successfully breastfeed.[28]

Using the keyword "cesarean" on www.4women.gov links to nongovernment Web sites with contradictory information regarding VBAC. One link leads to this statement, "Studies show that VBACs are more risky for the woman and baby than a repeat C-section."[29] Another links to, "Vaginal deliveries have fewer risks for you and the baby than cesarean delivery. Vaginal deliveries require fewer blood transfusions and result in fewer infections."[30]

Information about Epidurals for Labor

Also posted on the MedlinePlus Web site using key words "vaginal birth" is biased and inaccurate information that favors the use of drugs and anesthesia. It states, "Most women require some form of anesthesia to help relieve the pain of labor and delivery. There are many ways to control pain experienced with delivery. These include: (1) medication, (2) regional anesthesia, and (3) epidural block. The most common way to control pain during delivery is the epidural block. It is used for vaginal deliveries and cesarean sections...It does not affect the baby." No risks are mentioned and no information about the impact of medication and regional anesthesia on the progress of labor, nor the effect on initiation of breastfeeding. No other nonpharmacological options for pain relief are mentioned. This educational program also states that an epidural block "does not affect the baby."[31] This is an incorrect statement.

A patient education pamphlet from the American Association of Anesthesiologists posted on the Web is detailed, easy to understand, and includes rare side effects of both epidural analgesia for labor and anesthesia. However, the names of the drugs used are never mentioned. And there is no information about the possibility of needing extra time to push the baby out, since epidurals slow down the pushing phase.[32]

Another authoritative Web site on epidural anesthesia associated with an Ivy League medical school is comprehensive, educational, and designed to make women feel comfortable with the procedure. However, it includes this statement, "Both general and regional anesthesia are safe and have no significant effects on the baby."[33]

Drugs commonly used today for epidurals in labor include a "local" anesthetic (bupivacaine, mepivicaine, or ropivicaine) and an opioid (narcotic). Both "caine" drugs and opioids cross the placenta, and are transferred to the baby. They are also found in colostrum, the yellowish fluid rich in antibodies and minerals that a mother produces after birth and before her milk comes in. A common synthetic opioid used in the United States today for epidurals is fentanyl. As are several other drugs, fentanyl is not approved by the Federal Drug Administration (FDA) for use in pregnancy and childbirth. Fentanyl is a fat-soluble opioid with addictive potential. It has an analgesic potency of about eighty times that of morphine[34] and fifty times that of heroin. It is typically used to treat patients with severe pain, or to manage pain after surgery. It is also used to treat cancer patients who are already physically tolerant to opiates.[35]

The impact of any drug on an individual and the unborn baby is complex and dependent on factors such as fetal maturity, dose, formula, body weight, length of exposure, and other drugs that are already in the system. Because we don't have any comprehensive evidence about short- or long-term effects of the drugs used for epidurals, it is inaccurate to state that epidurals are "safe" or that "they do no affect the baby."

Giving birth by cesarean and the dose of fentanyl administered during labor and birth has an effect on whether or not first-time mothers with healthy newborns are able to establish breastfeeding before leaving the hospital. The dose of fentanyl given to mothers in one study ranged from 8 to 500 micrograms. The authors concluded that fentanyl might impede the establishment of breastfeeding, particularly when administered at higher doses.[36]

All opioids are transferred to the baby and transfer is faster and more complete for fat-soluble[37] drugs such as fentanyl, and fentanyl derivatives. The Academy of Breastfeeding Medicine (ABM) recognizes that longer labors and instrumental deliveries increase difficulty with the initiation of breastfeeding and recommends good breastfeeding support and close follow-up after postpartum hospitalization when mothers use epidural analgesia.[38]

Epidurals also increase the risk for complications in labor. Compared to women who did not have an epidural for pain relief in labor The Cochrane Pregnancy and Childbirth Group found that women who had an epidural had greater pain relief but were also at higher risk for fetal malposition, and a longer first and second stage of labor. They were also more likely to need oxytocin (to augment contractions) and an instrumental delivery (forceps or vacuum extractor).[39] This information related to epidurals is rarely mentioned in patient education brochures or on authoritative Web sites. Mothers should have access to this information to evaluate their options for pain relief to make an informed decision about choice of pain relief and to access appropriate resources to support, facilitate, and maintain breastfeeding if they plan to do so.

Information about Home Birth

Posted on www.4women.gov, a federal Web site, is this statement about home birth, "The American College of Obstetricians and Gynecologists (ACOG) is against homebirths. ACOG states that hospitals are the safest place to deliver a baby. In case of an emergency, says ACOG, a hospital's equipment and highly trained physicians can provide the best care for a woman and her baby." [40] There is absolutely no study that concludes that hospitals are the safest place to give birth for women with an uncomplicated pregnancy. In fact studies have shown that home births and giving birth in birth centers is as safe or safer and reduces the risk for complications, including a cesarean section.[41]

Posting this statement on a federal Web site discriminates against other maternity care providers such as family physicians, midwives, and doctors of osteopathy, which are all licensed and trained to assist women in childbirth. It also provides the public with biased information about the safety of hospital births and denies them safe alternative choices. Evidence shows that the routine use of medical interventions used in hospitals increases complications and cesarean rates. These include inductions, use of epidurals, and electronic fetal monitoring.[42]

Accessing Information Mandated by Law

Only two states in the United States mandate hospitals to disclose their medical interventions rates to the public: New York and Massachusetts. In New York State the Maternity Information Act requires every hospital to make public its rate of birth-related procedures including induction, episiotomy, electronic fetal monitoring, and cesareans. In 2004 the New York city hospital cesarean rate ranged from 18.3 percent for North Central Bronx Hospital to 39.6 percent for Presbyterian Hospital, affiliated with Columbia University in Manhattan. Women who planned to give birth in a New York City hospital had no access to this information.

In 2004, Choices in Childbirth, a nonprofit maternity care advocacy group called hospitals to inquire about their cesarean section rates. They found that the hospital staff they contacted could not provide that information. In June 2005 the Office of the New York City Public Advocate, concerned about the increasing cesarean rate in the city's hospitals, many of them above 30 percent, conducted an investigation and tried to obtain that information. Despite the law, forty-three out of forty-four hospitals in New York City failed to provide that information to the Public Advocate's Office when requested in June 2005.[43] A follow-up investigation in July 2006 determined that once again hospitals failed to provide site-specific maternity information to the public.[44]

WHAT CAN WE LEARN FROM OUR COUNTERPARTS ABROAD?

In 1993, the government of Great Britain's policy document on maternity care, *Changing Childbirth*, mandated that all women have access to evidence-based information to make informed choices about their care. One initiative that resulted from this recommendation was the Informed Choice Initiative that now provides evidence-based information in the form of clear, easy-to-read pamphlets for consumers. Maternity care professionals have a more detailed fully referenced companion leaflet. Unlike in the United States, consumers and many other stakeholders are involved in the development of all the Informed Choice leaflets.

The Informed Choice educational pamphlet on cesarean section and subsequent births is forthright when comparing vaginal birth with cesarean delivery and clearly informs women of their right to accept or refuse recommended procedures. "A 'normal' or vaginal birth has always been safer for the mother than a cesarean and this is still the case . . . Although the decision is made by the doctor, whether you agree to this is your decision. You and your partner need to understand what is likely to be involved, so that if you decide to give your consent, it is based on both of you understanding the major issues."[45] The consumer pamphlets are meant to be discussed with care providers.

A 52-page evidence-based consumer education document on cesareans developed by the independent, government funded, National Institute for Clinical Excellence (NICE) is available at no cost worldwide through the Internet.[46]

The document includes comprehensive information on what mothers can expect from their caregivers and what precautions should be taken to avoid complications. Women are informed that the most common problem affecting babies born by cesarean is breathing difficulties and that this risk is 35 per 1,000 cesareans as opposed to 5 per 1,000 for a normal birth. Women are informed about factors that *increase* and *decrease* their odds for a cesarean. Mothers are informed that they have the right to refuse a cesarean section even if this will harm them or their baby's health.

This Is the Information Available to All Women from the National Institute for Clinical Excellence

With a cesarean you are more likely to experience:

Pain in the abdomen
Bladder injury
Injury to the tube that connects the kidney and bladder
Needing further surgery
Hysterectomy
Admission to intensive care unit
Developing a blood clot
Longer hospital stay
Returning to the hospital afterward
Death of the mother
Having no more children
In a future pregnancy, the placenta covers the entrance to the womb (placenta previa)
Tearing of the womb in a future pregnancy
In a future pregnancy, death of the baby before labor starts
More likely to have another cesarean in the future.[47]

With regard to an epidural for pain relief in labor, women are informed that they will probably need an additional hour to complete labor, drugs to speed up their contractions, a catheter to empty their bladder, and their mobility will probably be restricted. They are also told that about half of first-time mothers are likely to need an assisted birth with forceps or a vacuum extractor. An evidence-based pamphlet is also available for nondrug methods of pain relief. It includes a full range of options from opioids to hypnosis, intradermal water injections to maternal positioning, one-to-one continuous labor support, and acupuncture. Mothers are given the benefits and disadvantages of each option and its impact on the mother and her baby.[48] Regardless of whether patient education information is posted on the Internet or available in a printed format, the messages that women receive are consistent, evidence-based, and respect women's values and right to make their own decisions.

In New Zealand the government health service provides free access for their residents to the "Plain Language Summaries," research findings from The Cochrane Library. These are easy-to-read conclusions of the best available evidence on a variety of health and maternity care subjects.[49]

Women have the right to make informed decisions about a cesarean delivery. But in fact accurate and comprehensive information is not easy to come by. Given that the United States does not have a national health care system, who then is responsible for providing evidence-based comprehensive information about maternity care practices? The federal health service? State health services? Private professional associations? What oversight measures are in place to assure that childbearing women have access to accurate information that directly affects their health and the health of their babies? When it comes to information about the country's foremost surgical procedure, women are likely to be confused and misinformed.

A RIGHT TO KNOW ABOUT MATERNITY OUTCOMES FROM HOSPITALS

Preceding the publication of *Crossing the Quality Chasm*, the Institute of Medicine published an extensive and revealing report on the safety of health care in America, *To Err Is Human*. The report estimated that at least 44,000 and as many as 98,000 people die in U.S. hospitals each year as a result of medical errors that could have been prevented. Adverse drug events, improper blood transfusions, and surgical injuries occur regularly and high error rates with serious consequences are more likely to occur in intensive care units, operating rooms, and emergency departments. Cesarean sections are performed in the United States more than any other surgical procedure, yet mothers have little knowledge about cesarean-related quality of care.[50] Hospital reporting on infection rates, surgery-related complications, and maternal mortality is currently voluntary, required in some states, but not in others. Women need access to this information before they can make a truly informed decision about a cesarean birth.

ESPECIALLY FOR MOTHERS

Women's values, preferences, and experience of childbirth are different and all women should not be treated the same way. Today, care provided to childbearing women varies from one provider to another and one place of birth to another. When caregivers provide you with information that is comprehensive and easy to understand together, you are more likely to make better decisions about your care. You are also more likely to make informed decisions that are right for you.

What Does Informed Choice/Consent Mean?

In pregnancy and childbirth, by communicating openly with your caregiver, together you can make decisions that best meet your needs. Because all decisions will ultimately affect you and your baby, you have the right to make the final decision about your care. You should know that every woman has the right to fully participate in all decisions regarding her own health care and that of her child. This legal doctrine is called the right to informed consent. The World Health Organization, the European Parliament, the American Hospital Association, and many other organizations support and endorse the right of women to make their own health care decisions in consultation with their caregivers. In the United States, the Health Insurance Portability and Accountability Act of 1996 (HIPAA) makes it a federal requirement for your caregivers to provide you with full and accurate information regarding any aspect of your care and to respect your choice. Your care provider should provide you with the following:

A description of the treatment or procedure that is recommended.
The risks, benefits, and available alternatives to what is recommended.
The likely result of no treatment at all.
The probability of success.
Any major problems that may be anticipated while recovering from a procedure.
Any additional information you wish to have.

What Is a Consent for Treatment Form?

When you give birth in a hospital or birth center, you are asked to sign a consent to treatment form. Your signature gives permission to the staff to care for you and your baby. Usually this form includes common procedures such as vaginal exams, fetal monitoring, use of IVs, pain medication, breaking the bag of water, and the use of forceps or vacuum extractor. All procedures have benefits and risks. The form may also include use of an epidural for pain relief in labor. You do not have to agree to everything on the form. You can delete from or add statements to the form. A separate consent is sometimes required for an epidural and always required for a cesarean delivery. You can change your mind at any time by making your wishes known to your caregivers. If you choose not to agree with a treatment or procedure you may be asked to sign a waiver of liability acknowledging that you are taking responsibility for your decisions. You can at any time express verbally what you wish to consent to and what you don't.

What Is Informed Refusal?

Women also have a right to refuse any drugs, test, treatment, or procedures including a cesarean section. All competent adults are entitled to an "informed refusal." When a care provider has clearly explained the benefits and risks, a woman has the right to choose among the options available to her or refuse them altogether. ACOG states that patients may decline a physician's advice or recommendation, even during treatment, based on "religious beliefs, personal preference, or comfort." You have a right to receive care that respects your personal values, culture, and religion. All medical care is received by choice. Health care providers must have your informed consent before going ahead with a procedure, test, or surgery.

You have the right to choose where and with whom you want to give birth. You can choose a hospital, a birth center, or a home birth. You can choose an obstetrician, a family physician, an osteopath, or a midwife. If you are not satisfied with the care you receive you have the right to change your care provider or the place of birth you have chosen. You have the right to move freely and use any position that is comfortable for you during labor and birth. At any time you have the right to obtain your medical records from your individual care provider or from the hospital or birth center in which you received your care.[51, 52]

How Can I Find Out More about Tests and Procedures?

As a mother-to-be, you have the responsibility of obtaining early prenatal care, living a healthy lifestyle, and finding out as much as you can about the process of labor and birth. Your caregiver will give you information and advice. You will probably feel better about making decisions regarding tests, procedures, or treatments, inducing your labor, or scheduling your cesarean if you ask questions. These may help you to get the information you need to make an informed choice:

Can you explain what will happen?
Where can I get more information?
Can you write this down? Draw me a picture?
Can you tell me about the risks involved?
How will this affect my baby?
I want to think about this before I make a decision.
I don't feel comfortable with this recommendation. Is there anything else I can do or try?

If a Cesarean Is Recommended in Labor You Can Ask the Following Questions

Is this an emergency? Is my health or the health of my baby compromised at this time?
How is this helpful to my baby or me?

What can I expect?

Are there any risks involved?

Do I have time to think about this and give you my answer later?

I would like more time to think about this. If I choose not to go ahead with this recommendation, what would the consequences be for my baby and me?

Can you recommend a safe alternative?

What You Should Know about Giving Birth in a Hospital

You will find it helpful and you will receive more appropriate care if you take the time to find out about childbirth and discuss issues you are concerned about with your care provider. Despite what many people believe, no patient is ever obligated to comply with medical advice given by any member of the staff in a hospital. As a childbearing woman you have the right on your behalf and on behalf of your baby to say "yes" or "no" to any procedure, drug, test, or surgery recommended by the staff. It is against the law for any member of a hospital staff to go ahead with any procedure at all without your consent. That includes nurses, physicians, midwives, medical, nursing, or midwifery students, and laboratory technicians. George J. Annas, Professor of Health Law, Bioethics, and Human Rights at Boston University School of Public Health writes, "Hospitals . . . are not isolated islands, and physicians are not foreign diplomats with legal immunity. Nor do patients check their legal rights at the hospital door. Medicine must be practiced within the framework of the law of the United States and the state in which the hospital is located . . . Public facilities, in addition, must assure that those human rights guaranteed by the U.S. Constitution are afforded to all patients."[53]

There are thousands of Web sites that provide information about childbirth. To get the best quality information on the science behind childbirth and cesarean section look for Web sites that post evidence-based information. The sites often will state that the information is "evidence-based" or based on the "best available evidence," or is "best practice." Here are a few reliable sources:

RESOURCES

Finding Reliable Nonbiased Information on the Internet

The American College of Nurse-Midwives promotes the health of women and babies through the development and support of the profession of midwifery, http://www.midwife.org (last accessed on July 6, 2008).

Center for Healthcare Rights, http://www.healthcarerights.org (last accessed on July 6, 2008).

Childbirth Connection (formerly Maternity Center Association) provides trusted pregnancy and childbirth guidance to women and their families as well as their babies. Read The Rights of Childbearing Women at http://www.childbirthconnection.com (last accessed on July 6, 2008).

Coalition for Improving Maternity Services, Promoting the Care and Well-Being of Mothers, Babies, and Families. Read, Having a Baby? Ten Questions to Ask, http://www.motherfriendly.org (last accessed on July 8, 2008).

The Cochrane Collaboration, an international not-for-profit organization, providing up-to-date information about the effects of health care, http://www.cochrane.org (last accessed on July 8, 2008).

Informed Choice is for maternity professionals, pregnant women, their families, and carers, http://www.infochoice.org/ (last accessed on July 8, 2008).

International Childbirth Education Association, available for purchase. The Pregnant Patient Bill of Rights and Responsibilities, http://www.icea.org (last accessed on July 8, 2008).

Lamaze International envisions a world of confident women choosing normal birth, http://www.lamaze.org (last accessed on July 8, 2008).

Patient Rights at Your Fingertips, http://www.patient-rights.org (last accessed on July 8, 2008).

Vbac.com provides childbearing women and maternity care professionals access to research-based information, resources, continuing education, and support for VBAC (vaginal birth after cesarean), http://www.vbac.com/informedconsent.html (last accessed on July 6, 2008).

Your Right to Your Hospital/Medical Records, http://www.nwhalliance.org/YOURRIGHTTOYOURRECORDS.htm (last accessed on July 8, 2008).

3

PATIENT CHOICE OR PHYSICIAN CHOICE CESAREANS?

What is happening is that the threshold for doing a cesarean has dropped....
There are now a million women a year giving birth with a scar in their bellies—
you can do the math and count how many women are going to have accreta,
how many are going to have placenta previa, how many babies will be still-
born,...Rather than focusing on the less than one percent of this that may be
attributable to cesarean by choice, it's time to reopen the question that hasn't
been looked at in 25 years, when the section rate was roughly half of what it is
now.[1]

As the number of cesareans continue to rise in several countries women are
being increasingly held responsible for "choosing" to have a surgical birth. The
subject of "cesarean on demand," and "maternal choice" cesareans has been
researched and debated in medical journals, reported on by the media, and
was recently the focus of a U.S. National Institutes of Health-sponsored State-of-
the-Science Conference.[2] Mother-driven cesareans or cesareans-on-demand is
a seemingly reasonable explanation. Given today's climate of fear about giving
birth, the buzz about damage to the pelvic floor, and the perception that cesareans are easy and very safe procedures. If one adds the dimension of women's
right to make their own decisions about how they want to give birth, the issue becomes an even more important focus for a heated debate. Despite the
fact that the issue of "maternal choice" cesareans has been prominent in the
United States for several years, there is no credible data to support the assumption that a substantial number of women are simply choosing to have a
primary (first birth) cesarean delivery without a medical indication.

Many physicians have said that it is their patients who "demand" cesareans
without medical justification. Although that may be the case, several studies
found that women are choosing cesareans based on incomplete information
about the risks, or because they were persuaded by their physicians over the
course of the pregnancy.[3, 4, 5]

Some researchers suggest that it is the providers' perceptions, own bias, or assumptions of the mothers' wants and needs that is being expressed or reported.[6] To say that women "choose" to have a cesarean implies that they have access to the best available evidence. They understand the short- and long-term benefits and risks of the surgical procedure. They have discussed the issue with their care provider and made an *informed choice* to have a cesarean rather than go through labor. There is no data to show that this is the case in the United States. Reports from several countries do no support the view that a majority of women are "choosing" cesarean sections.

Studies of "maternal choice" cesareans in various parts of the world, including Brazil, Taiwan, Australia, Sweden, Italy, Turkey, Hong Kong, Chile, the United States, and Britain found that a very small minority of women actually request a cesarean. The mothers may believe or have been told that a cesarean is the safest way to give birth to avoid trauma to themselves or their baby.[7] Sometimes it is social and cultural factors that influence women to perceive a cesarean delivery as a more favorable birth option available to women of a higher economical and social class.[8] In a questionnaire researchers in Kingston (Ontario, Canada) asked women attending prenatal clinics at Kingston General Hospital in 2005 whether all women should be offered the choice of having an elective primary cesarean. Women were given information about the risks and benefits of the procedure. Although one in two women pregnant for the first time and about one in four women with previous children felt that women should be offered the choice, the majority of them would not request a cesarean for no medical indication.[9]

Some mothers have an extreme fear of labor that may be associated with a previous traumatic experience, psychological problems, or abuse. When their fear of labor is addressed through professional counseling the majority of women go on to have a normal birth.[10, 11]

In Brazil cesarean rates in private hospitals can run as high as 80 percent to 90 percent. About one quarter of all women in Brazil give birth in private hospitals paid for by private health insurance. Well-to-do women in Brazil have been blamed for choosing cesareans as their preferred mode of birth. Contrary to this perception one study of women interviewed in two cities in Brazil found that the majority of women do not prefer to have a cesarean, especially first-time mothers. Rather researchers found that physicians use their position of power and their medical expertise to influence women to "choose" a cesarean. Three out of four first-time mothers interviewed in private hospitals wanted to have a normal birth, but ended up having a cesarean. Eight out of ten women in public hospitals did not anticipate that they would have a surgical delivery.[12] Another study conducted in four separate cities in Brazil found that 70 to 80 percent of women in both the private and public sector preferred to have a vaginal delivery. But 31 percent of women who gave birth in a public hospital and 72 percent of the women who gave birth in a private hospital had a cesarean section. For two out of three women with private insurance and for one out of four women who gave birth in a public hospital the decision to have a cesarean was decided upon before admission to the hospital.[13]

Recently, women and birth activists in Brazil have called for public hearings to denounce the abuse of cesarean sections in the private health sector. In September 2006 the Federal Public Prosecutor's Office in Sãu Paulo held a public hearing requested by Parto do Princípio (a network of more than 250 women active in sixteen states) to investigate the excessive cesarean rates for women with private health insurance. Parto do Princípio saw the public hearings as an important opportunity to discuss a problem that has been harming thousands of women and babies in Brazil. The group presented evidence and testimony on the risks of cesareans and on how women in Brazil were being deceived to accept unnecessary surgeries. Present at the hearings were representatives from the Ministry of Health, the National Health Agency, the Federal Council of Medicine, the Association of Private Hospitals, the Federal Council of Nursing, the Paulista School of Medicine, and representatives of health care plans. As a result of these hearings there is now a formal public process in place for women to report physicians whom they think misled them into having an unnecessary cesarean section and appropriate sanctions are in place. No statute of limitations has been placed on this process.[14]

"MATERNAL REQUEST" CESAREANS IN THE UNITED STATES

Despite common perceptions about cesareans on "maternal request" a United States national survey of women's birth experiences found only 0.2 percent of women who had a primary cesarean (first cesarean) requested one without a medical indication. More importantly one in four women surveyed who had a cesarean reported being pressured by their care provider to have one.[15] There has been a growing trend in the number of planned primary cesareans performed on healthy low-risk women at term without a medical indication as noted on U.S. birth certificate or hospital discharge records. Planned cesareans performed on healthy low-risk women increased by 67 percent between 1991 and 2001. In 2001 over 80,000 women gave birth by cesarean with no clear medical indication. These cesareans were performed for "no indicated risk." No indicated risk (NIR) is a specific category recently created to more accurately reflect those operations performed before labor has begun and for which there is no medical indication such as breech, preeclampsia, or placenta previa, marked on the birth record.[16]

The number of women having their first baby by cesarean is increasing for women of all ages. The CDC estimates that primary cesareans with "no indicated risk" to be between 3 percent and 7 percent. According to researchers and statisticians at the U.S. National Center for Health Statistics one cannot infer from current birth records that pregnant women are actually *choosing* to have a cesarean for no medically indicated reason.[17]

In 2007 expectant mothers who received their prenatal care at the Montefiore Medical Center in Bronx, New York, were surveyed and asked about their attitudes toward cesarean delivery on maternal request (CDMR). Ninety-five percent were not in favor of a medically elective cesarean and felt that vaginal delivery was safer for the mother (93 percent) and the baby (88 percent).[18]

The term "maternal request" cesareans has been used extensively, but inaccurately, as a substitute for the "no indicated risk" cesarean data and as such has created the *perception* that mothers are indeed asking to have a cesarean for reasons other than medical necessity, and are pushing up the cesarean rate. However, serious discussions among U.S. physicians about offering elective cesareans took place as early as 2000. At a Kansas City conference sponsored by the American College of Obstetricians and Gynecologists (ACOG) maternity care experts and researchers debated whether or not healthy women at term should be offered an elective cesarean and if cesareans at term (38 weeks) were cost-effective. Fifty per cent of conference attendees who participated in this debate favored the resolution that healthy pregnant women should be offered an elective cesarean at term.[19] An editorial that same year from ACOG's then President suggested that the time was right for maternal choice cesareans.

In July 2003 Health Grades Inc., a publicly traded company that provides performance reports, ratings, and profiles of hospitals, physicians, and surgical procedures to the health care industry, liability insurers, employers, and consumers released a report entitled, *First-Time Preplanned and "Patient Choice" Cesarean Section Rates in the United States*. Health Grades relies on public records for their reports.[20] Health Grades identified "patient choice" (the two words always in parentheses in their documents) cesareans as preplanned, first time cesareans with no medical indication performed on a woman who has not labored and had no prior cesareans. If none of the twelve medical indications for cesarean section were marked on the birth record it was "hypothesized" that the operation was performed as a result of "patient choice." Health Grade reported that nationwide from 1999 to 2001 about 62,000 cesareans were performed for "patient choice." In reality there was no way that anyone could confirm from public records that it was the mothers who requested these operations. Only that the birth record showed that the surgery was performed for "no indicated risk." Following the release of the report major media sources reported on the increasing trend of choice cesareans without further investigation. "More Women are Choosing to Have Caesarean Sections," said a CNN report. An article in *USA Today* stated, "More Moms Opt to Undergo C-Section Birth."[21] Health Grades issues its own press releases.

The following October ACOG issued a press release regarding ACOG's Committee on Ethics' opinion, "Surgery and Patient Choice: The Ethics of Decision Making."[22] Unlike an editorial, commentary, memo, or update that would circulate within the membership of the organization or in its publications, a press release is distributed to thousands of media outlets worldwide. ACOG stated that "medical evidence is still limited" regarding the benefits and risks of elective cesareans, consequently in "the case of *elective cesarean delivery*, if the physician *believes* that cesarean delivery promotes the overall health and welfare of the woman and her fetus more than does vaginal birth, then he or she is ethically justified in performing a cesarean delivery." The press release reiterated that, "An increasing number of women are requesting elective cesarean instead of a vaginal delivery in the belief that the surgery will prevent future pelvic support or sexual dysfunction problems, or for other reasons." ACOG presented no evidence to substantiate either of these statements. But it may have planted a seed suggesting that "patient choice cesarean" and "cesarean on demand" were a real phenomenon worth considering. An option to discuss with their physicians.

The American College of Nurse Midwives,[23] the Society of Obstetricians and Gynecologists of Canada,[24] the Canadian Association of Midwives,[25] The Royal College of Obstetricians and Gynecologists of Britain,[26] The Royal College of Midwives in the United Kingdom,[27] and the International Federation of Obstetricians and Gynecologists,[28] do not support patient choice cesareans when there is no evidence that it is more beneficial than a normal birth.

In June 2004 Health Grades sent out a press release reporting that "patient choice" cesareans had increased by 25 percent between 2000 and 2002.[29] This time the press release included a quote from its vice president of medical affairs, "Now we see that this increase is continuing, and that the overall in-hospital complication rates for 'patient choice' C-sections may be lower than that of vaginal deliveries."[30] No evidence supported this statement. The report cited ACOG's press release about patient choice cesareans. It also suggested that C-sections were probably more cost-effective over time since they protected women from pelvic floor problems, which would require treatment and further surgery in the future. A questionable assumption. Evidence shows that in the short-term a cesarean without labor will reduce the likelihood of urinary incontinence in approximately 6 percent or less of women at 1 year after childbirth and will protect about 3 percent of women from anal incontinence at 1 year. There is no strong evidence that planning a cesarean instead of having a normal birth protects women from experiencing incontinence beyond the age of 50.[31]

Health Grades makes their data on hospital quality measures available to the employees of 125 companies including more than fifty Fortune 500 companies, via their corporate intranets. The "Hospital Quality" reports according to Health Grades "help women choose a high-quality hospital" by posting complication rates for "patient choice" cesareans. It is easy to see from what sources women would learn that a cesarean will protect them from future pelvic floor problems and to be sure to ask their doctor about a "patient choice" cesarean. The reports also serve to reinforce the *normality* of elective cesareans for reasons other than medical indications.

In September 2005 Health Grades released a *third* report on "patient choice" cesarean section rates in the United States. In fact the company saw the "exponential growth" of "patient choice" cesareans as an example of "empowerment and consumerism among selected women in the United States."[32] With direct intranet access to thousands of employees, the company raised the stakes on "patient choice" cesareans, framing the issue as a reproductive right. An issue that employers could not question if they were considering not reimbursing for non-medically indicated cesareans. Health Grades does not report on the risks associated with cesarean section. Following this third report on "empowered" women who can choose how they want to give birth, the media once again reported on the so called "patient choice" cesareans. A CNN report indicated that elective C-sections increased by 36 percent in a 3 year period. (September 12, 2005).[33] In its June 2007 *HealthGrades Maternity Care Report* the company included a list of hospitals in nineteen states which received the HealthGrades Maternity Excellence Award and a list of HealthGrades Five-Star Maternity Care Hospitals; those with the lowest rate of complications (best performing hospitals) associated with "patient choice" cesareans.[34]

THE NIH STATE-OF-THE-SCIENCE CONFERENCE: LOWERING THE BAR FOR SCIENCE

The national cesarean rate in 2006 had climbed to 29.1 percent, the highest ever. Despite any hard evidence that women in the United States were demanding cesarean sections, in March 2006 the National Institutes of Health cosponsored a State-of-the-Science Conference in Bethesda, Maryland, entitled, "Cesarean Delivery on Maternal Request."[35]

The objective of the conference was to report on the extent of cesarean delivery on maternal request defined as a planned primary cesarean with no indicated medical risk. An independent panel had been charged with reviewing the available evidence on several questions related to cesareans by choice in advance of the conference. The results of their findings were presented at the conference in Bethesda. Curiously, *not one single study* was included by the panel to substantiate that in the United States mothers were requesting cesareans without a medical reason. Moreover, the panel was aware that a recent national survey of women's birth experiences found that less than1 percent of women who had a primary cesarean had actually chosen to do so without a medical indication.[36, 37] For one and a half days, researchers and practitioners discussed the issue of cesarean delivery "on maternal request" now coined, CDMR. The panel recommended that until quality evidence became available, a mother's request for a non-indicated risk cesarean can be considered by her physician so long as she is informed of the benefits and risks of the procedure. The panel cautioned that a cesarean should not be planned before 39 weeks (an assessment that is difficult to accurately make) and is not recommended for women who want a large family (accumulating cesareans increase health risks), both of which are extremely difficult to assess.

At the time of the NIH Conference in 2006 there was extensive evidence about the risks of cesarean section. A systematic review comparing outcomes from cesarean with a normal birth was published by Childbirth Connection in New York and posted on their Web site. The evidence showed that the procedure itself, not a medical condition, was associated with increased short- and long-term health problems for the mother and the baby.[38] A World Health Organization study had reported that the higher the number of cesareans among 124 Latin American hospitals, the higher were the rates of maternal complications and deaths. So too was the number of babies who died or who needed to be admitted to intensive care for 7 days or longer following birth.[39]

The NIH panel recommended that consistent with ethical principles, a doctor could honor a mother's request for a primary cesarean section for no medical indication provided she was informed about the benefits and risks of the operation. Basically, the recommendation reiterated ACOG's position in its October 2003 press release and the majority view at the 2000 Kansas City conference. It seemed clear for many attendants at the conference that something was amiss. Cesarean section, a major abdominal surgery with documented health risks, was being promoted by a panel of experts at the highest level of the federal health service without any strong evidence to substantiate it.

Participants at the NIH State-of-the-Science Conference (researchers, medical journal editors, physicians, midwives, nurses, lactation specialists, and consumer advocacy groups) were given the opportunity to comment in an open discussion forum, and to present their views and provide their own evidence to contribute to the debate. Audience participants questioned the validity, quality, and limitations of the panel's research findings. They found the evidence presented at the conference to be weak and inconclusive. Leading authors of two studies on "no indicated risk" cesareans present at the conference clarified to the panel that their studies could not be used to infer that these cesareans were performed on "maternal request." Furthermore the NIH panel recommendations put into question the physicians' ethical imperative to first do no harm by supporting non-medically indicated cesareans based on the presentation of weak evidence and the omission of existing contrary valid evidence.[40, 41]

Diony Young, Editor of *Birth: Issues in Perinatal Care*, who was present at the conference wrote, "The cesarean delivery rate continues its alarming increase in many parts of the world. Again, however, it must be emphasized that *this is not women's doing*—many factors contribute, of which requests by women in the absence of medical indications comprise an extremely small number.... As many noted it (the NIH Conference) seems to have been conceived and conducted based on a faulty premise."[42]

The Media Perpetuates "Maternal Request" Cesareans

Immediately following the NIH conference national newspapers and major media networks repeated the NIH panel's position regarding cesareans on "maternal request." Many media reports only included comments by NIH panel participants without presenting a different point of view. *The Washington Post* reported, "NIH Panel Finds No Extra Risk in Caesarean Section," and choosing the option of cesarean section "continues to grow in popularity."[43] It also reported that the panel reached its conclusions "after studying the most current scientific evidence." The article included quotes from three high-profile obstetricians who support "maternal request" cesareans. The Associated Press repeated the panel's conclusion, "there's too little research to say definitely whether it's a good or bad idea."[44] Reporting on this critical issue without further investigation propagated the false assumption that cesareans are as safe as a vaginal birth and that a substantial number of women are asking for cesareans for no medical reason. *USA Today*[45] and National Public Radio[46] were two news media outlets that presented a more balanced view of the issue.

The American College of Nurse Midwives stated that "Inaccurate or misleading headlines and reporting about the recent NIH panel on cesarean delivery for maternal request will exacerbate the harm unnecessary surgery causes women."[47]

In an essay in the *Annals of Family Medicine*, family physicians Lawrence M. Leeman and Lauren A. Plante noted, "In recent years we have seen a decline in women's choices for vaginal birth as vaginal birth after cesarean (VBAC) becomes less available and vaginal breech birth is rarely performed. The question of patient-choice cesarean delivery asks only whether a woman should have the right to choose a cesarean delivery in the absence of a medical indication. A woman's right to choose a vaginal delivery is not addressed.... Why advocate for patient choice only when that choice is a cesarean delivery?"[48]

Studies on Risks of Cesarean Delivery on the Heels of the NIH Conference

Soon after the NIH conference several studies were published adding to the body of evidence on the risks related to cesareans. In August 2007 ACOG reported on a French study confirming that cesareans whether performed before or during labor were associated with increased risk for fatal blood clots, infection, complications from anesthesia, and a three-fold increased risk of postpartum maternal death when compared with vaginal birth.[49]

In September 2006, the CDC had published their findings on infant and neonatal mortality for first cesareans with "no indicated risks," more popularly known as cesareans "on maternal request." Researchers found that neonatal mortality rates for full-term infants were almost twice as high among infants delivered by cesarean section for "no indicated risk" when compared with vaginal delivery. The planned cesareans were performed between 37 and 41 weeks,[50] the time frame within which the NIH panel recommended performing a cesarean on "maternal request."

Randomized Control Trials or Medical Experiments?

Some have argued that there are no randomized controlled studies (considered the gold standard of research design) regarding planned low-risk term cesareans compared to planned vaginal birth, and therefore we don't have enough information on the risks of cesareans by choice. Others have rightly questioned the ethics and value of such a study. This kind of trial would theoretically expect thousands of participating pregnant women to agree at random to a have a planned cesarean for their first birth without a medical indication or proceed with a planned vaginal delivery at term. Since 90 percent of U.S. women now have a routine repeat cesarean, women would have a repeat operation if they became pregnant again. Given what is already known about the short-term and long-term health risks for both mothers and babies, one could anticipate more infections, blood clots, readmission to the hospital, uterine ruptures, hysterectomies, adhesions, ectopic pregnancies, and major hemorrhage from placental problems. More babies are likely to be born preterm, of low birth weight, and more likely to experience respiratory problems serious enough to require intensive care.[51]

Cesarean section outnumbers any other major surgical procedure in the United States. Cesareans performed on healthy women carrying healthy full-term babies are increasing for women of all ages and all races, regardless of medical indicators. To imply that all these women are making an *informed choice* to have a surgical delivery for "convenience" or to avoid pelvic floor problems in the future is, at best, misleading.

ESPECIALLY FOR WOMEN

All women have the right to make the best decision for themselves and their babies. This requires that you have full and accurate information about the benefits and risks of the surgery for yourself and your infant, both the short-term effects and the long-term impact. If you are thinking about scheduling a cesarean for non-medical reasons, try to find out as much as you can about it before making up your mind. You should be given information about the short and long-term risks for you and your baby, and how a cesarean would affect any future pregnancies.

RESOURCES

H. Goer, Cesarean Section: Everything You Need to Know, at IVillage.com, http://parenting.ivillage.com/pregnancy/plabor/0,,8wvj,00.html (last accessed on May 25, 2008).

March of Dimes, If You're Pregnant: Cesarean Birth by Request, http://search.marchofdimes.com/cgi-bin/MsmGo.exe?grab_id=4&page_id=1900800&query=cesarean&hiword=CESAREO+cesarean+, (last accessed on May 25, 2008).

PART II

CESAREAN DELIVERY AND ITS IMPACT ON MOTHER AND BABY

4

ABOUT CESAREAN SECTION

Cesarean section is a major operation, with great potential benefit, but also with substantial risks for both mother and baby. The hazards can be kept to a minimum, first, by avoiding unnecessary operations, and, second, by meticulous attention to proper anesthetic and surgical techniques.[1]

The number of cesarean sections performed in any one country or community varies according to medical risk factors, socioeconomic status, cultural norms, the influence of malpractice, health insurance coverage, reimbursement rate, geographic location, type of hospital, ready access to staff and surgical supplies, physician convenience, ethical norms, and individual physician practice patterns.[2]

Surgical techniques for cesarean section and materials used during the operation vary among physicians and countries. Several methods have been suggested to reduce the risk of blood loss, infection, complications, actual operating time, and hospital costs. Some of these techniques and their long-term health effects have been thoroughly evaluated.[3,4,5,6,7] These issues are important because they impact the mother's postpartum health and recovery. They also impact the health of her baby, early mother-infant attachment, and her ability to establish and maintain breastfeeding. Birth by cesarean, even when mothers and babies are healthy, increases maternal and neonatal mortality. With a scheduled cesarean mothers are at least twice as likely to die and babies almost three times as likely to die as a consequence of the surgical procedure itself.[8,9]

WHAT IS THE DIFFERENCE BETWEEN AN ELECTIVE AND AN EMERGENCY CESAREAN?

A cesarean can be planned weeks or months in advance or can become necessary during labor and birth. An elective or scheduled cesarean is one that is planned in advance. An elective cesarean is usually performed before labor begins, before the membranes have ruptured and before labor is induced. With a scheduled cesarean the medical staff, the mother, and her family have time to make preparations for the birth of the baby. The term elective has also been used to mean a medically unnecessary cesarean.

The terms "emergency" or "crash" cesarean can be misleading and are interpreted in several ways. They usually refer to an unscheduled cesarean section that has been decided upon during labor or birth. Sometimes mothers wait minutes or an hour or two before the surgery actually begins. When time is of essence, every effort is made to move as quickly as possible. The consensus among clinicians is that a cesarean should begin within 30 minutes of the time the decision is made. The common term is "decision to incision." In Britain, four levels of urgency guidelines have been established to assist care providers on how best they can respond when an operation is needed. Level 1: If there is an immediate threat to the mother's or baby's life. Level 2: If the mother's or baby's health is compromised, but is not immediately life threatening. Level 3: Neither the mother nor baby's health is compromised, but there is the need for an early cesarean delivery. Level 4: The cesarean is timed to suit the mother, the physician, and the operating room staff schedule.[10]

Reasons for Planned Cesarean

A planned cesarean is often the safest choice for mothers who have a medical condition (such as diabetes), with a very large baby, HIV (human immunodeficiency virus), a genital herpes outbreak close to their due date, uterine tumors that obstruct the birth canal, or a low-lying placenta. The baby may be a footling breech, or positioned in a transverse lie (horizontally). Recently, in the United States, an increasing number of planned cesarean sections have been performed with no medical indication recorded on the birth certificates.[11]

Reasons for a Cesarean in Labor

For some women who labored for many hours, the thought of having to give birth by cesarean can be very disappointing. For others, a cesarean signals the end of a long, painful, and exhausting process. Serious unexpected complications such as hemorrhage from the placental site, a prolapsed umbilical cord, or nonreassuring fetal heart tones (baby's heart rate is abnormal), make a cesarean the safest option.

Consent for Surgery

If the cesarean is scheduled, mothers can take the time to review the consent for surgery document before the operation. Often, if the cesarean has been decided upon during labor, mothers have very little time if any to review the forms or ask questions. Some hospitals combine the consent for surgery (cesarean) documents with a general consent form given to all mothers when admitted to the labor and delivery unit.

Preparation before Surgery

Intravenous fluids (IV) are necessary before regional anesthesia and during surgery. The mother may be given an antacid about 30 minutes before surgery to reduce the risk of aspiration of any stomach content into her lungs, should she require general anesthesia. She may also be given medication for nausea. Research shows that all women should be given prophylactic antibiotics before surgery to reduce the risk of infection-related complications, including fever, endometritis (infection of the endometrium), wound infection, urinary tract infection, and serious postoperative infection. Antibiotic prophylaxis reduces infectious by about two-thirds.[12]

To further reduce the risk of infection the nurse will clip the pubic hair along the incision line and apply an antiseptic. Because any anesthetic used will affect the mother's ability to control her bladder and to keep it empty, a catheter will be inserted in her urethra. The bladder is located close to the uterus. When it is empty it can be kept out of the way during surgery and the risk of bladder injury can be reduced. The catheter remains in place till the mother regains control of her bladder functions, usually within 24 hours. Additional fluids, before the anesthetic is given, help to prevent a fall in blood pressure. The mother may also be given oxygen. Her blood pressure and the baby's heart rate will be monitored. A pediatrician and the newborn nursery staff will be notified that a cesarean will be performed. The staff will make sure an infant warmer is available and working and that resuscitation equipment is in place. The anesthesiologist or nurse anesthetist will talk to the mother about her options for anesthesia. The safest options are an epidural or a spinal although not all hospitals provide regional anesthesia. General anesthesia poses the highest risks for both the mother and her baby. In case of emergency, general anesthesia works faster.

Anesthesia

Anesthesia may be given by a general anesthesiologist, an anesthesiologist whose specialty is obstetrics and neonatal care, or it may be administered by a nurse anesthetist. Before and after surgery the anesthesiologist monitors the mother's heart rate, blood pressure, body temperature, and body fluid balance. He controls the mother's level of pain and monitors her medical condition. Anesthesia and surgery affect the mother's entire system so it's important for the anesthesiologist to find out as much as possible about her medical history and any medications she may be taking. If the mother has a medical condition such as asthma, diabetes, or heart problems, he takes this into consideration. Time permitting, he will discuss with the mother the anesthesia choices available to her, their risks and benefits, and describe the procedure.[13]

There are two anesthesia options for a cesarean section: regional anesthesia or general anesthesia. Regional anesthesia, an epidural or a spinal, allows the mother to be awake during surgery, talk to her partner, communicate with the surgical staff, and hear her baby's first cry. The mother can have eye-to-eye contact, speak to her baby, and hold her close to her chest for a few moments if one of her arms is freed from restraint. Some mothers prefer not to be awake during a cesarean. General anesthesia today is usually used in cases of emergency, when medical conditions of the mother warrant it, or if there is no anesthesiologist on staff trained in administering regional anesthesia.

Lumbar Epidural Block

There are two common types of regional anesthesia used for a cesarean. Epidural anesthesia, (a stronger form of the epidural analgesia used for labor pain), and a spinal block. Both block pain sensation in the nerves in the lower part of the body and result in loss of muscle function. A lumbar epidural blocks the nerves that register pain sensations from the uterus and cervix to the spinal cord and to the brain. Before the anesthesiologist administers the epidural, the mother's back is wiped with an antiseptic solution and a sterile drape placed over her lower back. She will be asked to lie on her left side or in a sitting position with her chin on her chest and her knees close to her belly.

A local anesthetic is first injected into her skin before inserting the epidural needle. After a minute or two the epidural needle is inserted into her lower back between two vertebrae. The needle guides a small catheter to the epidural space located outside the dura, the membrane that covers the spinal canal. A test dose of medication will be given through the catheter to confirm that it has been placed at the correct site. The needle is then removed but the catheter stays in place to administer additional medication if needed and is taped to the mother's back. The mother usually begins to feel the numbing effects throughout her lower body and in her legs in about 3 to 5 minutes.[14]

Common drugs used today for epidurals include a combination of anesthetic agents and narcotics. Anesthetics include bupivacaine and ropivacaine. Fentanyl, or sufentanil are common narcotics. After the birth, morphine (Duramorph) may be inserted into the epidural catheter to allow the mother to be pain-free for a few hours. If the epidural is not effective before the surgery begins, the mother may need to have spinal anesthesia or a general anesthetic.

Spinal Anesthesia

With spinal anesthesia the anesthetic is injected with a needle directly into the spinal canal. A mother will feel numb from her lower chest down to her feet. A needle thinner than a larger needle can reduce the chances of a spinal headache caused from leaking of spinal fluid when the membrane covering the spinal canal is punctured. Because spinal anesthesia numbs the chest area also, sometimes the mother will feel short of breath or feels she is having difficulty breathing. Spinal anesthesia lasts about an hour or two.[15]

Which Regional Anesthetic Is More Effective?

Spinal anesthesia is sometimes preferred for cesarean section. The technique is less complicated than for an epidural, and it takes less time to administer (about 8 minutes less), and the spinal block delivers a deeper level of pain relief. However, women who have a spinal for a cesarean section tend to have a higher risk for hypotension (low blood pressure). Researchers of the Cochrane Library found no difference between the two methods with regard to failure rate, the need for postoperative pain relief, or the need to switch over to general anesthesia, and could not reach a conclusion regarding the relative incidence of intraoperative side effects of each.[16]

General Anesthesia

When time is of the essence or in countries or facilities where regional anesthesia is cost prohibitive and skilled personnel are unavailable, general anesthesia is used. General anesthesia poses the most risks. Complications such as pulmonary aspiration (acidic stomach content are diverted to the trachea and the lungs), and neonatal depression is more likely. Aspiration of stomach content can cause pneumonia and breathing problems.[17]

With general anesthesia the medication is given into a vein and results in a rapid loss of consciousness. The mother is first brought into the operating room where the anesthesiologist monitors her blood pressure, oxygen level, and heart rhythms. She is placed on her back on a slightly tilted operating table, and as she begins to breathe oxygen through a mask placed on her nose and mouth, the anesthetic is injected through an IV. After the baby has been born additional pain medication can be given to the mother to alleviate her pain. With general anesthesia the mother becomes unconscious almost immediately, and an airway tube will then be inserted into her mouth and down her windpipe to assure that she and her baby are getting enough oxygen. The tube is removed when the surgery is complete. The tube also serves as a safeguard to protect any stomach regurgitation from entering the lungs.[18] With any type of anesthesia mothers may experience nausea, vomiting, or a headache after the delivery.

IN THE OPERATING ROOM

The mother will be assisted onto the operating table and a hip wedge placed under her right hip to tip the uterus slightly and lower the risk for compression of the blood vessel returning blood to the mother's heart. Being at an angle also lowers the chance of the mother feeling nauseous. To achieve the same effect the operating table can be tilted sideways to a 15 degree angle. Her abdomen will be washed down with an antiseptic and covered with sterile drapes leaving an open window for the physician to make the incision and deliver the baby. A screen is placed across the mother's abdomen and she does not see the surgery taking place.

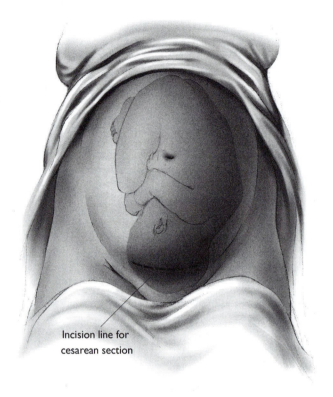

Incision line for
cesarean section

Photo 4.1. Incision line for cesarean section (low transverse).
Source: © Martens & Kiefer 2007.

Skin Incision

The skin incision for a cesarean birth is usually transverse and made just below the pubic hairline (Pfannenstiel incision). If it heals properly it will not be noticeable. This is called a "bikini incision." Occasionally a physician will make a vertical skin (midline) incision if the baby is large, or if the mother or baby's condition is critical and there is not much time to spare. This incision begins above the mother's pubic bone and extends to the mother's umbilicus (belly button) (see Photo 4.1).

Uterine Incision

Below the skin lie fatty tissue and the abdominal fascia (see Photo 4.2). Separating the abdominal muscles from each other instead of cutting them allows the mother to heal better (see Photo 4.3). The most common type of uterine incision is transverse and is made in the lower part of the uterus (low-segment incision). Occasionally a low vertical incision may be made for a preterm baby, or

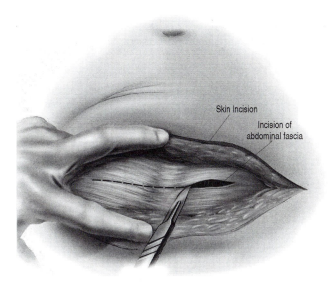

Photo 4.2. Incision of skin and incision of abdominal fascia.
Source: © Martens & Kiefer 2007.

for an abnormally positioned placenta. An incision in the lower part of the uterus bleeds less, heals stronger, and results in a lower risk for complications (see Photo 4.4). With a low-segment transverse scar it is safe to plan a VBAC with a future pregnancy. Rarely, an extension of the transverse incision is made, a J-shaped, or inverted T-shaped incision to make additional room. With these incisions the mother may not be able to labor for a VBAC.

If there are uterine fibroids or dense adhesions from a prior uterine scar a vertical incision (classical) will be made in the upper part of the uterus. A vertical incision is also used in case of extreme emergencies or if a large baby needs additional room to be born. This type of incision is also made for preterm babies in a breech position and for mothers who are obese. With a classical incision bleeding is extensive and additional blood can be lost if the placenta (usually positioned in the upper part of the uterus) is accidentally cut. With this incision infection and adhesions are more likely. Planning a normal birth with a prior classical uterine incision is not recommended.

The mother should not be able to feel pain but only pressure or a tugging feeling. She may feel nausea as the uterus is being handled, will hear the suctioning of the amniotic fluids and will notice a slight burning smell when the blood vessels are being cauterized.

When the uterine incision is made the amniotic fluid (bag of waters) is suctioned. The blood vessels that have been cut are cauterized to reduce blood loss. The physician brings the baby out of the uterine cavity while another physician applies pressure on the mother's abdomen (see Photo 4.5).

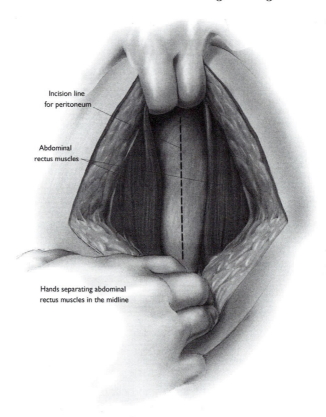

Photo 4.3. Incision line in peritoneum and abdominal rectus Muscles. *Source:* © Martens & Kiefer 2007.

The amniotic fluid is quickly suctioned from the baby's mouth and nose. With a vaginal delivery the baby's chest is compressed by the uterine contractions and its airways are cleared of most of the fluid by the time it is born.

The umbilical cord is clamped and the baby covered to avoid body heat loss. At birth the nursing staff and perhaps a pediatrician assess the baby's vital signs and when they are stable the baby can be placed on the mother's chest. A staff member trained in infant resuscitation may also be present, especially if the mother has had general anesthesia. If there are complications the staff may need to take the baby for evaluation and monitoring.

When the cord has been clamped, the placenta will need to be separated from the uterine wall and taken out of the uterine cavity. With a normal birth, the contractions take care of this function. Current evidence-based surgical techniques suggest that the placenta should be pulled away from the uterine wall very gently rather than forcefully. The physician then examines the uterus and begins closing the incision. The uterus and other layers will be closed with

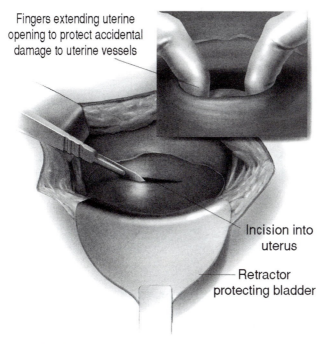

Fingers extending uterine
opening to protect accidental
damage to uterine vessels

Incision into
uterus

Retractor
protecting bladder

Photo 4.4. Entering the Uterus by a Lower Segment Incision.
Source: © Martens & Kiefer 2007.

dissolvable sutures, the skin is sutured or stapled, and a bandage will be placed over the scar (see Photos 4.6 and 4.7).

After the delivery, the mother will most likely feel herself trembling and perhaps also nauseated for a short while. When the surgery is complete the mother's abdomen will be wiped down, she will be given a clean gown, and covered with a warm blanket. To make the mother comfortable she may be given a sedative or an additional pain medication through her IV. The mother can ask to delay the medication until she has had time to spend a few minutes with the baby.

POST-OPERATIVE RECOVERY

As with any other major surgical procedure, the mother will be taken to a recovery area or the room she labored in where her vital signs will be monitored. In recovery, a nurse will assess the mother's vital signs every 5 minutes until they are stable; then every 15 minutes for an hour, and then every 30 minutes, until she is well enough to go to the postpartum unit. The nurse will check her perineal pad every 15 minutes for at least an hour and check for any excessive bleeding. She will palpate the fundus to check for firmness. A firm fundus means the uterus is contracting and controlling

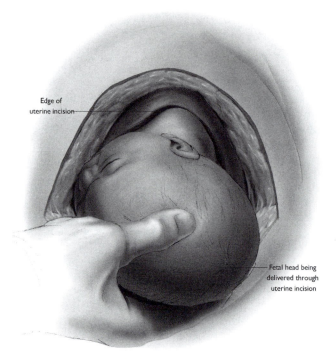

Edge of
uterine incision

Fetal head being
delivered through
uterine incision

Photo 4.5. Delivering the fetal head through the uterine incision.
Source: © Martens & Kiefer 2007.

bleeding from the placental site. Oxytocin is usually administered through the IV to make the uterus contract. If the mother was under general anesthesia she will be positioned on her side to help with drainage of secretions, turned, and helped with coughing and deep breathing. Breathing deeply to remove secretions is important when any type of anesthesia is used. If she has had a spinal or an epidural, her level of anesthesia will be checked every 15 minutes until full sensation has returned. Fluid intake and urine output is measured for volume and the presence of a bloody tinge (bladder trauma). The mother may be given additional medication to relieve pain and nausea, as needed.

The nursing staff will also watch the baby if her baby is with her in recovery. They will check the baby's temperature, breathing, skin color, and heart rate. When the mother is ready, she can begin breastfeeding her baby. The mother may wish just to hold her baby, hear his voice, stroke his head, and talk to him, depending on how alert she may be and how much pain she feels. Sometimes mothers are extremely tired, especially if the cesarean was performed after many hours of induction and labor. If the mother can't be with her baby, her partner can provide a verbal account of the first few hours in the nursery. Every effort should be made to keep the mother and her baby together

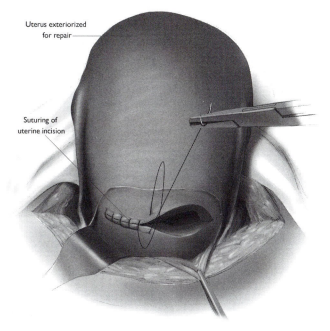

Uterus exteriorized
for repair

Suturing of
uterine incision

Photo 4.6. Suturing of uterine incision. *Source*: © Martens &
Kiefer 2007.

right after birth. Skin-to-skin contact facilitates mother-infant attachment and
breastfeeding. It is easier for a mother to begin breastfeeding before the anesthesia has worn off.

Postpartum Recovery in the Hospital

Surgery makes the mother vulnerable to pulmonary infection due to the
use of narcotics and sedatives and her altered immune response. The mother
will be encouraged to walk as soon as she is able to, and to cough and breathe
deeply every 2 to 4 hours when she is awake. Walking stimulates the digestive
system, increases circulation, and reduces the odds of developing a blood clot.
The urinary bladder catheter will be removed when the mother is able to
walk. Gas pain is usual for the first few days. To minimize her discomfort, the
nursing staff will help her to move her legs, tighten her abdomen, and walk
slowly as soon as she is able to do so.

To help the mother with postoperative pain she may have had narcotics
placed in her epidural after the surgery or she will be offered analgesics. She
may have patient-controlled analgesia (PCA). With PCA the mother can control
the amount of pain medication she needs. With PCA mothers tend to use less
medication overall. Usually morphine or meperidine is used, and the mother
can self-administer small doses of medication through an intravenous pump,

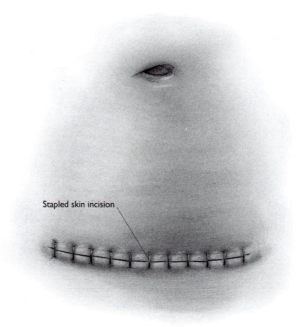

Photo 4.7. Stapled skin incision. *Source*: © Martens & Kiefer 2007.

as needed. The pump is preset to dispense the drugs to avoid overmedication. If there are no complications, the dressing over the skin incision is usually removed 24 hours after surgery. The skin sutures will be removed after discharge.

The nursing staff will assist the mother into comfortable positions and help her with the challenging task of breastfeeding after surgery. For mothers who have had a cesarean, a lactation consultant can be very helpful in assisting them to initiate and establish breastfeeding, despite the pain and discomfort from surgery. The mother may be ready to shower on the second day. In the United States, if there are no complications, most mothers are discharged by the end of the third day after the cesarean surgery.

ESPECIALLY FOR MOTHERS

A cesarean may become necessary at some point during your pregnancy or during labor, even if you have done all you could to prepare for a normal birth. If you plan ahead and think about what is important to you, you can have a positive birth experience. Find out what options are available to you, talk to your doctor or midwife, and ask that important requests be honored and included in the admitting orders if the cesarean is scheduled. You may want to give a copy of your cesarean birth preferences to your nurses as well as your preferences for a normal birth. Of course, if a cesarean is decided upon during labor, it may not be possible for the staff to honor all your requests. It is important for you and for the staff to communicate openly about the options available to you. Find out if you can have a copy of the consent for surgery to review during your pregnancy. Here are some issues that may be important for you. It is helpful to discuss them with your partner and your care providers. If the cesarean is planned:

- Is it possible to wait to begin surgery after your labor begins? This will reduce the baby's risk of being born premature and having breathing problems.
- Can the anesthesiologist give you a spinal or epidural so you can be awake during the birth, see your baby's face, hear your baby's first cry, and start breastfeeding sooner?
- Can your baby have her first exam (Apgar Score) in the operating room?
- Can you hold your baby on your chest while the team completes the cesarean? You can see, feel, and speak to your baby while your doctors complete the surgery.
- Can the anesthesiologist delay giving you sedatives after your baby is born to allow you to interact with your partner and your baby and be alert during recovery?
- Can the anesthesiologist give you pain medication through your epidural to extend your pain relief for the first 24 hours after your baby is born? This allows you to feel better without being drowsy.
- Can you record your baby's first cry? Videotape or take pictures of your newborn?
- Can your partner go with the baby to the nursery during observation? Your partner can then tell you about your baby's first moments.
- Can you have your baby in the recovery room? Can family or friends visit you and the baby in the recovery area?
- Can your partner stay with you overnight in your postpartum room? Can the hospital provide a cot to sleep on?
- Can you have rooming in? Keep your baby with you rather than in the nursery?
- Is a lactation specialist available to help you get started with breastfeeding? Babies born by cesarean need extra help to initiate breastfeeding. Mothers who had surgery need additional support and guidance to initiate and continue breastfeeding successfully.
- Do you have any other concerns you wish to discuss with your care providers?

Potential Complications of a Cesarean: What You Should Know

Since a cesarean delivery is major abdominal surgery as well as the method of birth of your baby, there are some general effects from a cesarean that may lengthen your recovery and affect your ability to be with your baby as much as you would like soon after the birth. They may affect your ability to care for your baby in the first few weeks at home. You may have some health problems down the road that you did not anticipate. Knowing about these potential complications may help you make an informed decision about having the surgery and may help you cope better if they do develop. *Compared to a vaginal birth, the following are more likely for mothers with a cesarean section:*

- Complications from anesthesia
- Pelvic pain
- Bladder injury
- Injury to the ureters (tubes that connect the kidneys to the bladder)
- Developing a blood clot
- Higher risk for infection
- Admission to the intensive care unit
- Returning to the hospital due to complications from the cesarean
- Emotional well-being and overall mental health may be compromised.

Give Yourself Time to Recover

A cesarean section is major abdominal surgery. Pain medications and the anesthesia will affect how you feel. You may experience extreme pain (when the anesthesia wears off), nausea, vomiting, uncontrollable shaking, extreme tiredness, and the need to sleep. Medications that you need to calm your pain will likely make you feel drowsy. You may feel a deep sense of disappointment that your birth did not go as planned. It is normal and important for mothers to take care of their own physical and emotional needs so that they can be prepared to welcome and care for their baby. With no other major surgery is a patient ever expected to assume full responsibility of providing for the basic needs of another vulnerable and totally dependent human being.

Recovering from major surgery, caring for your baby, and adjusting to your new family all at the same time will take quite a bit of energy. Every mother is different. How you feel and when you are ready to welcome your baby will depend on many things. Some mothers recover quickly, others take several weeks. You may be very pleased with how everything turned out or you may be upset and disappointed that your baby was born by cesarean. You may find it easy to initiate breastfeeding or may need additional help from a lactation consultant. Friends or family may be ready to help out when you come home, or you and your partner may be caring for your baby alone or with the help of a postpartum doula. This baby may be your firstborn in which case there will be much to learn about parenting and caring for an infant. Or you may have had a cesarean before and know what to expect and what the normal path to recovery is like. Perhaps your baby needs to stay in the nursery for special care after you have gone home. Your feelings about your cesarean birth will take time to sort out.

For Partners of Mothers Having a Cesarean

If the birth of your child by cesarean section is planned you will probably have the time you need to discuss your concerns with your partner, physician, and family before the operation. You will probably receive specific information about the procedure and your partner and your baby's path to recovery. Having this knowledge ahead of time will give you time to think about how involved you want to be, and how you can best support your partner and meet her needs.

If your partner has a cesarean at some point during labor your experience may be very different. Partners always feel thankful and excited when their child is born, even by cesarean. But, not all fathers cope well witnessing the mother's surgery. Some partners feel reassured and grateful to be present and involved, while others may feel stressed, shocked, confused, or helpless. Often all the attention is on the mother and the baby; the staff moves quickly and may not have the time to explain what is happening. Taking initiative to communicate with the staff and asking the questions you need to will be very helpful. Partners feel more reassured when their concerns are addressed.

Many fathers want to accompany their partners to the surgical suite and be present for the birth of their child. Others feel very uncomfortable being present when their partner is having major surgery. The decision to go into the operating room or wait outside to welcome your baby may not be an easy one to make. Although the medical staff will take care of your partner and your baby's medical needs, you are the one who can best meet the mother's emotional needs. You are the one who knows her best. She will need to feel safe, talk about how she feels, and know about the baby's care after the birth. During the surgery you can sit beside her at the head of the table, talk to her, share with her what you see happening in the room, and welcome the birth of your baby together. If the baby needs medical attention, the staff may need to take your baby to the nursery right away. Your partner may want you to go along and come back to let her know how your baby is doing.

Breastfeeding after a Cesarean

Many mothers can successfully learn about and initiate breastfeeding after a cesarean. However, they need a lot of support before they leave the hospital. Many hospitals make a concerted effort to make sure mothers and their babies have established a healthy breastfeeding pattern before leaving the hospital. You are most likely to succeed with breastfeeding after a cesarean if the hospital has been designated as Baby Friendly. The staff at a Baby Friendly hospital talks to mothers about the importance of breastfeeding and help mothers and babies have skin-to-skin contact and initiate breastfeeding as soon as possible after birth, usually within 30 minutes to 1 hour. They encourage mothers to keep their babies with them at all times (rooming in) and feed their babies only breast milk whenever the baby wants it. To maintain a good breastfeeding pattern they will show you how to keep your milk coming in even if you need to be away from your baby. They will also give you a list of resources and support groups in your community. Many hospitals are working toward becoming Baby Friendly. Ask what your hospital is doing to help mothers establish breastfeeding, especially after a cesarean birth.

Hiring a Postpartum Doula

Mothers who have had a cesarean birth may benefit from the services of a postpartum doula. A postpartum doula comes to your home and provides whatever the family needs to make their recovery and adjustment to parenting easier. Doulas can help families learn about newborn baby care, comfort and care for the mother, assist with breastfeeding, light meal preparation, and baby laundry. She can help parents gain confidence in caring for their new baby or help older children welcome their new sibling and help comfort their mom. Some families benefit from a few visits from a postpartum doula; others use the services for a few months. Doulas work days, evenings, overnight, or on weekends.

RESOURCES

Baby Friendly Hospitals, http://www.BabyFriendlyUSA.org, (last accessed on March 15, 2008).

Birthrites, Caesarean Birth, Making Informed Choices Information Booklet, http://www.birthrites.org, (last accessed on March 15, 2008).

Centers for Disease Control and Prevention, Breastfeeding, http://www.cdc.gov/breastfeeding, (last accessed on May 25, 2008).

DONA International, Postpartum Doula, http://www.dona.org.

La Leche League International Is It Possible to Breastfeed After a Cesarean Birth? http://www.llli.org/FAQ/cesarean.html, (last accessed on May 25, 2008).

National Collaborating Centre for Women and Children's Health, *National Institute for Clinical Excellence. CG 13 Caesarean Section, Full Guidelines* (London: Royal College of Obstetricians and Gynecologists Press, April 2004, http://guidance.nice.org.uk/CG13/guidance/pdf/English, (last accessed on May 25, 2008).

Penny Simkin, The Best Cesarean Possible, Pennysimkin.com, http://pennysimkin.com/acticles/Best_Cesarean_Possible.pdf, (last accessed on May 13, 2008).

U.K. Midwifery Archives. From Radical Midwives Homepage. Planning a Good Cesarean, http://www.radmid.demon.co.uk/csgood.htm, (last accessed on May 25, 2008).

U.S. National Library of Medicine, Health Information in Multiple Languages, http://www.nlm.nih.gov/medlineplus/languages/languages.html (July 5, 2008).

5

How Safe Are Cesareans?

Pregnant women should be offered evidence-based information and support to enable them to make informed decisions about childbirth. Addressing women's views and concerns should be recognized as being integral to the decision making process.[1]

Concerns about Cesareans Are Not New

Throughout the 1960s the U.S. cesarean birth rate averaged 5 to 7 percent. By 1978 it had increased by 300 percent and one in six mothers were giving birth by cesarean. Concerned about the rapidly rising cesarean rate, the U.S. Department of Health and Human Services and the National Institutes of Health (NIH) sponsored a multidisciplinary *consensus conference* on cesarean section. The 1981 *consensus report, Cesarean Childbirth,* published the findings of this investigation.[2] More than 25 years ago this widely disseminated report made it clear that a cesarean delivery put women and newborns at increased risk for complications.

The report cautioned that a cesarean is a major surgical procedure and as such was associated with several complications less likely to be experienced in a vaginal birth. Complications of a cesarean delivery were substantially higher (five to ten times higher) than complications related to a vaginal birth. The risk for complications varied widely between institutions in different parts of the country—from 4.2 to 50 percent. Maternal mortality also varied widely between institutions and was related to the surgeons' and the anesthesiologists' level of skill, and the availability of adequate hospital resources. Despite these wide variations, however, the NIH report concluded that although maternal mortality was extremely uncommon, 10 maternal deaths per 100,000 births, overall a birth by cesarean carried about four times the risk of maternal mortality compared to a vaginal birth.

Cesarean-associated risks for newborns include fetal lung immaturity and respiratory distress syndrome (RDS) when cesareans are scheduled before term. RDS is a serious life threatening complication. The fetal lungs are the last major organs to mature before birth. A protein called surfactant is needed to allow the small air sacs in the baby's lungs to inflate and deflate allowing the intake of oxygen. Babies born too early have immature lungs, which tend to collapse and require treatment with surfactants to improve their condition. The 1970s saw a considerable increase in the number of babies born by cesarean section in the United States who developed RDS, and consequently needed admission to neonatal intensive care units. A number of these newborns died. An evaluation of this phenomenon indicated that many of these complications and deaths were ill-timed and iatrogenic (physician caused). In one study reviewed by the NIH, obstetricians scheduled cesareans at what they estimated to be 38.9 weeks of pregnancy. After birth, however, pediatricians' independent assessment of the same newborns placed the maturity of the infants at about 36.6 weeks. Similarly, in another study the obstetricians estimated the length of pregnancy to be 39.0 weeks as opposed to the post-birth evaluation of 35.4 weeks. A significant difference in the potential for preterm birth, low birth weight, breathing difficulties, health complications, and death.

THE CRUX OF THE ARGUMENT TODAY

For years proponents of the safety of cesarean section have argued that climbing cesarean rates were justified. Studies that indicated cesarean-related health risks were biased. They argued that researchers had not separated complications of the surgery itself from the diagnosis for which they were performed. They contended that overall cesarean rates needed to be risk-adjusted. There is now a large body of evidence to support the position that cesarean surgery, planned for low-risk women, increases the risk for complications and death for both mothers and babies. Ironically, because of the ongoing worldwide increase in planned cesareans for healthy women without prior labor, it is possible to identify risks associated to the surgery itself.

How Does a Cesarean Birth Affect the Mother?

Studies on the impact of planned low-risk cesareans from several different countries, varying healthcare systems, and socioeconomic societies have found similar significant risks for mothers and babies associated with cesarean section. Researchers in France,[3] Latin America,[4] and Canada[5] compared the outcomes of low-risk women who planned a cesarean with the outcomes of a similar group of low-risk women who had a vaginal birth. Their findings show that cesareans expose mothers and newborns to the risks of major abdominal surgery and increase the risks for maternal and fetal death. Cesareans by "choice" and routine repeat cesareans warrant serious reconsideration.

Compared to a vaginal birth, a cesarean delivery exposes women to several complications: surgical injuries, a higher rate of infection, complications from anesthesia, longer hospital stays, and readmission to the hospital sooner after discharge and for a longer duration of time. Cesarean section puts women at risk for deep venous clots, pulmonary embolism (blood clot in the lungs), and stroke. Giving birth by cesarean increases the severity of pain and the length of time mothers experience it. All abdominal surgeries cause adhesions (scar tissue) over time that are more likely to continue to cause chronic pelvic pain. Adhesions can also cause bowel obstruction and complicate future surgeries including elective repeat cesareans. Women who have a cesarean birth are more likely to experience poor overall mental health and self-esteem and poor overall functioning. More women are at risk for death with a cesarean delivery.[6] The significance of these complications warrants a more detailed examination.

Surgical Injuries

During surgery inadvertent injuries to the gastrointestinal tract, and urinary tract can occur.[7] A prior cesarean also puts women at increased risk for injuries with future pelvic surgeries. A study conducted in France found that compared to women who never had a cesarean delivery women who once gave birth by cesarean experienced significantly higher incidences of hemorrhage and injuries to the bladder and intestines after a vaginal hysterectomy performed years later for non-pregnancy-related reasons. The risk for complication for women with one or more prior cesareans was 18.3 percent compared to 3.58 percent for women without a prior cesarean.[8]

Infection

Infection is the most common side effect of cesarean delivery. According to a report from the American College of Obstetricians and Gynecologists (ACOG) endometritis (the inflammation of the inner lining of the uterus caused by infection) occurs in 10 percent to 50 percent of women who give birth by cesarean compared to 1 percent to 3 percent of women who have a normal birth. Women who are obese or who are diabetic run a higher risk for of infection.[9] The infection can develop within 48 hours or up to 6 weeks after the birth. Women can also suffer from wound and urinary tract infections. Infection is a much more critical issue in less affluent countries with high cesarean rates where cost for routine use of prophylactic antibiotics may be prohibitive. All women who have a cesarean should be given antibiotics to prevent infection,[10] but many are not. A Canadian study of women who had a planned elective cesarean found that only 25 percent of the women who had a postoperative surgical site infection were administered a preventive dose of antibiotics.[11]

Although care providers prescribe antibiotics as a preventive measure, antibiotic-resistant infections are not uncommon in many hospitals and are becoming more prevalent. Nosocomial (hospital acquired) infections are a serious threat to patient health. The Centers for Disease Control (CDC) estimates that each year, nearly 2 million people in the United States acquire an infection while in a hospital. More than 70 percent of the bacteria that cause these infections are resistant to at least one of the antibiotics commonly used to treat them.[12]

Currently the most common multidrug-resistant strain of staphylococcus is methicillin-resistant staphylococcus aureus (MRSA). MRSA is about two-and-a-half times more lethal than infections that are treatable with methicillin. In 2005, there were 300 MRSA infections among the 1.3 million C-sections and 600 MRSA infections among the 2.9 million vaginal deliveries.[13]

Blood Loss

Serious blood loss during and after a cesarean birth is more likely compared to a vaginal delivery.[14] At times a blood transfusion may be necessary. A rare potential complication of severe childbirth or postpartum hemorrhage is Sheehan's Syndrome. Severe blood loss deprives tissues and organs of oxygen, causing tissue death. With childbirth severe blood loss can affect the pituitary gland (a small bean-shaped gland at the base of the brain), which produces hormones that regulate metabolism, fertility, healing of wounds, breastfeeding, and other vital functions. This results in a permanent lower than normal production of pituitary hormones (hypopituaterism). The effects can be seen immediately (such as in the difficulty or inability to breastfeed), or slowly, perhaps months or years later in life.[15]

Complications from Anesthesia

Three commonly available options for anesthesia for a cesarean section are an epidural, a spinal, and general anesthesia. With epidural anesthesia milder reactions can include heart palpitations, feeling confused or apprehensive, and a metallic taste in the mouth. Low blood pressure, shivering, nausea, vomiting, and backache are more serious side effects. With an epidural, the needle can unintentionally be pushed in farther than intended, past the dura, the membrane that encloses the spinal cord (a lumbar puncture). A small amount of spinal fluid can leak out and cause a severe headache. If the anesthetic enters the spinal fluid it can affect the mother's chest muscles and make it difficult for her to breathe. Rare complications can include neurological problems, a toxic drug reaction, problems in breathing, and death.[16] Sometimes the anesthesia fails to take its full effect. A British survey of several methods and techniques used for cesarean section reported an overall failure rate of 7.1 percent for epidurals, 2 percent for combined spinal-epidurals, and 1.9 percent for a onetime injection of spinal anesthesia.[17]

Postpartum Pain

Although women who have a cesarean birth are often told that they will fully recover in 6 weeks, eight out of ten women who had a cesarean in a

U.S. hospital experienced pain as a problem within 2 months of their surgery. One-third considered the pain to be a major problem. For 18 percent of the women the pain persisted for at least 6 months.[18]

Post-Surgical Adhesions

Long after giving birth, women can experience pelvic pain from internal scar tissue. After a cesarean section there is a high risk of developing pelvic adhesions. According to the National Women's Health Resource Center, adhesions occur when bands of scar tissue adhere to pelvic or abdominal organs. The process resembles plastic wrap that clings to itself. Scar tissue forms as a result of trauma or injury to the peritoneum, the clear membrane (or sheath) that covers the abdominal and pelvic organs. The membrane is slippery when healthy but when injured the immune system response causes inflammation and the production of fibrin matrix, a sticky scar tissue. Adhesions may not form for months or even years after a cesarean section. Adhesions that bind organs and tissues together cause the pain. Repeat cesareans sections have a very high risk for adhesions.[19]

Bowel Obstruction

Mothers who give birth by cesarean are almost three times more likely to have major bowel problems than mothers who have a vaginal delivery. Months or even years after a cesarean 1 to 9 per 1,000 women will be at risk for an intestinal or bowel obstruction due to adhesions.[20] Based on the U.S. 2005 cesarean birth rate of 30.2 percent at least 1,242 and as many as 11,179 mothers would potentially be at risk for intestinal or bowel obstruction as a result of adhesions from the surgery.[21]

Blood Clots

A blood clot or thrombus can form in a vein as a result of a surgical procedure. Most blood clots occur in the deep veins of the legs (deep vein thrombosis or DVT). The clot can potentially detach from its original site and cause a pulmonary embolism that can be fatal. According to an Agency for Healthcare Quality and Research (AHRQ) report on patient safety, deep blood clots occur relatively frequently in hospitalized surgical patients.[22] A study of over 1 million women who gave birth in Sweden between 1987 and 1995 found that the risk of pulmonary embolism (blood clot in the lungs) at birth and in the postpartum period was seven times higher for women who had a cesarean when compared to women who had a spontaneous vaginal birth.[23]

Deep vein thrombosis and pulmonary embolism are the leading causes of maternal death associated with a cesarean section.[24] The risk of stroke from a blood clot for mothers who have a cesarean is relatively rare, 1 to 9 per 10,000. But it is four times higher than for mothers who have a normal birth.[25] In 2005, 1.2 million women in the United States gave birth by cesarean.

Approximately 124 and as many as 11,179 mothers who had the operation would potentially be at risk for developing blood clots related to the surgery.

The Need for Intensive Care

In developed countries it is rare for women to need intensive care following childbirth. However, it is more likely after a cesarean section than a vaginal birth. The risk is approximately 9 per 1,000 cesarean deliveries.[26]

The Need for Rehospitalization

Women who have a planned cesarean are five times more likely to need an extended hospital stay or rehospitalization for complications related to the surgery or to anesthesia.[27] A study conducted by the Maternal Health Study Group of the Canadian Perinatal Surveillance System found that compared to women who had a vaginal birth women who had a cesarean were three times more likely to be readmitted to the hospital within 60 days of their initial discharge. The complications that required rehospitalization included obstetric surgical complications, pelvic injury/wounds, blood clotting problems, and major infection.[28]

Unsatisfactory Birth Experience

Women who give birth by cesarean are more likely to report less overall satisfaction after their surgery and over a longer period of time than women who have a vaginal birth. An unplanned cesarean has a greater negative impact on the mother's feelings. Women who gave birth in a U.S. hospital in 2005 were asked how they felt while giving birth. Compared to women who had a vaginal birth more women who had a cesarean felt overwhelmed, frightened, weak, agitated, groggy, and helpless.[29] Especially with unplanned cesareans, women are more likely to have feelings of lower self-esteem, a sense of failure, disappointment, and loss of control.[30] Childbirth experiences make a deep and lasting impact on women's lives.[31,32] Distressing feelings of a cesarean delivery are remembered many years after the birth. Mothers have expressed feelings of fear, panic, shock, helplessness, disempowerment, pain from anesthesia that was not effective, being denied information, and not being treated with respect.[33]

Maternal Death

Although maternal death resulting directly from a cesarean section is rare in developed countries today, it is three to seven times greater than for women who have a vaginal birth. In France, researchers found the risk of postpartum death was 3.6 times higher after a planned cesarean birth for breech than after a vaginal birth. The deaths were a result of complications of anesthesia, birth-related infection, and venous thromboembolism (blood clots).[34] Cesarean deliveries have been increasing much faster in Latin American countries than in other regions in the world. A World Health Organization 2005 survey of cesarean delivery rates and pregnancy outcomes based on twenty-four geographic regions and eight countries in Latin America found that increasing cesarean delivery rates were positively associated with maternal and neonatal mortality.[35]

ESPECIALLY FOR MOTHERS

Every mother will ultimately make the best decision for herself based on her interpretation of the information she receives, in the context of her own philosophy of birth, and her own personal life circumstances. Take the time you need to find out about the benefits and risks of cesarean section, talk it over with your partner and your caregiver. You will then be better prepared to make an informed decision.

- To reduce the risk of premature birth and respiratory complications for the baby, a scheduled cesarean should not routinely be carried out before 39 weeks.
- Make sure you are given prophylactic antibiotics before the surgery.
- Ask if your physician uses a double layer of sutures to close the uterine incision. A double layer of sutures reduces the risk for a uterine rupture in a future pregnancy.
- Make sure you have access to pain medication when your anesthesia begins to wear off.
- To reduce your risk for blood clots after the surgery ask your care provider about compression/antiembolism stockings or an intermittent pneumatic compression device. If you are at increased risk for blood clots you may be offered heparin (an anticlotting medication).[36]
- If you have a cesarean at some point during labor, take the time to talk to your care providers about why you needed the surgery and what implications this may have for future pregnancies.

RESOURCES

W. Ponte, Cesarean Birth in a Culture of Fear, *Mothering Magazine*, October 2007, http://www.mothering.com/articles/pregnancy_birth/cesarean_vbac/cesarean-birth-in-a-culture-of-fear.html.

What Every Pregnant Woman Needs to Know about Cesarean Section, Childbirth Connection, http://childbirthconnection.com/article.asp?ck=10164.

6

BREAKING THE SILENCE: BIRTH TRAUMA, CESAREANS, AND POSTTRAUMATIC STRESS

> Pregnancy, birth, and the postpartum period are milestone events in the contin-
> uum of life. These experiences profoundly affect, women, babies, fathers, and
> families, and have important and long-lasting effects on society.[1]

For many women childbirth is a joyous, fulfilling, and empowering experience. For others it can be one of the most traumatic events of their lives. Memories of childbirth can be vivid, deeply felt, and can last many years, perhaps even a lifetime. Women who express a long-term satisfaction with their births feel a sense of accomplishment. They have positive memories of their caregivers. They feel they were in control of their birth and their experience contributed to their feelings of self-confidence and self-esteem.[2,3]

Other mothers have long-term memories of a childbirth gone awry. An experience that left them feeling distressed, confused, and angry. Although much is now known about the physical health risks associated with a cesarean delivery, formal knowledge about the psychological impact of a cesarean birth is beginning to gain ground. A U.S. survey of women's first births in 2005 revealed that women who had a cesarean birth were more likely to feel fright-ened, helpless, and overwhelmed, and less likely to feel capable, confident, powerful, and unafraid while giving birth.[4]

Many new mothers are familiar with the common symptoms of the baby blues, which may last for a week or two: The sadness, anxiety, mood swings, difficulty in sleeping, trouble concentrating, and not feeling like oneself. In-creasingly we are learning about the frequency and impact of depression during or after pregnancy. One in eight new mothers in the United States suf-fers from postpartum depression, a condition that can develop anytime within a year of childbirth.[5] Remarkably, current research tells us that some women experience childbirth as a traumatic event and up to 6 percent meet the clinical criteria for posttraumatic stress disorder (PTSD).[6,7]

Childbirth can be an extremely painful experience, sometimes associated with feelings of being out of control, so it is understandable that some women may experience the birth itself as a psychological trauma.[8] Women who have a "normal" vaginal delivery can also experience birth as traumatic.[9] Unwanted, invasive, and painful interventions together with a perception of inadequate care are also risk factors for a traumatic birth.[10, 11] British researchers found that 3 percent of women who had an uncomplicated hospital birth displayed clinical symptoms of posttraumatic stress at 6 weeks postpartum and 24 percent displayed at least one of the three components of PTSD.[12]

Researchers have also identified feelings of numbness, lack of mobility from epidural anesthesia, and not being involved in making decisions regarding their care, as risk factors for a traumatic birth.[13] Invasive procedures such as vaginal exams, use of IVs, and bladder catheters can also trigger a traumatic response from survivors of early childhood sexual abuse and women who live with domestic violence.[14, 15, 16] Women who may lack support from their partner or family, or who have an unplanned pregnancy, or a previous history of stillbirth, are also more vulnerable.[17]

HOW WOMEN FEEL ABOUT THEIR CESAREAN BIRTH VARIES WIDELY

A cesarean section (although not an uncommon procedure these days) is an invasive procedure that is often initiated unexpectedly at some point in the process of labor or birth. Emotional reactions and adjustments to a cesarean birth vary widely. Some women recover quickly from a cesarean. They resolve and integrate their cesarean birth as one step toward becoming a mother. Other women, especially mothers who had an unanticipated cesarean (perhaps after long hours of labor), can experience sadness, disappointment, and loss of self-esteem, guilt, and anger. A woman's experience of her cesarean birth and her perceptions of the event are influenced by multiple complex factors: the reason for which the cesarean was performed; her cultural values; her beliefs and expectations of her birth experience; prior traumatic events in her life; the social support available to her during pregnancy and childbirth; her own perception of how she was treated by her caregivers; her involvement in making decisions regarding her care; and her personal sense of control of her birth.[18, 19, 20, 21]

That birth by cesarean can have an adverse psychological impact on some mothers was already a concern in the mid-1970s and early 1980s, as the cesarean rate in the United States was climbing rapidly.[22] Research, anecdotal reports, and personal testimonies helped to increase awareness about the negative psychological repercussions that some women experience following a cesarean birth.[23, 24, 25]

More than a decade ago social scientists already recognized that birth by cesarean could have a powerful negative psychosocial impact on some women. The effects were significant and far-reaching. Birth by cesarean can impact self-esteem, mother-infant attachment, spousal relationship, and the new mother's ability to respond to her newborn's needs.[26,27,28] The risk seemed to be greater when women had an "emergency" cesarean, had general anesthesia, or were separated from their newborns after the birth.[29] A negative experience of a primary cesarean birth may last years and affect a woman's future pregnancies.[30] A difficult first birth that leads to an emergency cesarean or an instrumental birth can be so terrifying that some women in a subsequent pregnancy would rather have a cesarean delivery than experience labor again.[31]

CESAREAN DELIVERY AND POSTTRAUMATIC STRESS

Women who have a surgical birth are more likely to experience feelings of loss, grief, personal failure, and lower self-esteem.[32] Cesarean section is major abdominal surgery and often the emotional impact of a cesarean is misunderstood, dismissed, or overlooked. The outcome of the pregnancy and birth, the new baby, is validated, but not the process of the birth or the negative feelings the mother may have experienced. Some women who experience a cesarean, especially if it was not an anticipated, can suffer from posttraumatic stress.[33,34] Current evidence suggests that the incidence of posttraumatic stress disorder after childbirth ranges from 1.5 percent[35] to 6 percent.[36]

Phyllis H. Klaus, CSW, MFT, is a psychotherapist and international consultant who specializes in medical and psychological concerns of pregnancy, birth, the postpartum period, trauma, and abuse issues. She explains,

> Events are traumatic and create feelings of powerlessness when they are dangerous. When they are actually or appear to be life-threatening to oneself or a loved one. When they are sudden (the situation changes quickly from "normal" to dangerous), they are experienced without explanations, and when the situation appears overwhelming. There is no time to prepare, no way to plan an escape, or to prevent something from happening. A number of events during labor or birth such as an emergency, unexpected or unwanted interventions, serious problems in the mother, physical damage, a sick or compromised infant, and separation from the baby, can be classified as traumatic, with a capital T. Major trauma for a woman occurs in childbirth when she has inordinate fear and is in a situation where she has no control. Other aspects of trauma are more subjective and relate to how a woman is treated. How she perceives her experience, and how she feels about the experience. These experiences are often man-made and cause shame, humiliation, and stigma.[37]

Some mothers experience their cesarean as a physical assault and a form of institutional violence. For some mothers the surgical birth is experienced as a rape.[38] A growing body of psychosocial literature and increasing personal testimonies from mothers themselves in books, on e-lists, Web sites, and personal blogs also suggest that some women suffer from Posttraumatic Stress Disorder after their cesarean section. They experience the same physical and psychological symptoms as those experienced by combat veterans, major disaster victims, or plane crash survivors.[39,40]

The symptoms of birth-related PTSD may emerge weeks, months, or years after the event.[41,] Posttraumatic Stress (PTSD) is a diagnostic category used to describe symptoms arising from an emotionally traumatic experience. It may involve an actual or *perceived* serious injury or actual or *perceived* threat to the physical integrity of oneself or others. Individuals with posttraumatic stress experience feelings of intense fear, helplessness, or horror in response to the traumatic event. PTSD is also a well-known reaction to other medical experiences such as open heart surgery or cancer. Women who suffer from a postpartum hemorrhage or a preterm birth and women who undergo infertility treatments may also suffer from PTSD. When symptoms occur in the first 30 days of the traumatic event it is called an acute stress response. The diagnosis of PTSD is made when the clinical symptoms persist.[42] The stress response symptoms include:

Intrusive thoughts and re-experiencing of the event in flashbacks or nightmares.
Avoidance of places or people that might trigger a reminder of the event. Symbolic or real reminders of the event bring out intense feelings of distress.
Numbing of emotions and general responsiveness.
A sense of hyper vigilance or increased arousal. Disturbed sleep, anxiety, lack of concentration, feeling irritable or angry.

Women with clinical symptoms of posttraumatic stress re-experience the birth and the emotions associated with it in dreams or thought intrusions. They avoid places or people that remind them of the event. Mothers will also exhibit symptoms of hyperarousal, such as difficulty in sleeping or concentrating, irritability, and an excessive startle response. Untreated posttraumatic stress often leads to clinical depression.[43] A traumatic birth of any kind can leave a woman feeling disempowered, violated, or betrayed. While experiencing such clinical symptoms, depending on their individual condition, mothers are more likely to have difficulty tolerating their infant's vulnerability and establishing an emotional closeness. Their capacity for feeling tender and warm toward their infants and people close to them is directly affected. Mothers who feel fearful, sad, and withdrawn will have difficulty with the process of mother-infant attachment.

Some Mothers' Feelings about Their Cesarean Birth

Because I had a previous c-section...a c-section was arranged...As I was wheeled away...I felt like I was an animal led to the slaughter with no mind of my own and doing as I was told...No real consideration was given to how I felt. I was lying there having the epidural inserted, screaming out inside, why, why, I don't want this.[44]

I signed papers giving them permission to do the caesarean....I felt sacrificial. I was crying and holding my partner's hand and telling him that I loved him. I felt lost. I remember staring up at the glare of the quadruple-headed theatre (operating room) lamp that seemed to sear its clinical, alien rays across my cut-open body. I remember the light's protruding handle becoming covered in my blood from the surgeon's glove.[45]

When my son was three years old I was nine weeks pregnant... I became terrified: terrified of doctors, hospitals, everything. I hadn't seen a doctor; I was too scared to get shafted again. The terror and pain came back to me. I began to relive the experience again.[46]

Recently, I was the victim of date rape: afterward I started having flashbacks of the last few minutes of consciousness before my daughter was delivered by cesarean section. Finally, it became crystallized for me what those awful indescribable feelings were since the c-section.... I hope that other women can get in touch with those feelings of rage, betrayal, loss, etc., and start the healing process even if it comes three years after the assault like it has in the case of my c-section, or should I say, their c-section.[47]

Inadequate anesthesia—my epidural wore off during surgery and the anesthesiologist didn't believe me. It was dosed high enough pre-op but started wearing off towards the end. I could feel the stitching and then the stapling. Finally, to stop my screaming, the anesthesiologists pretty much put me completely out, but only because the surgeon told him to. I still have nightmares—six years later.[48]

What bothered me the most about my sections was the way they were acknowledged by the rest of the world I guess. I mean, yes, I had a wonderful baby, and wasn't I happy, and the answer was no. I actually felt assaulted and violated and out of control. Also with both sections, even though they were 10 years apart, I didn't feel there was anything out there really to help me deal with getting it together psychologically. To most of my family and friends it is like, it happened, it's over, get on with it, and I have ... twice, but there is sadness there and I think there needs to be some way of addressing and handling that.[49]

Despite my rational mind recalling the surgery, and a memory of the perfect baby's lustily wailing reality, my body and heart are giving me a different message. No child came from my body. There is no child. Wait—there IS a child? I am confused. I am hallucinating. I am grieving. For the next several weeks, my heart stops whenever there is a knock on our apartment door, because I am irrationally convinced that it's the newborn's real mother, the one who birthed him, who has come to take him home. It has taken me months, years, to overcome my body's messages of a missing child.[50]

Before my son was born, I was unaware of the underbelly of grief and anger associated with the unwanted, and often unnecessary surgical extraction of our children. I was amazed to find many women who felt the same way about their cesarean birth experience. It is kept quiet not only by the medical community, but by the mothers as well. Many women think that the feelings they have after a cesarean are wrong and they are afraid to share them with others, even loved ones. It has inspired me to create a place where these women can vent, share poetry, artwork, cesarean and VBAC birth stories, and anything else that helps them through those painful feelings.[51]

What is so bad about c-sections? They are not as nature intended for women to give birth. They take so much away from healthy women, and brand us for life. Anytime we become pregnant again, anytime we write down any medical information, we will have to write down c-section. We are branded as "broken" by the medical community and often by ourselves. I feel like my scar is like a cattle brand. Look at me, I couldn't do it. Well, I could have! I just didn't have all the support I needed and information necessary to. Next time, I will not make that mistake.[52]

BREAKING THE SILENCE–THE IMPORTANCE OF SUPPORTIVE COMMUNITIES

Research and experience strongly suggest that providing women with the opportunity to make sense of their traumatic birth is vital for their emotional well-being.[53, 54] Penny Simkin, PT, coauthor with Phyllis Klaus CSW, MFT, of *When Survivors Give Birth* counsels many women who have had a traumatic birth. She tells us,

> The childbirth experience lives on in the new mother's thoughts and emotions as she integrates her prior expectations with all the rewarding, challenging, painful, frightening, exhausting, and demanding aspects of it. She needs to make sense of her childbirth by reconstructing it and putting it into words to understand what happened and how she felt. Of course, if she feels triumphant, powerful, and fulfilled by her child's birth, having a chance to recall the details and relive the joy will reinforce the positive aspects, enhance her self-esteem, and deepen her satisfaction. Negative or mistaken impressions, however, do not go away if they remain unresolved; in fact, they tend to fester and grow. If the birth was traumatic for her or her baby, early processing and reframing may even prevent later Post-Traumatic Stress Disorder or Postpartum Depression. If she is angry at or disappointed in herself, in people who were there, or over the events that occurred, she will benefit from a caring, empathic listener who acknowledges and validates her feelings. When the time is right, this person can help her to a more comfortable or positive perspective.[55]

Since the late seventies and early eighties women have created their own safe and supportive communities to help them make sense of a traumatic birth.[56] A place where mothers can openly share their feelings of their cesarean birth validates their experience. Supportive networks that address birth trauma issues, Web sites, and warm lines where mothers can write or phone in and talk about their birth, have formed in several countries including the United States, Britain, Canada, New Zealand, and Australia. Peer self-help support groups provide emotional support and a nonjudgmental place where mothers can feel understood and respected. A place to express their grief, confusion, disappointment, guilt, or anger about their cesarean births. It gives mothers an opportunity to reconstruct the events around their cesarean birth, and hopefully to eventually integrate their experience in the context of their lives. They are also a source for community resources, education, and counseling services. Support groups, above all, provide mothers with a safe place where other mothers with similar experiences can affirm that having those feelings is normal and does not make them bad mothers. These supportive communities also testify to the need for a better understanding of the impact of the medicalized model of care on women's psychological well-being and consequently on their ability to care for their babies.

Sharon Storton, MA, LMFT, has worked extensively with women who have experienced birth trauma. She tells us,

> Our culture can give women the clear message that discussing these experiences aloud is shameful and unacceptable. Women often report that any emotion other than gratitude or joy is silenced. Social and family pressures tell women, "just get over it and move on." Sometimes moving on requires understanding what happened, mastering the story and the experience, and even breaking the silence about what occurred. At times, a woman is ready to take these steps toward healing immediately after her delivery. For some individuals, this process can come years after the experience. Challenging childbirth can have a sense of "freezing in time" until the silence can at last be broken.[57]

ARE SOME WOMEN BEING FORCED TO REPEAT THE TRAUMA?

Currently in the United States more than 90 percent of women who had a prior cesarean have a repeat operation. Some hospitals and care providers support women's choice for a planned VBAC, but thousands of other women are basically having a forced repeat cesarean because hundreds of hospitals have decided they cannot or will not for financial or malpractice reasons meet ACOG's controversial recommendations (issued first in 1999) for a planned VBAC.[58] (See chapter on VBAC.)

How have these guidelines affected women's mental health? It's been 9 years since the guidelines were issued in 1999. To date we have no information on the impact of that policy on the thousands of women who had no choice but to repeat a major abdominal surgery they most likely didn't need. Medical societies, policymakers, researchers, employers, mental health professionals, and the media have yet to investigate the ethical, moral, legal, financial, and health issues regarding forced repeat cesareans in the United States.

ESPECIALLY FOR MOTHERS

Healing from a Traumatic Experience

Some women experience their birth as a traumatic event. Often they are not aware of how the trauma has impacted their life, their sense of self, and their feelings about mothering. Because a newborn demands so much care and attention, mothers often do not have the time to process these feelings and they can linger for a long time. It is normal for a mother to appreciate the fact that her birth by cesarean resulted in a healthy baby, while still feeling sad, confused, or angry about the experience itself. Friends, family, and even partners of mothers who have had an emotionally difficult cesarean or vaginal birth often do not understand why mothers don't just "move on," or why they "obsess" about their birth experience.

It is important that, whenever you are ready, you find the right time, a safe place, and a person you trust to resolve some of these feelings. It might be weeks, months, or years after your cesarean birth, or even during a subsequent pregnancy, before you will be able to talk about your birth experience. If you are planning to have another baby and plan to labor for a VBAC or have a planned repeat cesarean, you will feel better about your pregnancy and birth if you first process your feelings about the difficult cesarean you've already experienced. Find out how you might be able to avoid the reoccurrence of those events.

These are some suggestions that may provide insight into your birth experience, begin to normalize your feelings, and eventually integrate it into your life.

- Know that you are not alone; many other mothers have felt the same way.
- Trust yourself to know that you are a good mother, even though you may have very confusing feelings about your cesarean-delivered baby.
- Talk to your partner about how you feel without placing blame on his or her role in your baby's birth. Ask your partner to share his or her feelings and perceptions (he or she may be feeling powerless, or angry, or distressed). It may help you to forgive each other for events neither of you could control and realize that both of you did your best at the time.
- Share your experience with others who understand. This is an important step in moving away from a sense of isolation. Talk to a friend or family member you trust—one who is likely to validate your feelings. A support group should validate your feelings and actions, and respect your individual point of view. Consider using the resources at the end of this chapter.
- Write or draw your feelings in a journal.
- Write letters to the people who affected you negatively. You don't have to mail them.
- Join a cesarean/VBAC support group, or become part of an on-line group of mothers who feel as you do.
- Reconstruct your birth experience. Remembering your birth in detail using words (speaking into a tape recorder, or writing about it) helps to reduce your feelings of anxiety and distress, change the way you see yourself (as a victim or a failure), and helps you to understand what actually happened as opposed to what you wished had happened.
- Hold your baby or child in your arms and share the positive feelings and events of your birth experience. Obtain and go over your medical records, or just the operative report if you need to so you can better understand the sequence of events.
- Gather as much information as you need to help you understand your birth experience and to make the changes you want for your next birth.
- Consider having a doula at your next birth.
- Remember that others may not understand your very real and normal feelings and may feel helpless or frustrated in trying to help you feel better.

- Unresolved issues can sometimes lead to clinical depression. You might want to seek professional mental health counseling.

RESOURCES

Birth Crisis Network, Britain, http://www.sheilakitzinger.com/birthcrisis.htm.
Birthrites, Australia, http://www.birthrites.org.
Birth Trauma Association, Britain, http://birthtraumaassociation.org.uk.
International Cesarean Awareness Network, United States, http://www.ican-online.org.
Mind, Britain, http://www.mind.org,uk.
Solace for Mothers, http://www.solaceformothers.org.
Trauma and Birth Stress, PTSD After Childbirth, New Zealand, http://tabs.org.nz

7

How Does a Cesarean Birth Affect the Baby?

We are increasingly learning that common birth practices and maternity unit hospital protocols have a significant impact on maternal and infant health outcomes. We are learning more and more that what affects the mother ultimately affects her baby. That it is essential for optimal health outcomes that mothers and babies should not be separated at birth, but that every effort should be made to support and maintain the mother-baby dyad.[1]

Birth by cesarean poses several challenges for a baby. Compared to babies born vaginally, babies born by cesarean are at risk for health complications they are less likely to face with a normal birth. Cesarean babies are more likely to have difficulty breathing on their own, especially if the mother did not labor. With a scheduled cesarean, babies are more likely to be born preterm, before the lungs have fully developed. Respiratory complications can be serious enough to require admission to a special care nursery. With a cesarean, mothers and babies are less likely to have skin-to-skin contact immediately after birth. Skin-to-skin contact has several adaptive benefits for the newborn.[2] Pain medications that sedate the mother can affect the newborn's ability to latch on and breastfeed. Drugs used for anesthesia, including epidurals, cross the placenta[3] and can make it more difficult for babies to initiate breastfeeding. The American Association of Pediatrics encourages all maternity care providers to collaborate to support breastfeeding. This includes avoiding common but often unnecessary procedures that interfere with breastfeeding and that may traumatize the newborn. Routine procedures following a cesarean birth, such as suctioning the newborn's mouth, esophagus, and airways can also make it more difficult for babies to begin and continue breastfeeding.[4]

Late Pre-Term Birth and Planned Cesareans

Preterm birth is defined as a live birth before 37 completed weeks of gestation. A baby born between the 34th and 36th week of pregnancy is considered as a late preterm birth. When cesarean sections are scheduled there is a margin of error in pinpointing fetal maturity. Being born only 1 week earlier can make a difference in terms of complications babies are likely to suffer. The March of Dimes (MOD), is concerned that increasing inductions and planned cesareans may be contributing to the rising number of babies born preterm. Late preterm births account for 70 percent of all premature births in the United States and are the fastest growing subgroup of premature babies.[5]

According to a National Institute of Health (NIH) report on the nation's children, the number of low birth weight infants (less than 5 pounds. 8 ounces) in the United States increased to 8.2 percent in 2005, up from 8.1 percent 2004, and 7.9 percent in 2003. Low birth weight infants are at higher risk of death or long-term illness and disability than are infants of normal birth weight. This increase is partly due to the increase in twin, triplet, and higher order multiple births, but the NIH also noted that a change in obstetrical practice, such as increased inductions and cesarean delivery, might have also played a part.[6] In 2005 about 31,000 hospital-born infants were identified as low birth weight.[7]

LATE PRE-TERM BIRTH AND BRAIN DEVELOPMENT

In July 2005 the National Institute of Child Health and Development (NICHD) convened an invitational conference with the March of Dimes Foundation to address national concerns about infants born late-preterm (3 to 6 weeks before their due date).

Late/preterm infants are at increased risk for several health problems related to prematurity. Emerging research also suggests that they have more less mature brains compared with term infants. Because babies born late-preterm are also *physiologically* and *metabolically* less mature than babies born at term, they tend to have difficulty with digestion, dehydration, infection, regulating their blood glucose, and body temperature. Their liver function is immature putting them at risk for accumulating high levels of bilirubin (a neural toxin), and becoming jaundiced. Their central nervous system is not fully developed and at 35 weeks of gestation their brains are about two-thirds the size of a term infant's brain. In the last 4 weeks of gestation brain growth (the cerebral cortex) is dramatic. There is rapid growth in the area of the brain responsible for cognition, learning, perception, reason, fine motor control, language, and social functioning. The brain mass of a late preterm infant is about 70 percent that of the full term baby. It is also underdeveloped in terms of myelinization, the developmental process in which protective fatty material wraps around nerve cells. Babies born late/preterm are more likely to have learning and behavior problems at school age than babies born at 40 weeks.[8, 9, 10, 11]

The March of Dimes Prematurity Campaign has developed and is disseminating several publications for expectant mothers and health professionals recommending not inducing labor or scheduling a cesarean before 40 weeks.

"If your pregnancy is healthy, it's best if your baby is born at 40 weeks," states their Late-preterm Brain Development Card prepared for health care providers (March of Dimes Foundation, February 2008). The Association of Women's Health, Obstetrics, and Neonatal Nursing (AWHONN) has also developed an educational consumer and health professional resource center to help meet the specific needs of infants born late-preterm, which they have posted on their Web site.

Infant and Neonatal Death and Planned First Cesareans

Increasingly, in many countries around the world, women are having a planned cesarean without a medical indication. These are considered low-risk cesareans. In the United States the number of healthy women who have a primary cesarean (first cesarean delivery) at term (37–41 weeks and a singleton pregnancy) without any medical indication increased 49 percent from 1996 to 2001. These are cesarean deliveries for which no medical diagnosis was reported on the birth certificates. How do these planned cesareans affect neonatal (the first 28 days of life) and infant (less than 1 year of life) health? In 2006 researchers at the CDC examined live births between 1998 and 2001. They reported that newborns of mothers who had a planned cesarean were more likely to die in the first 4 weeks of life (1.77 per 1,000 births) than newborns of mothers who had a vaginal birth (0.62 per 1,000 births) that is, almost three times the risk. The infant mortality rate for first-time mothers with a planned cesarean was 2.85 per 1,000 compared to 1.83 for mothers who had a vaginal birth, that is, a 56 percent higher rate. For mothers who had one or more children before their planned cesarean the infant mortality rate was 4.51 per 1,000 compared to 2.18 for a similar group of women who had a vaginal birth, that is, more than twice the increase.[12]

Breathing Difficulties and Admission to Intensive Care Unit

Birth by cesarean increases the risk for breathing problems. Infant respiratory distress syndrome, a complication related to scheduled cesareans, was the most expensive condition of all hospital stays in 2005. The cost for each stay with this diagnosis was $114,200. Newborns with this condition were hospitalized for an average of 25.7 days. The cost and length of hospital stay surpassed those for spinal cord injury, heart valve disorders, and leukemia.[13]

Contractions of labor help to prepare the baby's lungs for respiration at birth. In her article on the role of stress, pain, and catecholamines (produced by the body in response to stress), Simkin explains that during each contraction of labor there is temporary reduction in the amount of oxygen that is available to the fetus. Contractions reduce the amount of oxygenated blood that is passed through to the placenta. This causes the baby's heart rate to slow down. To adapt to this level of stress the baby increases her production of catecholamines, which shunts the blood going to her vital organs, and preserves her energy stores. This adaptive response allows the baby to receive the same amount of oxygen as before labor contractions. This increased surge of catecholamines accumulated during labor also helps to prepare the baby's lungs to breath on their own at birth by absorbing the liquid in the baby's lungs. Babies born by a scheduled cesarean have lower levels of catecholamines than babies born vaginally.[14] A scheduled cesarean (without labor) is likely to make it more difficult for the baby to breathe on her own initially.

Babies born before term have a higher risk of persistent pulmonary hypertension, a potentially life-threatening condition. To facilitate the transition from the uterine environment to the outside world, the blood vessels in the baby's lungs relax and allow blood to flow through them with the first breaths after birth. This function allows the blood to exchange carbon dioxide for oxygen. When this adaptation fails, the blood vessels do not relax and pulmonary high blood pressure (hypertension) prevails. Newborns who experience persistent pulmonary hypertension and low blood oxygen levels can suffer from damage to vital organs and the brain. Persistent pulmonary hypertension is four times higher for babies born by elective cesarean than for babies born vaginally.[15]

Mother-Infant Attachment Is More Likely to Be Delayed

Holding, touching, and caring for healthy, sick, or premature infants, or infants with congenital problems, enhances attachment between mothers and babies. Minimizing or avoiding separating babies from their mothers after birth reduces stress in healthy newborns and mothers.[16] The World Health Organization and the American Academy of Pediatrics encourage skin-to-skin contact between mother and baby as soon as possible after the birth for at least 1 hour and until the newborn has successfully completed the first breastfeed.[17] Placing the newborn belly down directly on her mother's chest has several important health benefits. Skin-to-skin contact calms the mother and her baby and helps to stabilize the baby's heartbeat and breathing. The mother's body heat keeps the baby warm, reduces the newborn's crying, stress, and energy use. Skin-to-skin contact helps with the baby's metabolic adaptation and stabilizes its blood-glucose level. If the mother is the first person to hold the baby rather than a staff person, it helps to colonize the baby's gut with her mother's normal body bacteria gut.

The Lamaze Institute for Normal Birth recommends no separation of mother and baby after birth with unlimited opportunity for breastfeeding. "Nature prepares a mother and her baby to need each other from the moment of birth. Oxytocin, the hormone that causes a woman's uterus to contract, also causes the temperature of her breasts to rise and helps her feel calm and responsive. This hormone stimulates "mothering" feelings as the woman touches, gazes at, and breastfeeds her baby. More oxytocin is released as she holds her baby skin-to-skin. Endorphins, narcotic-like hormones, are also released and enhance mothering feelings. High levels of adrenalin, which are normal in babies at birth, make the baby alert and prepare him to look for his mother, find his way to her breast, and breastfeed."[18]

The Listening to Mothers II U.S. national survey of women's childbearing experiences revealed that only 14 percent of mothers who gave birth by cesarean had their baby in their arms immediately after birth, compared to 43 percent of the mothers who had a vaginal delivery.[19] With a cesarean delivery babies are more likely to be taken to the nursery for observation and monitoring for potential problems during the first hour of life. They are also more likely to spend time in a nursery for newborns than rooming in with their mothers. The separation seems to have an impact on the mother's initial ability to respond to and care for her infant. When mothers and babies stay together, babies cry less, the mother's perception of her infant improves, and it enhances the mother's confidence in her mothering skills.[20] Babies are more likely to be breastfed and for a longer period of time if they have early skin-to-skin contact.[21]

A Swedish study found that the baby's father could provide skin-to-skin contact with his newborn and offer the same calming and comforting benefits as the baby's mother, when the mother is not able to receive her infant immediately after a cesarean birth. This skin-to-skin contact between the father and his baby also facilitates the newborn's pre-breastfeeding behavior. A calm newborn is better prepared for breastfeeding when mother and baby are together for the first time. The researchers of this study recommend that the fathers should be the primary caregivers for their newborns when mothers and babies are separated.[22]

With an Epidural Breastfeeding Is Likely to Be Delayed

The U.S. Healthy People 2010 goal is for 75 percent of mothers to initiate breastfeeding at birth, for 50 percent to breastfeed until at least the fifth or sixth month of life, and one-fourth of mothers to breastfeed through the end of the first year.[23] In 2007 the CDC reported that less than half of the states met the Healthy People goals for initiating breastfeeding.[24] A cesarean birth makes it more difficult for mothers to initiate and establish breastfeeding. The CDC established that hospital birth practices have a significant impact on the initiation and continuation of breastfeeding. The use of medications during labor and cesarean birth has a negative effect on breastfeeding, and so does the separation of mother and baby after birth and during the hospital stay. The maternity care experience exerts a unique influence on both breastfeeding initiation and later infant feeding behavior. Although the hospital stay is typically very short, events during this time have a long and lasting impact. Medications and procedures administered to the mother during labor affect her infant's behavior at the time of birth, which in turn affects her infant's ability to suckle satisfactorily at the mother's breast.[25] If hospitals provide mothers with the support, guidance, and education from a lactation specialist, mothers are more likely to initiate and continue breastfeeding.

Advantages of Breastfeeding for Babies and Young Children

The U.S. Agency for Healthcare Research and Quality (AHRQ) recently reviewed the evidence on the short- and long-term health impacts of breast-feeding in industrialized countries. The researchers found that breastfeeding reduced an infant's risk of ear infections by up to 50 percent, serious lower respiratory tract infections by 72 percent, and a skin rash similar to eczema by 42 percent. Children with a family history of asthma who had been breast-fed were 40 percent less likely to have asthma, and children who were not prone to asthma had a 27 percent reduced risk compared to those children who were not breastfed. The likelihood of developing type 1 diabetes was reduced by about twenty percent. These benefits were seen in infants who were breastfed for 3 or more months. Breastfeeding also reduced the risk of type 2 diabetes by 39 percent compared to infants who were not breast-fed. For premature infants, breastfeeding decreased the occurrence of necro-tizing enterocolitis, a serious gastrointestinal infection that often results in death.[26]

Advantages of Breastfeeding for Mothers

Immediately after birth, breastfeeding increases levels of oxytocin, the hor-mone that stimulates uterine contractions. Effective uterine contractions are essential to prevent postpartum bleeding from blood vessels that were once attached to the placenta. Breastfeeding also helps with weight loss. The AHRQ study on the benefits of breastfeeding found that women who breastfed their infants had up to a 12 percent reduced risk of type 2 diabetes for each year they breastfed. Breastfeeding also decreased their risk of ovarian cancer by up to 21 percent, and decreased the risk of breast cancer by up to 28 per-cent in mothers whose lifetime duration of breastfeeding was 12 months or longer.[27]

The Cost of Not Breastfeeding

Breastfeeding for at least 6 months provides significant health, developmen-tal, and psychological advantages for infants. It also has significant economical advantages. The United States Breastfeeding Committee estimates private and government health insurance spend $3.6 billion a year to treat diseases and conditions that can be prevented by breastfeeding. Compared to treating 1,000 infants who were exclusively breastfed, hospital costs for treating 1,000 infants who were never breastfed (with lower-respiratory infections) range from $27,000 to more than $31,000. Necrotizing enterocolitis, NEC (a serious disease affecting the gastrointestinal tract during the first 3 weeks of life) occurs ten times more often in formula-fed infants. The cost of treating each infant with NEC is about $200,000.[28]

The Baby-Friendly Hospital Initiative

Collaborative care and support from all maternity care professionals is important for helping mothers establish breastfeeding, especially mothers who give birth by cesarean section. The Baby-Friendly Hospital Initiative (BFHI) is an effort by UNICEF and the World Health Organization to ensure that all maternity care facilities, whether free standing or in a hospital, become centers of breastfeeding support. With expert counseling and breastfeeding support based on the WHO/UNICEF Ten Steps of the Baby-Friendly Hospital Initiative to promote successful breastfeeding (BFHI), mothers are more likely to initiate breastfeeding, to be exclusively breastfeeding at 3 and 6 months, and more likely to maintain breastfeeding at 12 months. Birthing facilities that meet all Ten Steps of the BFHI guidelines are designated as Baby-Friendly. According to Baby-Friendly U.S.A., a mother's experience of birth and the care she receives can affect breastfeeding and how she cares for her baby. Even facilities that are not yet designated Baby-Friendly can support mothers in many ways.[29] Birth practices and institutional protocols, while maintaining the safety and well-being of both mothers and babies, can at the same time help mothers to feel supported, confident, and ready to relate positively with her baby. With a cesarean birth, every effort should be made to initiate skin-to-skin contact between the mother and her newborn and help mothers who choose to breastfeed to initiate and establish breastfeeding before they leave the birth facility.

ESPECIALLY FOR MOTHERS

Birth by cesarean affects you as well as your baby. A long labor preceding a cesarean, pain from the surgery, complications such as developing a fever, your reaction to medications, or developing an infection, may make it difficult for you to be with your baby right after birth. Holding, feeding, and soothing your baby may be more painful than you anticipated. You and your baby will benefit from skin-to-skin contact and rooming in (having the baby in your room as opposed to the nursery) as soon as possible. But, you should take the time you need to feel ready to welcome your baby. Should you have a cesarean delivery, the following suggestions can help you and your baby get off to a more healthy and satisfying start together.

- Ask to have an epidural or spinal anesthesia instead of general anesthesia. Regional anesthesia has less side effects and gives you both a chance to be together sooner after birth.
- In the operating room, after your baby has been born and if you are feeling well, ask that one of your arms be released and your baby be placed belly down on your chest as soon as it is safe. You can also ask that the baby be placed skin-to-skin with your partner as soon as it is safe. Your baby will be less fussy and more ready to breastfeed.
- Ask that a lactation specialist help you to recognize your baby's hunger signs, to position your baby to latch on correctly at your breast, to support you to continue to breastfeed while in the hospital, and to provide you with a list of community resources that you can access once you are home.
- Your health insurance may reimburse you for the services of a lactation consultant once you are home and for the rental of a breast pump if you need one.
- You may want to draft a birth plan to communicate your needs and wishes for staff support with breastfeeding.
- You will be in pain after the initial anesthetic wears off. Ask about the safest pain medication available for breastfeeding.
- Ask for your partner, friend, or doula, to stay with you in the room to help you lift your baby, change positions in bed, change the baby's diapers, and help you get out of bed.

RESOURCES

American Academy of Pediatrics, Parenting Corner, Q & A, Breastfeeding, http://www.aap.org/pubed/ZZZORSNYKRD.htm?&sub_cat=1 (last accessed on July 10, 2008).

American Womens' Health, Obstetric, and Neonatal Nurses (AWHONN), Late-Preterm Infant Initiative, http://www.awhonn.org (last accessed on July 10, 2008).

Centers for Disease Control, Breastfeeding, http://www.cdc.gov/breastfeeding (last accessed on July 10, 2008).

La Leche League International, Is It Possible to Breastfeed after a Cesarean Birth?, http://www.llli.org/FAQ/cesarean.html (last accessed on July 10, 2008).

March of Dimes, Cesarean Birth by Request, http://modimes.org/prematurity/21239_19673.asp (last accessed on July 10, 2008).

March of Dimes, Prematurity Campaign, http://www.marchofdimes.com/prematurity/prematurity.asp (last accessed on July 10, 2008).

United States Breastfeeding Committee, Frequently Asked Questions, http://www.usbreastfeeding.org/breastfeeding/faq.htm (last accessed on July 10, 2008).

8

IMPACT OF A CESAREAN DELIVERY ON A FUTURE PREGNANCY

A placenta that grows in a uterus with one or more scars from a previous cesarean section may not do as well at providing oxygen and nutrients to the developing fetus compared with a placenta growing in an unscarred uterus. This may cause life-threatening problems.[1]

In the last several years researchers have taken a closer look at the aftermath of cesarean delivery on women's subsequent pregnancy and birth. The health of younger siblings of children born by cesarean is also affected. When women become pregnant after a cesarean delivery they are at higher risk for developing problems in a future pregnancy and birth; even if they schedule a repeat cesarean section. The current controversial ACOG guidelines for laboring after a prior cesarean have resulted in a repeat cesarean rate of over 90 percent. Research is clear about the increasing risks of multiple cesarean sections. A vaginal birth after a prior cesarean (VBAC) reduces the risks for complications for mothers and babies compared to a repeat operation.

Placental abnormalities that increase the odds for miscarriage, poor fetal growth, bleeding during the pregnancy, and premature birth are higher for women with a previous cesarean delivery. The risk for placenta previa (a low-lying placenta that covers part or all of the inner opening of the cervix), placenta accreta (a placenta that implants itself too deeply and too firmly into the uterine wall), and placenta increta and percreta (more deeply imbedded placenta that involves the entire uterine muscle and sometimes other organs such as the bladder), are much more common with additional cesarean sections. The risk of uterine rupture in future labors is increased. In a future pregnancy babies are more likely to be low birth weight and be born preterm. They are also more likely to have a congenital malformation, or a central nervous system injury. A prior cesarean is associated with increased risk of perinatal death and unexplained stillbirth at term. With a prior cesarean women are more likely to have difficulty conceiving and more likely not to want additional pregnancies.[2]

INFERTILITY, REDUCED FERTILITY

Women who have a cesarean are more likely to have difficulty becoming pregnant again. It is estimated that up to 10 percent of women who give birth by cesarean will experience this problem. Several studies have found that women who have a cesarean have fewer children subsequently, but it is not clear at this time whether this decreased fertility is associated with the surgery itself or to other factors that lower the odds for fertility and increase the odds for a cesarean delivery. A report by the National Collaborating Centre for Women's and Children's Health in Britain found that compared to women who had a vaginal birth, women who had a cesarean were less likely to want additional children and more likely to have difficulties becoming pregnant.[3]

Ectopic Pregnancy

A prior cesarean is a risk factor for an ectopic pregnancy. With an ectopic pregnancy the fertilized egg implants itself and grows outside of the uterus, usually in one of the fallopian tubes. Because an ectopic pregnancy is life-threatening for the mother, the pregnancy must be terminated. An ectopic pregnancy can, although rarely, also implant on one of the ovaries, or in the cervix. With a prior cesarean the embryo can become attached at the site of the previous uterine scar (cesarean scar pregnancy). Although there are other reasons why women have an ectopic pregnancy, the odds for an ectopic pregnancy for women with a prior cesarean are 1 to 9 per 1,000.[4] An untreated ectopic pregnancy eventually leads to internal hemorrhage. According to the U.S. Centers for Disease Control, hemorrhage that results from an ectopic pregnancy is one of the leading causes of maternal deaths in the United States.[5]

Uterine Scar Rupture

A cesarean birth puts women at risk for a uterine rupture (separation of the uterine wall at the site of the prior cesarean scar) in a subsequent pregnancy. For women with no uterine scar the risk of a uterine rupture is 1 in 10,000. For women who plan a repeat operation it is 1 in 500 and about 1 in 200 for women who labor for a VBAC. The risk for uterine rupture is higher when labor is induced with oxytocin or a prostaglandin gel. Cytotec, a drug developed to treat ulcers, has been used in the United States (without prior approval from the Food and Drug Administration (FDA) or from the drug's manufacturer) as an agent to induce labor in women with an uterine scar. For many women the results have been devastating, leading to maternal death, fetal death, or severe neonatal neurological problems.[6]

Placenta Previa

As the cesarean rate continues to climb, physicians worldwide are bracing themselves for the anticipated increase in severe complications associated with placental problems and a prior uterine scar.[7, 8]

For the majority of women the placenta implants itself at the top of the back wall of the inner lining of the uterus. A placenta previa is implanted in the lower segment of the uterine wall, partially covering the os or internal part of the cervix. Placenta previa occurs in about 1 to 9 out of 1,000 women with one prior cesarean and a low-horizontal scar.[9] Mothers who have one prior cesarean birth and become pregnant again are four times more likely to have a placenta previa compared to women who give birth normally. With two or three cesareans mothers are seven times more likely to have a placenta previa in a subsequent pregnancy. With four or more cesareans the risk for placenta previa is forty-five times higher.[10]

A placenta previa puts a woman at higher risk for complications during her pregnancy and during childbirth. She is more likely to suffer from hemorrhage and blood clots, go into shock, or require a blood transfusion. Depending on the location of the placenta, women are more likely to need another cesarean to prevent hemorrhage and injury or death to the baby. A placenta previa also puts the fetus at risk because babies are more likely to be born preterm.

Placental Abruption

A placenta previa increases the risk for placental abruption (premature separation of the placenta), one of the leading causes of death for pregnant women in the third trimester. Normally, within a few minutes of the birth of a baby the placenta naturally separates from the inner wall of the uterus with contractions and is pushed out by the mother. A placental abruption is the premature partial or full separation of the placenta during pregnancy or during labor before the baby is born. It causes the uterus to bleed and decreases the oxygen and nutrient supply to the baby. The risk for a placental abruption with a placenta previa after a prior cesarean is 1 to 9 per 1,000.[11]

Placenta Accreta, Increta, and Percreta

Placenta previa increases the odds for severe life-threatening hemorrhage and for three additional complications of pregnancy: placenta accreta, placenta increta, and placenta percreta. A placenta accreta grows into or through the muscular uterine wall too firmly to detach normally from the uterine lining after the birth of the baby. It is a potentially life-threatening condition even if the mother plans a scheduled repeat operation. With a placenta accreta a pregnant woman is likely to experience vaginal bleeding during the third trimester and give birth to a premature baby. When the pregnancy goes to term, a cesarean is planned. There is a high risk for hemorrhage after the baby is born. The placenta needs to be removed surgically to stop the bleeding. Sometimes a blood transfusion is needed. If the bleeding cannot be controlled, the mother will need a hysterectomy (removal of the uterus). The risk of placenta accreta is 1 per 1,000 for women with one prior uterine scar and 1 in 100 with more than one prior cesarean.[12] A publication by the ACOG states that the occurrence of placenta accreta is ten times higher than it was 50 years ago.[13]

With placenta increta and placenta percreta the placenta is even more deeply rooted in the uterus and through the thickness of the muscular uterine wall. At times a placenta percreta extends to other nearby pelvic organs such as the bladder. An ACOG report on cesarean section warned in 2000 that "institutions must be prepared to manage the potential complication of severe hemorrhage associated with higher rates of placenta accreta."[14] Even U.S. hospitals designated as a Level III Neonatal Intensive and Maternal Care Unit and as a Level I Trauma Center may not be able to prevent maternal deaths from major obstetric hemorrhage due to placenta previa and placenta accreta.[15]

Hysterectomy

A cesarean birth makes it more likely that a woman will need an emergency hysterectomy in a subsequent pregnancy. A hysterectomy (removal of the uterus) becomes necessary to save the mother's life when massive bleeding cannot be controlled. The bleeding is the result of placenta accreta, placenta increta, or placenta percreta. Complications from a hysterectomy may include infection, pulmonary embolism, gastrointestinal difficulties, and cardiovascular and neurological problems. After having a hysterectomy many women also develop psychological problems.

Preterm Birth

With a placenta previa babies are more likely to be born with low birth weight, prematurely (before the end of the 37th week), have congenital anomalies, and suffer from neonatal complications. These preterm babies are more likely to suffer from jaundice, anemia, infections, apnea (interrupted breathing), intraventricular hemorrhage (bleeding in the brain), heart failure, vision problems, and respiratory distress syndrome, a potentially life-threatening condition. Preterm babies often require special care nurseries. They are also at greater risk for learning and developmental disabilities and cerebral palsy. Although there are several other risk factors that contribute to premature birth, according to the March of Dimes preterm birth contributed to more than one-third of U.S. infant deaths in 2004. The organization is concerned that the increasing rate of late preterm births (34–36 weeks) is increasing in relation to the increase in inductions and scheduled cesarean sections.[16] In 2001 health care costs during the first year for a preterm baby was approximately $42,000, compared to $3,000 for a healthy full-term baby.[17]

Stillbirth and Neonatal Death

Researchers at Cambridge University in the United Kingdom compared health outcomes of second pregnancies for women who had one prior cesarean delivery with women who had a vaginal delivery. They found that a prior cesarean was associated with an unexplained almost two-fold increase in stillbirth or neonatal death. For women who reached their 39th week of pregnancy the absolute risk of unexplained stillbirth was 1.1 per 1,000 women with one prior cesarean delivery compared to 0.5 per 1,000 women with a prior vaginal birth. The authors of the study cautioned that women thinking about future pregnancies should take these findings into consideration.[18]

Multiple Cesareans Increase Harm

The risks for serious complications for mothers increases with each additional cesarean. Lack of access and choice for planned VBAC in the United States has forced thousands of women to undergo an avoidable repeat cesarean. A U.S. study of 30,000 mothers who gave birth by cesarean in nineteen academic medical centers found that complications from a cesarean delivery increase progressively with each additional surgery. For mothers who had one to six cesarean deliveries, with each additional cesarean the risk for complications increased.[19] Researchers in Israel found similar results. Mothers who had three or more cesareans experienced more complications including dense adhesions, which made it more difficult to deliver the baby.[20] Denying women the option to labor for a VBAC is likely to put women and their babies at additional risk for life-threatening complications.

ESPECIALLY FOR MOTHERS

The risks and benefits of any surgical intervention are ultimately assessed and evaluated in the context of each woman's personal life and circumstances. Although research regarding these risks can provide a mathematical probability of their occurrence, in the end, a woman's own perceptions of these risks, her medical condition, her relationship with her partner and family members, her philosophy and expectation of her birth, her trust in her care providers, and her feelings for each unique pregnancy, are the factors that will influence whether or not she will have a cesarean.

RESOURCES

March of Dimes, Pregnancy and Newborn Education Center, Placenta Previa, http://search.marchofdimes.com/cgi-bin/MsmGo.exe?grab_id=4&page_id=13893888&query=placenta+previa&hiword=PLACENTAE+PLACENTAL+PLACENTAS+PLACENTATION+placenta+previa+ (last accessed on July 5, 2008).

March of Dimes, Preterm Labor Assessment Tool Kit, http://www.marchofdimes.com/prematurity/21326_23788.asp (last accessed on July 5, 2008).

National Library of Medicine, MedlinePlus, Placenta Previa, http://www.nlm.nih.gov/medlineplus/ency/imagepages/17122.htm (last accessed on July 5, 2008).

PART III

COMMON REASONS FOR CESAREAN

9

I'm Laboring as Fast as I Can: Prolonged Labor, a Highly Variable Diagnosis

Many aspects of the birth environment in hospitals can induce stress. The setting and the people in it may be strange to the laboring woman. Common procedures, such as restriction of fluids and food, vaginal examinations, electronic fetal monitoring, and confinement to bed, can further add to the stress. Fear, pain, and anxiety may be increased and this can have potentially adverse effects on the progress of labor."[1]

The term, dystocia is derived from the Greek word tokos (childbirth). Dustokia means difficult childbirth. Dystocia is also known as dysfunctional labor, prolonged labor, or failure to progress. Dystocia is the most common reason why women have their first baby by cesarean section. Most healthy women begin and end their birth journey safely. Given enough time, the right support, freedom of movement, and unrestricted by routine medical interventions the overwhelming majority of low-risk mothers will give birth safely without needing a cesarean section for failure to progress. A North American study of over 50,000 home births attended by professional midwives reported a cesarean rate of 3.7 percent. For nearly 12,000 low-risk women who gave birth in a freestanding birth center in the United States the cesarean rate was 4.4 percent.[2]

For some women labor will be unusually prolonged and without an intervention both the mother and her baby are likely to suffer severe complications. In countries where access to a cesarean is limited it may result in death. When is a woman really in labor? How long can she safely labor before she is diagnosed with dystocia? Which interventions are appropriate? Can dystocia be avoided altogether? Is a cesarean always the best option for "failure to progress"? These are controversial issues.

Dystocia has been called the "wastebasket" diagnosis that leads to unnecessary surgical intervention. One that is often inappropriately made based on a subjective interpretation of what constitutes "abnormal" labor.[3] In the

English language medical literature there was at one time more than sixty terms to describe a difficult labor or more specifically a *disorder* of labor.[4] Many reasons can cause labor to progress slower than expected. Contractions may be inefficient and the cervix may not dilate to 10 cms (cervical dystocia). The baby may be malpositioned in the mother's pelvis (fetal dystocia). The mother's pelvic shape or size (pelvic dystocia) may not easily accommodate the baby. Or the mother's fear of labor, severe pain, or stress, can interfere with the progress of labor (emotional dystocia). A prolonged labor can also be caused by how labor is "managed" (iatrogenic dystocia).[5] For example, we know that the use of epidural analgesia in labor and inducing labor when the cervix is not favorable and ready to dilate slows down the progress of labor making "failure to progress" a likely diagnosis.

OVERDIAGNOSIS AND MISDIAGNOSIS OF DYSTOCIA INCREASE CESAREAN SECTIONS

In 1980, when the cesarean rate was about 16 percent, a report by the National Institutes of Health (NIH) identified dystocia as one of the four main indications for cesareans. One in three women had a cesarean due to a difficult labor. The NIH report found that the diagnosis of dystocia was being made more frequently and often managed by cesarean section. Failure to progress was often classified as *abnormal* or *dysfunctional* when in fact women were in the early phase of labor (before 4 cm dilation) when the cesarean was performed. And labor progress was in fact normal. Primary cesareans (women having their first surgical birth) were performed for dystocia for babies of *normal* birth weights. The NIH concluded that these cesarean deliveries did not provide "survival advantage" when compared with vaginal birth. The NIH recommended walking while in labor, rest, hydration, sleep, emotional support, and lastly oxytocin augmentation as viable options to helping labor progress before resorting to a cesarean section.[6]

In 1988 the Public Citizen's Health Research Group in Washington, DC, a national, nonprofit consumer advocacy organization, published the first of four reports on what it called a rapidly growing national epidemic of unnecessary cesarean sections. Based on public birth records obtained from state departments of health, Public Citizen reported that the diagnosis of dystocia (fetopelvic disproportion [FPD], big baby/small pelvis) had increased nationally by 42 percent between 1980 and 1985. Since mothers' pelvises "have not gotten smaller and babies heads had not gotten bigger" in those 5 years the authors of the report reasoned, the increase was "due to subjective factors on the obstetricians' part." Public Citizen reported that individual physician rates for dystocia ranged from 0 percent to 57 percent. The diagnosis also varied between clinic patients and private patients. Among several university-affiliated hospitals in the Denver, Colorado, metropolitan area dystocia was the diagnosis for 0.5 percent of women in the public clinic service and 13.7 percent for private patients.[7]

In 1996 a report on the rise of cesarean sections commissioned by the Medical Leadership Council, an association of over 2,000 U.S. hospitals revealed that 50 percent of cesareans for dystocia were unnecessary. The operations could have been avoided without compromising the health of the mother or her baby. Dystocia-related cesareans were much more likely to be performed between 6 P.M. and midnight than during any other time of the day. Over one-third of primary cesareans (first cesarean) for dystocia were more likely to be performed on a weekday. The time bias was a powerful nonclinical influence on the cesarean rate.[8]

In 1997 the Institute for Healthcare Improvement, a Boston-based leading organization in improving the quality of health care, was consultant to a collaborative of several health care organizations who wanted to reduce their cesarean section rates. The Institute recognized that several longstanding hospital practices initiated a chain of unnecessary interventions that eventually lead to cesareans that could have been avoided. The way that labor was managed increased the odds that women would need a cesarean. Women were admitted to the labor and delivery unit when they were not in active labor. Once admitted, they were expected to progress according to arbitrary time limits. When labor progress was perceived as "slow," their bag of water was broken and women were "allowed" 24 hours to complete their labor. If progress was still "slow," labor was augmented with oxytocin making electronic fetal monitoring and laboring in bed necessary. Because an induced labor is more intense and more painful women were more likely to request an epidural. Epidural analgesia slowed the progress of labor and sometimes led to an instrumental delivery (with forceps or vacuum extraction) or a cesarean section. The routine induction of labor with an unripe cervix (closed and noneffaced cervix) for women who did not go into labor by their due date often led to failed inductions and consequently a cesarean. The Institute cautioned that "the more you do, the more you do."[9]

The way labor is managed today is even more technologically intensive. Cesareans for dystocia, continues to be performed in some hospitals when women are not in "true" labor (active phase of labor). Women also have cesareans in second stage (pushing phase) for unprogressive labor based on arbitrary time limits. The U.S. Agency for Healthcare Research and Quality examined cesarean deliveries from thirty hospitals in California and Iowa. It found that 68 percent of the cesareans included failure to progress as one of the indications for the surgery. At least 16 percent of these operations were performed too early, in the latent phase of labor when the cervix was dilated from 0 to 3 cms. Active labor had not yet begun. For women who had a cesarean in second stage (pushing stage), 36 percent did not have a prolonged pushing stage according to established guidelines. ACOG guidelines allowed 2 hours for women to give birth the first time without an epidural and 3 hours with an epidural. Multiparas (women who gave birth before) could have up to 2 hours with an epidural. In the study authors speculated that either physicians were not aware of the ACOG criteria, which they deemed unlikely, or they simply disagreed with ACOG's definition of what constituted lack of progress in labor.[10]

All Women Don't Labor the Same

In obstetrics textbooks, the current standards of measuring the progress of "normal" labor are still based on Friedman's Curve—a method of charting the progress of labor pioneered in the 1950s by Dr. Emmanuel A. Friedman. For first births cervical dilation is expected to progress at 1.2 cms per hour for women in active labor. For women who have given birth before, progress is measured as 1.5 cms per hour. Friedman had explained that the "active" or true phase of labor could begin at any stage of cervical dilation, when contractions consistently become stronger and closer together. For second stage (pushing phase) progress according to Friedman's Curve is 1.0 cm per hour for first-time mothers and 2 cms per hour for multiparas. Labor progress was considered "abnormal" if there was no progress for more than 2 hours in the active phase (secondary arrest of dilation) and no progress for more than 1 hour in the second stage.[11]

Researchers have since challenged the 50-year-old standard of expecting all women to labor at a predetermined number of centimeters per hour. Several studies have found that "normal" variations of labor exist outside of the traditional time line of Friedman's Curve and health outcomes for both mothers and babies are not compromised when women take longer to give birth, that is, if their labor is not induced and they do not have an epidural for pain relief. In one study of nearly 1,500 low-risk women attended by nurse-midwives at the University of New Mexico Hospital, two out of ten women had a longer than normal active phase and 4 percent a longer second stage. All had uncomplicated normal births.[12] When labor begins on its own, the active phase of labor can take more than twice as long as the norm established by Friedman's Curve. Larger babies can safely be born if women are given more time to complete their labor. Sometimes labor can stall for more than 2 hours without compromising maternal or infant safety.[13]

The World Health Organization (WHO) recommends that caregivers not intervene to speed up labor before the cervix has dilated to at least 4 cm dilation. No medical interventions such as breaking the bag of waters, or augmenting labor with oxytocin should be introduced in this phase. Using these guidelines helps to reduce the misdiagnosis of prolonged labor. Inductions are less likely to be started and physicians are less likely to perform a cesarean for failure to progress or a failed induction.[14]

All Women Don't Push the Same

It is a common concern that if a mother's efforts to give birth exceed the standard time line the baby is more likely to suffer brain damage or death. Mothers are more likely to suffer from severe perineal tears, infection, and increased hemorrhage. Caregivers often shorten the second stage by using forceps, a vacuum extractor, or performing a cesarean section. As with normal variations of labor, women differ in how long they need to give birth. For some first time mothers it can safely take as long as $3^1/_2$ hours to give birth.[15] For some African-American and Puerto Rican women cared for by midwives the pushing phase took about half the standard time by Friedman's standards.[16]

Most caregivers limit the mother's efforts to push her baby to 2 hours for first time mothers and 1 hour for women who had prior births. And start to time the beginning of second stage (pushing phase) when the cervix has dilated to 10 cms. However, evidence shows that it is safe to delay pushing until the mother actually feels the urge to push and allow her to follow her own instincts, letting her push as long and as often as she wants during a contraction. In the normal course of labor there is often a rest period between the first and second stage, when women do not feel the urge to bear down. Contractions come further apart and are less intense for a few minutes or as long as an hour. That rest period is usually longer for first time mothers. Eventually as the baby makes its way down through the pelvis, contractions become stronger and women have an involuntary urge to push. The urge to push is reflexive when the baby's head puts pressure on the mother's pelvic floor. To reduce stress on the baby, mothers can push with every second or third contraction. With an epidural women are often aggressively coached to push believing that these efforts will hasten the birth process when in fact they do not. Research suggests that babies tolerate the stress of labor better with a passive descent approach. That requires patience, encouragement, and support. When the mother and baby's vital signs are stable an intervention with forceps, vacuum extractor, or a cesarean is not necessarily the best approach for women who do not conform to an arbitrary time limit.[17]

In many hospitals women are instructed to push while lying on their back (lithotomy position). Pushing in this position makes contractions less efficient and causes the mother pain. It is also reduces blood flow to the placenta and limits the amount of oxygen available to the baby. This position is more likely to cause fetal distress (non-reassuring fetal heart rate) and consequently, a cesarean.

The WHO guidelines for normal birth describe two distinct phases for second-stage labor. The early non-expulsive phase where the cervix is fully dilated, the baby continues to descend through the birth canal but the mother feels no urge to push. And the late expulsive phase when the baby reaches the pelvic floor and triggers the mother's urge to push. The guidelines recommend that a woman should be encouraged to assume whatever position she prefers once she is in the expulsive phase.[18]

Freedom of Movement Helps Labor Progress

In traditional cultures and when giving birth at home or a birth center a woman rarely lies down at the beginning of labor and almost never gives birth on her back. Yet in the majority of hospitals today protocols restrict women's movements to the confines of a bed or a chair. The use of IVs, continuous fetal monitoring, and epidurals for labor limit women's ability to walk, move around, and change positions. Evidence shows that those restrictions can slow down labor, increase pain, and the need for pain medications. The majority of women who give birth in U.S. hospitals cannot take advantage of freedom of movement. Less than half move or change positions in labor. Over 80 percent have routine IV lines, over 70 percent have epidurals, and more than half have their labor induced. While pushing, over one-half of mothers do so on their back.[19]

Women who have the freedom to walk, move, and labor in an upright position have an easier labor. They experience less severe pain, have less need for narcotics or epidural anesthesia and have a shorter first stage of labor. Babies are less likely to have fetal heart problems. In an upright position gravity may improve the baby's descent through the pelvis and align the baby more effectively to move through the pelvis. Change of positions also changes the relationship of the baby's head to the mother's pelvic diameters, increasing the opportunities for a better fit or a better angle to move through the pelvis. Mothers are likely to have stronger and more efficient contractions to help dilate the cervix. Women who walk during labor are also less likely to have continuous fetal monitoring, a risk factor for cesarean section. They also have more spontaneous births. In the second stage, women who squat, kneel, rest on hands and knees, or lie on their side rather than on their back have a shorter and less painful second stage labor and fewer episiotomies.[20]

X-ray pelvimetry shows that in a squatting or kneeling position the pelvic diameters are wider by as much as 30 percent and can provide more space for the baby to pass through the pelvis.[21] Women who have freedom of movement have more control of their birth and more choices to better meet their needs.

Emotional Distress Can Slow Down Labor

Hormones play a significant role in the progress of labor. Dystocia or prolonged labor can be caused by fear, anxiety, or extreme pain. These feelings release high levels of catecholamine in the blood stream, which can interfere with the normal progress of labor. In effect, in a state of psychological distress, high levels of cathecolamines also reduce blood flow to the uterus and placenta, slow down contractions, and reduce the flow of oxygen to the baby. Labor can slow down considerably or stop. Women may not feel safe and may be fearful of invasive procedures, a previous difficult birth, the baby being harmed, or of loosing control.[22] Emerging knowledge of the psychological factors that can impact the normal progress of labor suggests that women who may have had a prior traumatic birth or who may have suffered from physical, sexual, or emotional abuse may be more vulnerable to emotional dystocia. Women may have an unusually extreme fear of labor (tocophobia) based on personal or secondary knowledge of difficult births.[23]

Emotional support and comfort, encouragement, reassurance, and providing a sense of safety and calm can be very effective in increasing a woman's self-assurance and her ability to cope effectively with her labor. Respecting her individual needs and including her in all decisions related to her care can increase her sense of well-being.

Epidurals Can Slow Down Labor

Several studies have shown that an epidural can increase the risk for a cesarean section.[24,25,26] Caregivers are beginning to understand that women who still feel the effect of an epidural during second stage need more time to push their baby out. Epidurals can slow the progress of labor and birth. Although they provide excellent pain relief they can complicate and prolong the pushing phase. With an epidural the muscles of the mother's pelvic floor are numbed and muscle tone is weakened by the anesthesia. Mothers do not feel the urge to push and do not respond to it reflexively. Mothers need guidance to push effectively.

Epidurals can prevent the baby from completing the normal internal rotation on the pelvic floor, which facilitates the baby's birth. A study conducted at Boston's Brigham and Women's Hospital showed that with an epidural for labor, babies were four times more likely to be in the occiput posterior position (OP) just before birth.[27] When babies are in the OP position labor is more difficult and birth often requires an instrumental delivery or a cesarean section. A review of seven studies that included almost 3,000 women who had an epidural for pain relief in labor found that women who used passive pushing instead of pushing immediately after full dilation were more likely to have a spontaneous birth. They pushed for a shorter period of time, were less fatigued, and were less likely to need an instrumental delivery with forceps or vacuum extractor. Without an instrumental delivery women were less likely to suffer from perineal damage, fecal incontinence, anal sphincter damage, and damage to the pudendal nerve.[28]

A mother who has been given an epidural in labor should be allowed an additional hour to give birth to her baby. Some caregivers avoid the restrictions of a time line as long as the mother is progressing and vital signs are stable. Other caregivers recommend that active pushing be delayed until the top of the baby's head is visible.[29]

RESOURCES

A Guide to Effective Care in Pregnancy and Childbirth, Prolonged Labor, at Childbirth Connection, http://www.ChildbirthConnection.com, May 19, 2008.
Midwives Information and Resource Service, Informed Choice Leaflets, Positions
in Labour and Delivery, http://www.infochoice.org, May 19, 2008.

10

ESPECIALLY FOR MOTHERS: WALK, ROCK, SWAY, SQUAT, YOU CAN HELP YOUR LABOR TO PROGRESS

Having a Baby? Ask your care provider, "Can I walk and move round during labor? What position do you suggest for birth?" In mother-friendly settings, you can walk around and move about as you choose during labor. You can choose the positions that are most comfortable and work best for you during labor and birth. (There may be a medical reason for you to be in a certain position.) Mother-friendly settings almost never put a woman flat on her back with her legs in stirrups for the birth.[1]

During your pregnancy your baby grows and develops and prepares herself for her journey to birth. She needs no instructions to be born, but she will need your help. If you understand how you and your baby prepare and adapt for labor and birth together you are less likely to fear the overpowering and painful sensations of childbirth. You are also less likely to wonder if something has gone wrong and if your baby is still safe. Normal contractions of labor and birth can be painful, but they are not dangerous.

Toward the end of your last trimester your baby will position herself for birth with her head down close to your cervix. You will probably feel the weight of your baby deep down in your pelvis and pressing on your bladder. It will be easier for you to breathe and you will no longer feel your baby under your diaphragm. This is called lightening (see Photos 10.1 and 10.2). By that time your cervix has probably begun to soften. The weight of your baby, the placenta, and the amniotic fluid in your womb is suspended by three ligaments that have stretched along with your uterus during your pregnancy. If during labor you lie down on your back that weight will increase your pain, slow down the circulation to the baby, and make contractions less efficient in opening your cervix.

YOU CAN CREATE MORE SPACE FOR YOUR BABY TO BE BORN

Many women are told during pregnancy that they are carrying a "big" baby or that their pelvis is "too small," so they should have a cesarean section. But,

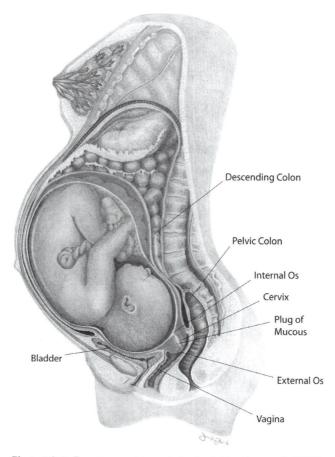

Photo 10.1. Pregnancy at term, baby is visible. *Source*: © 1985, 2006. Childbirth Connection. All rights reserved. Used with permission.

research shows that estimating the size of the baby, even with ultrasound, is inaccurate. Here is what you should know about your body and how it changes during pregnancy to make childbirth safe and easier for you and your baby.

During pregnancy you produce hormones that soften all the connective tissue (cartilage) in your body. Even your rib cage expands to increase your lung capacity. Your joints become more flexible. Muscle cells and connective tissue in the birth canal expand to make room for your baby to be born. Your pelvis has four separate bones, two hip bones (innominate bones) that join in front connected by a muscle called the pubic symphysis. The hip bones connect in the back to the sacrum (large triangular shaped bone at the end

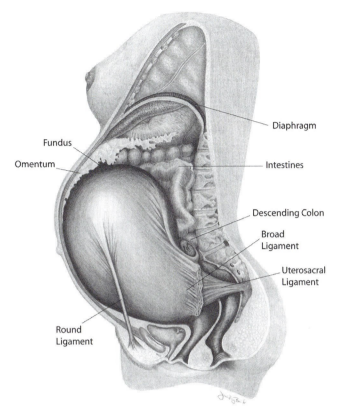

Photo 10.2. Pregnancy at term, external womb. *Source*: © 1985, 2006. Childbirth Connection. All rights reserved. Used with permission.

of the spine). The fourth bone, the tail bone (coccix) is connected to the sacrum.

Pregnancy hormones soften the pelvic joints (the sacro-iliac and the pubic symphysis) and makes them more elastic (see Photo 10.3). This flexibility helps your baby to adapt to the shape and size of your pelvis and allows the baby to pass safely through the pelvis making labor easier and less painful. The baby will be moving downward and through the open space inside these bones. Because your pelvic joints are very flexible during your pregnancy, the wideness of the space within your pelvis (pelvic diameters) changes shape and size when you move and change positions (see Photo 10.4). Your baby will have a snug fit as she moves through your pelvis but you can give her all the room she needs and you will experience less pain by making sure you have the freedom to move and change positions during labor.[2, 3]

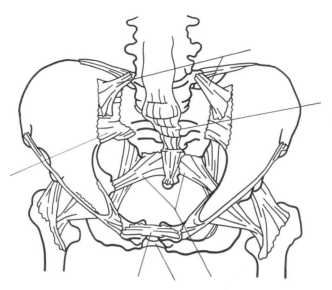

Photo 10.3. Female pelvis with indicated connective tissue that softens during pregnany allowing for maximum flexibility and more room for the baby during labor and birth. *Source*: Illustration by Shanna dela Cruz.

The majority of babies position themselves in the pelvic inlet in the safest and easiest way for their journey to birth. Head down, facing the mother's left or right side, and the back of the baby's head (occiput) towards the front of the mother's body. The positions are known as left occiput anterior (LOA)

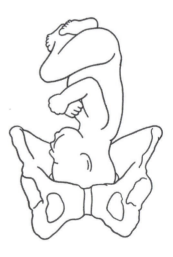

Photo 10.4. Baby's head engaged in the pelvis. *Source*: Illustration by Shanna dela Cruz.

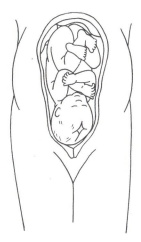

Photo 10.5. Baby in right occiput posterior position (ROP). *Source*: Illustrations by Shanna dela Cruz, copyright Ruth S. Ancheta (1994, 1999, and 2005). Reproduced by permission from Simkin, P. and Ancheta, R. (2000, 2005). *The Labor Progress Handbook: Early Interventions to Prevent and Treat Dystocia*. Oxford: Blackwell Publishing.

and right occiput anterior (ROA). Less often the baby will enter the pelvis facing the front of the mother's body and his head aligned toward the mother's spine. This position is known as occiput posterior (OP). With an OP position labor is slower, more difficult, and more painful since the mother feels the pressure of the baby's back in between contractions (see Photos 10.5 and 10.6).

The skull bones of your baby's head are also soft and flexible. They can mold to adapt to the space available in your pelvis. If needed they can slide over each other slightly (molding) as your baby makes her way down through the pelvis. Most babies will enter the pelvis in a head down position, with the chin tucked in on the chest (flexed). With a flexed chin the smallest diameter of the baby's head enters the pelvis (pelvic inlet). Most babies also enter the

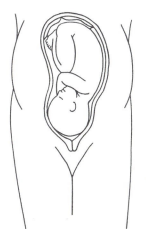

Photo 10.6. Baby in left occiput anterior position (LOA). *Source*: Illustrations by Shanna dela Cruz, copyright Ruth S. Ancheta (1994, 1999, and 2005). Reproduced by permission from Simkin, P. and Ancheta, R. (2000, 2005). *The Labor Progress Handbook: Early Interventions to Prevent and Treat Dystocia*. Oxford: Blackwell Publishing.

pelvis diagonally, where there is maximum room. The diameter of the part of the baby's head that enters the pelvis is about 9.5 cm, and the cervix dilates to 10 cms to accommodate the baby's head.

Upright Positions for Labor

Staying in an upright position, having the freedom to move and change positions makes labor shorter and less painful. It also reduces your need for pain medications and an epidural. If your baby is in a posterior position (OP) or its head is slightly tilted to the right or left (asynclitic) the freedom to move and help your baby to position herself better in your pelvis is even more important. For the first stage of labor, being upright allows gravity to help bring your baby down faster and easier. It also helps your cervix to dilate. It can help to align your baby at the best possible angle in the pelvis. Changing positions allows your partner or doula to give you a massage to reduce your pain where you need it and reduce your backache, because if you move and change positions to make yourself comfortable you will feel less pain. Being upright could be walking, sitting, kneeling, and supporting your upper body, sitting on a birth ball, moving side to side, swaying back and forth, leaning over and even climbing up or down stairs, supported, and at a slow pace. All these movements help to widen your pelvis. Raising one leg changes the amount of pelvic space on that side of your body. There are several different positions to facilitate labor and birth. Women choose what works best for them when they are in labor. However, it's best if you can try them out with your partner or doula before your labor so they feel comfortable for you. You are also more likely to remember them in labor. If you are planning to take a childbirth preparation class, make sure it includes education and practice time for different comfortable options for labor and birth (see Photo 10.7).

If Your Baby Is OP

Even if your baby enters your pelvis in a head down position, labor progress is slow, more painful, and more difficult when the baby is in an OP position. There are several ways to help your baby move out of an OP position. During the last part of your pregnancy, Jean Sutton and Pauline Scott, New Zealand midwives and authors of *Understanding and Teaching Optimal Foetal Positioning*, explain that with an OP baby, it is best to try to change his position before he enters the pelvis. Positions in which the mother leans or sits forward alters the angle and dimensions of her pelvis. That helps the baby enter the pelvis in a better position. These positions are done during pregnancy. You can find out more about optimal fetal positioning from http://www.homebirth.org.uk/ofp.htm.

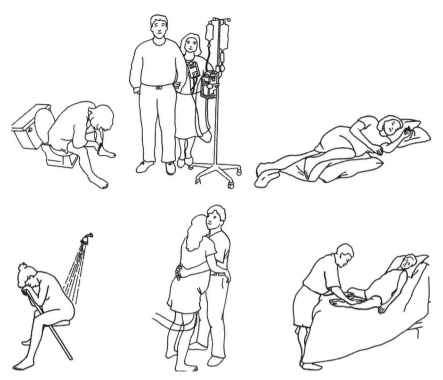

Photo 10.7. Helpful positions for "big baby-small pelvis." (They widen the pelvis, give the baby as much room as possible, and often reduce the pain.) *Source*: Illustrations by Shanna dela Cruz, copyright Ruth S. Ancheta (1994, 1999, and 2005). Reproduced by permission from Simkin, P. and Ancheta, R. (2000, 2005). *The Labor Progress Handbook: Early Interventions to Prevent and Treat Dystocia*. Oxford: Blackwell Publishing and by the International Childbirth Education Association.

With a baby in an OP in labor position mothers may have back pain even in between contractions. There are positions that are particularly helpful for "back" labor. Positions such as leaning forward, being on hands and knees, kneeling on one knee, resting one foot on a stool or chair change the level of the hips and the available space within the pelvis and are helpful during labor.[4] You can do many of them even if you are in bed. You may want to practice these positions a few weeks before your labor begins (see Photo 10.8).

Upright Positions for Birth

Your pelvis is wider side-to-side as your baby comes into the pelvis (pelvic inlet), but wider from front to back (pelvic outlet) as the baby moves down

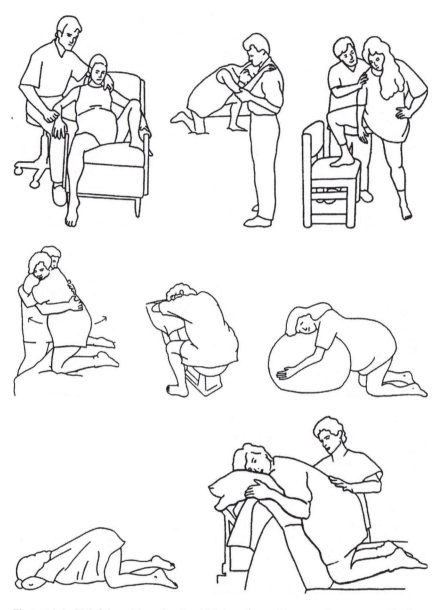

Photo 10.8. Helpful positions for "back" labor. (By raising one leg on one side they open the pelvis wider; leaning forward helps the baby rotate to an anterior position and reduces back pain.) *Source*: Illustrations by Shanna dela Cruz, copyright Ruth S. Ancheta (1994, 1999, and 2005). Reproduced by permission from Simkin, P. and Ancheta, R. (2000, 2005). *The Labor Progress Handbook: Early Interventions to Prevent and Treat Dystocia.* Oxford: Blackwell Publishing and by the International Childbirth Education Association.

and out of your pelvis. During labor the baby turns her body and head as she moves through your pelvis. When the top of your baby's head reaches and feels the resistance of the muscles of your pelvic floor, she will flex her chin even more and turn her head to face your tailbone to take advantage of the wider space of the pelvic outlet. Once her head has turned she will extend her head and neck to slide under your pubic arch (pubic bones) and move into the birth canal. Once her head is born with her chin facing your tailbone she will move her head sideways to rotate one more time so that her shoulders also turn and align themselves front to back to take advantage of the wider space of the pelvic outlet. These movements, flexing her chin (flexion), moving her head around (internal rotation), extending her neck (extension), and turning her shoulders around in the pelvis (external rotation) are called the cardinal movements. To help labor progress and facilitate the moves and positions of your baby as she goes through your pelvis, it is essential that your body and pelvis not be pinned down or restricted in any way. As your baby moves through your pelvis the flexible joints will allow your pelvic bones to widen side to side and your sacrum and tail bone to move backwards to give your baby the room she needs. Limiting your ability to move around is painful. Your contractions are less efficient in opening your cervix and labor will be longer (see Photo 10.9).

The Pushing Phase, Never on Your Back

When a pregnant woman at term lies down on her back the weight of the baby, the amniotic fluid, the placenta, and the uterus press down on major blood vessels, the inferior vena cava and the aorta. That pressure reduces blood flow and the oxygen supply to the baby. Contractions are not as effective. When pushing the baby out you give her more room if you are in a position that does not restrict the movement of your hips or tailbone. Your baby's head needs to slided own under your pubic bone and then back up again. So you will not be pushing against gravity, you can stand, lean over with support, squat, or kneel to push your baby out. Your baby will get all the oxygen she needs. Squatting opens the space within your pelvis by 20 to 30 percent.

Babies know how to take advantage of the space that opens up as they make their way down and through the pelvis. Pushing in an upright position means you are less likely to need forceps, a vacuum extractor, or a cesarean section. You are also less likely to tear your perineum since the tissues will not be stretched tightly as they would be if you were on a delivery table with your legs in stirrups. If you get tired, you may want to try lying on your side, supporting yourself on your hands and knees (helpful for rotating the baby from a posterior to an anterior position), or semi-sitting (see Photo 10.10).

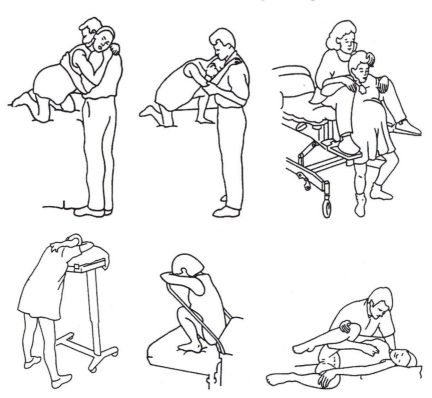

Photo 10.9. Helpful positions for pushing. (Leaning forward helps with "back" labor standing and squatting when the baby is engaged in the pelvis helps with a "big baby" lying sideways is an alternative comfortable position). *Source*: Illustrations by Shanna dela Cruz, copyright Ruth S. Ancheta (1994, 1999, and 2005). Reproduced by permission from Simkin, P. and Ancheta, R. (2000, 2005). *The Labor Progress Handbook: Early Interventions to Prevent and Treat Dystocia.* Oxford: Blackwell Publishing and by the International Childbirth Education Association.

Being in an upright position instead of on your back will shorten this phase of labor. You will feel less pain and are less likely to need an episiotomy. Not all mothers feel the urge to push when the cervix is fully dilated. It is safer for you and your baby if you push when you sense the urge to do so rather than pushing forcefully by holding your breath for a long time. Usually, women will normally hold their breath for about 5 to 7 seconds. If you have an epidural it will take you longer to push the baby out, so you will need more time. If you bear down and push when you feel the urge to do so your baby will be less likely to suffer from fetal distress (lack of oxygen), you won't get tired as easily, and you are less likely to suffer from perineal tears. Midwives are trained to support a mother in different positions for labor and birth. More and more labor and delivery nurses today also encourage mothers to use different

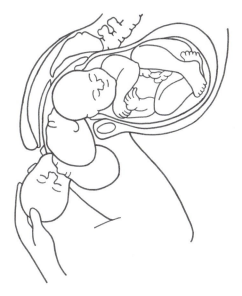

Photo 10.10. Cardinal movements. *Source*: Illustration by Shanna dela Cruz.

positions in labor and birth and work together with women who want to labor in an upright position.[5]

Impact of Routine Interventions on Freedom of Movement

Medical interventions such as continuous electronic fetal monitoring, IVs, and bladder catheters needed with epidurals, will affect your ability to move around and change positions. Some care providers are very comfortable monitoring the baby's heart rate electronically at specific time intervals (intermittently) or with a hand-held device such as a fetoscope or a Doppler. Research shows that this is the best way to monitor a low-risk mother and baby. However, with an induction or an epidural you and the baby will need to be monitored continuously with an electronic fetal monitor. If you allow your bag of waters to be broken early in labor (amniotomy) your baby will have a more difficult time changing positions in your pelvis. Also, the amount of time you will be "allowed" to labor will begin from the time your bag of waters breaks. This is often a maximum of 24 hours. If the baby is not born by then most caregivers will recommend a cesarean.

You will know what feels best for you when you are actually in labor. You will know when it is time to rest or lie down. Lying sideways rather than on your back is more helpful and less painful. Women in labor who are given the freedom to move and change positions to make themselves more comfortable feel more in control of their birth.

Your Feelings Can Affect the Progress of Your Labor

Labor and birth are not just physiological processes. The mind and body are closely intertwined and your feelings can slow down or stop your labor. If you are extremely afraid, anxious, feel unsafe, or intimidated, your body will produce hormones (catecholamines) that will interfere with the hormones that help labor progress. If you have had a prior traumatic birth or have experienced physical, emotional, or sexual abuse in the past, the physical sensations of labor and birth may consciously or unconsciously trigger an emotional response that may slow down or stop your labor. Sometimes women who have had those experiences ask to have a cesarean delivery rather than re-experience those events. With a cesarean delivery women may feel safer and more in control of their birth. A skilled and sensitive nurse, midwife, or doula can sometimes help women to cope with those feelings so labor and birth can progress. If you become aware of past traumatic experiences before you become pregnant or during your pregnancy you may want to consult a therapist that specializes in birth trauma or abuse issues.[6]

Progress in Labor Is Not Just about Cervical Dilation

Many first time mothers are anxious for labor to begin and sometimes are frustrated and worried that their labor is not progressing. Before the cervix begins to dilate (1 to 10 cms) its position moves from a posterior position to an anterior position. By moving forward it aligns better with the opening of the birth canal so that the baby can move down easily. The cervix needs to ripen and soften. Its texture is said to resemble the feel of the tip of the nose when not ripe and the feel of your earlobe when it is ripe. The cervix also needs to efface, become shorter and thinner. When the cervix is 10 cm dilated it is paper thin. Once there is enough room for your baby to move downward (10 cm) the baby will rotate internally on the pelvic floor, flex her chin, and her head will mold to accommodate the space within your pelvis. All these changes occur before your baby is born.[7]

Don't Rush to the Hospital as Soon as Labor Starts

If you have a healthy pregnancy and your labor begins at term (38–42 weeks) you are less likely to have a cesarean if you stay home until active labor has set in. Mothers pregnant for the first time often go to the hospital too early. Research shows that if you arrive at the hospital before you are in active labor, about 3 to 4 cms dilated with consistent contractions, you are more likely to end up with a cesarean. Signs of labor are not always clear. The early part of labor is highly variable and unpredictable. If your bag of waters breaks and the fluid is clear your labor is likely to begin with consistent contractions that will dilate your cervix within 24 hours. For some women labor begins with contractions that last several hours for others a few days before they are in active labor.

Mothers who are not knowledgeable about how their body works during labor are more likely to be anxious when they begin to feel the pain of early labor contractions. Some hospitals have a special area for women in early labor that allows them to pass the time until active labor has set in or when their bag of waters has broken. This way the staff is less likely to induce labor, use continuous monitoring, insert an IV, and break the bag of waters after admission to the labor and delivery unit so that labor progresses and birth takes place within a predetermined time limit. Mothers who give birth at home or at a birth center are often more closely in touch with their caregivers and more likely to have that information during pregnancy.

There are situations that make it necessary to contact your care provider as soon as possible and not wait until active labor: if you go into labor before term; if your bag of waters breaks and the liquid is not clear but yellow, green, brown, or black (that is meconium that can cause damage to your baby's lungs if inhaled) or has an odor; if you have vaginal bleeding. Your care provider will give you additional information specific to your needs.

Take a Childbirth Class

Women have many resources to learn about labor and birth. Unfortunately, today childbirth as seen by the media often focuses on what birth is rather than what birth can be. Most women who find out about childbirth only from television programs and some popular books on childbirth never get to find out about how their body is designed to give birth and how they can help themselves to make childbirth a more positive and empowering experience. They don't learn about patient rights, how to find out about the benefits and risks of procedures, or the many options that are available to them. Often, these issues are covered in quality childbirth education classes taught by certified educators credentialed by national professional associations. With a nationally certified educator you are more likely to learn about: the options that are available to you; the questions you need to ask your care provider; your rights as a patient; how to make labor and birth easier for you; the different methods of pain relief, with or without drugs; how to initiate and continue breastfeeding; and your newborn's innate qualities and behaviors that will help you to appreciate your role as a new parent.

Resources

To find out more about the benefits of movement, changing positions, and different ways to make yourself comfortable in labor, or to find out about childbirth classes in your community, visit these Web sites:

Childbirth Organizations, http://www.alace.org, http://www.bradleybirth.com, http://www.cappa.org, www.icea.org, http://www.lamaze.org, last accessed on May 18, 2008.

Lamaze International, http://www.lamaze.org/ExpectantParents/Pregnancyand BirthResources/MoreTipsandTools/FreedomofMovementTips/tabid/256/ Default.aspx, last accessed on May 18, 2008.

Tips for Maintaining Freedom of Movement, P. Simkin, Comfort in Labor, at Childbirth Connection, http://www.childbirthconnection.com, last accessed on May 18, 2008.

Watch women giving birth with freedom to move and in active positions, see Lamaze International, Everyday Miracles, http://www.lamaze.org/Expectant Parents/PregnancyBirthResources/WatchWomenGiveBirthWithConfidence/ tabid/183/Default.aspx, last accessed on May 25, 2008.

What Is Optimal Foetal Positioning?, http://www.homebirth.org.uk/ofp.htm, last accessed on May 25, 2008.

11

LABORING FOR A VBAC: A SAFE ALTERNATIVE TO A REPEAT OPERATION

can a hospital have a vbac policy which states no vbacs will be labored there? what happens when a vbac arrives in labor? does the vbac policy conflict with the right of the mother to receive care during labor? . . . this happened to my wife. she is a dr. who practices ob, and i was the only dr available to her. I am now accused of violating the vbac policy. she got stuck at 5 cm (she did not want a cesarean), so i drove her to the next hospital 70 miles away, where she delivered with some pit. (pitocin) . she had had 3 previous vbacs. . . . can you help me with the constitutionality of vbac policies or do you know a good lawyer? thx[1]

Vaginal birth after a cesarean—VBAC—a term coined by Nancy Wainer-Cohen, coauthor with Lois J. Estner of *Silent Knife: Cesarean Prevention & Vaginal Birth After Cesarean*. The groundbreaking book published in 1983 that shattered the myths that bolstered the wholesale of repeat abdominal surgeries for women who once gave birth by cesarean. The year the book was published 808,000 women gave birth by cesarean section despite the recommendation of a 1980 National Institutes of Health (NIH) consensus conference on cesarean section, urging for more VBACs.

Today, as 25 years ago, women in the United States are fighting for their right to labor and give birth rather than submit to a medically inappropriate major abdominal surgery. Many women pregnant after a prior cesarean birth, some in their last trimester, are shocked to find out that hospitals covered by their insurance plan have unilaterally banned VBACs from their labor and delivery units despite ample evidence and two definitive studies recently published by the NIH Maternal-Fetal Medicine Units Network, confirming the safety of VBAC even after more than one cesarean. History it seems is repeating itself.

A national goal of Healthy People 2010 is to improve the health and well-being of women, infants, children, and families. Included in its priorities to improve maternal and infant health is to reduce the number of repeat cesareans and increase the number of women who plan a VBAC (vaginal birth after cesarean). Its target is a national VBAC rate of 63 percent by the year 2010. Recent trends in routine repeat operations have been increasing contrary to these objectives.[2] VBAC was deemed a reasonable and safe option to routine repeat cesareans decades ago. But, in recent years misinformation about its safety and lack of scientific evidence behind current guidelines for VBAC has succeeded in increasing the routine repeat cesarean rate to more than 90 percent.

The single most controversial issue regarding birth after cesarean is the probability of a uterine rupture—the separation of the uterine scar from a prior incision during labor or birth. Overall studies have reported the risk to be less than 1 percent—the same risk as for any woman giving birth the first time. In recent years, the risk of a uterine rupture while laboring for a VBAC has overshadowed all other unpredictable obstetric complications likely to occur for any woman in labor—unpredictable emergencies such as a prolapsed umbilical cord, fetal distress (nonreassuring fetal heart rate), and hemorrhage from a placental abruption.

In fact the national fear about uterine rupture and its legal ramifications has had such a strong grip on maternity care providers that hundreds of U.S. hospitals are now refusing to provide care for women who want to labor for a VBAC. The only alternative that thousands of women with a prior cesarean birth have is a forced repeat operation, when no medical indication exists. Nine out of ten women with a prior cesarean had a repeat operation in 2005.[3] This national fear associated with VBACs is a relatively recent phenomenon associated more with medical malpractice suits and fixed reimbursement rates for childbirth rather than any recent scientific evidence. In fact laboring for a VBAC after a prior cesarean is not any more dangerous today than it was two decades ago. With support and proper care within safe guidelines about 75 percent of women will have a normal birth and avoid the complications of a repeat cesarean operation.

PLANNED VBAC AND REPEAT CESAREAN, HOW DO THE RISKS COMPARE?

After one cesarean delivery, each additional operation puts women and babies at added risks for complications. Compared with a planned vaginal birth mothers who have a repeat cesarean are at increased risk for maternal infection, adhesions, intestinal obstruction, chronic pain, cesarean scar, ectopic pregnancy, and placental problems. Placental problems from accumulating cesareans increase the risk for hemorrhage severe enough to require a blood transfusion. For the baby, a scheduled cesarean increases the risk of serious neonatal respiratory problems, sometimes requiring intensive care.[4]

With a planned VBAC there is the possibility that the uterine scar could separate partially or completely during labor or birth. Scar tissue in the uterus will expand and stretch as the uterus grows during pregnancy. Sometimes the scar stretches thin enough to cause a dehiscence or window. This is also known as a silent or incomplete rupture or an asymptomatic separation. A dehiscence can be seen when women have a scheduled repeat cesarean. It occurs in about 1 to 2 percent of mothers with one low transverse scar (side to side). A dehiscence heals on its own and does not need medical treatment.

A complete separation of the uterine scar is a tear through the thickness of the uterine wall at the site of a prior cesarean incision. Compared to a routine repeat cesarean the added risk of the separation of a cesarean scar is about 27 per 10,000 women who labor for a VBAC. Nearly 400 women would need to have a repeat cesarean to prevent one uterine rupture during labor. Compared to babies born by repeat cesarean deliveries there's the added risk that a baby would die as a result of a uterine scar rupture in 1.4 per 10,000 women laboring for a VBAC. Nearly 7,100 women need to have a repeat cesarean to prevent one baby from dying as a consequence of the separation of a scar. With a prior low horizontal uterine incision, a complete separation occurs in about 2 to 7 per 1000 women who labor for a VBAC. The likelihood that a woman would die while laboring for a VBAC is less than 1 in 100,000.[5] If the scar separates women will suffer from hemorrhage and may need a blood transfusion or a hysterectomy if the bleeding cannot be controlled. The baby may suffer from neurological complications or die.

Researchers from the Cochrane Pregnancy and Childbirth Group state that the risk of rupture with one prior low horizontal incision is not higher than any other unforeseen complication that can occur in labor, such as fetal distress, maternal hemorrhage from a premature separation of the placenta, and a prolapsed umbilical cord.[6] Uterine scar separations also occur in women who have never had a cesarean and women who have had an assisted birth with forceps. This type of rupture can also be caused by weak uterine muscles after several pregnancies, excessive use of labor inducing agents, or a prior surgical procedure on the uterus.

Two recently published studies by the National Institutes of Child Health and Human Development Maternal–Fetal Medicine Units Network confirm that VBAC is a safe alternative and may be safer than one or more repeat operations. Researchers reviewed the health records of women with one or more prior low transverse scars who labored for a VBAC. They found that the odds of having a vaginal birth increased with each labor after a prior cesarean. With no prior vaginal birth 63.3 percent of women had a normal birth. With one, two, three, and four VBACs 87.6 percent, 90.9 percent, 90.6 percent, and 91.6 percent had a vaginal delivery. The risk for a uterine rupture decreased after the first VBAC. With no prior vaginal birth the risk was 0.87 percent. With two, three, four, and five VBACs the risk was 0.45 percent, 0.38 percent, 0.54 percent, 0.52 percent. There was no increase in neonatal complications with increasing VBACs. The risk of uterine dehiscence was also reduced with increasing numbers of VBACs.[7]

In a study that looked at women who had repeat cesareans with each additional pregnancy researchers found that serious complications increased with each successive operation. Examining health risks with up to six repeat cesareans, the study found that placenta accreta, cystotomy (a surgical incision in the bladder), ileus (bowel obstruction), and injury to the bladder increased. The need for intensive care, ventilation after the surgery, hysterectomy, and blood transfusions also increased. With each repeat cesarean operating time was longer; so was the need for an increased hospital stay. The researchers recommend that women give serious consideration to having their first planned cesarean without a medical indication.[8]

THE FEAR OF VBAC IS A RECENT PHENOMENON

In 1981 the National Institutes of Health (NIH) consensus report, "Cesarean Childbirth," indicated that a prior cesarean delivery was one of the four major reasons why the surgery was performed. The other three were dystocia, fetal distress, and breech. Repeat operations accounted for 25 to 30 percent of the increase in cesareans from 1970, when the cesarean rate was 5.5 percent, to 1978, when it was 15.2 percent. More than 98 percent of women had a repeat operation in a subsequent pregnancy. With a low horizontal incision rather than the vertical (classical) incision on the uterus, a common practice in the early 1900s, the report found that the risk for complications when laboring after a prior cesarean was low—a less than 1 percent risk for a uterine rupture. The nineteen-member multidisciplinary task force, based on the available research at the time, made the following recommendations:

> In hospitals with appropriate facilities, services, and staff for prompt emergency cesarean birth, a proper selection of cases should permit a safe trial of labor and vaginal delivery for women who have had a previous low segment transverse cesarean birth...Informed consent should be obtained before a trial of labor is attempted. Patient education relating to cesarean birth and repeat cesarean birth should continue throughout pregnancy as an important part of patient participation in decisions concerning anesthesia, elective repeat cesarean birth, or trial of labor following previous cesarean birth.[9]

The American College of Obstetricians and Gynecologists (ACOG) supported the NIH consensus recommendations and drafted the first Guidelines for Vaginal Delivery After a Previous Cesarean Birth in 1982. In the 1984 revised issue, the ACOG stated that uterine rupture was rarely catastrophic when fetal monitoring, anesthesia, and obstetric support services were available. Since 50 to 80 percent of women with a low transverse uterine scar have successful vaginal births the ACOG recommended that women and their physicians discuss this option early during prenatal care. The guidelines also encouraged a planned VBAC for women who had had a prior cesarean for failure to progress. Up to 70 percent of this group of women had a safe VBAC. The ACOG recommended that institutions have the ability to respond to an emergency such as performing a cesarean delivery within 30 minutes from the time the decision is made until the procedure is begun.[10]

In 1988, based on additional research, the ACOG advised that the concept of routine repeat cesarean birth should be replaced. Barring medical contraindications, women "should be counseled and encouraged to attempt labor." Women with two or more prior cesareans who wished to labor for a VBAC should not be discouraged. Again, the ACOG recommended that an emergency cesarean be available "within 30 minutes from the time the decision is made until the surgical procedure is begun, *as is standard for any obstetrical patient in labor* [italics added]."[11] In the 10 years following the publication of the NIH cesarean report the national VBAC rate increased from less than 3 percent to 20.4 percent in 1990.

In the following years dozens of studies were published attesting the safety of VBAC. The majority of them reported a less than 1 percent risk of the opening or separation of a prior uterine scar that required an emergency cesarean.[12,13] In 1990, Dr. Bruce Flamm, author of the first world's largest VBAC study and several articles and books on cesarean and VBAC, summarized the findings of thirty medical reports on VBAC from seventeen countries including Germany, Zambia, Great Britain, Hong Kong, Indonesia, Ireland, Saudi Arabia, Sweden, Canada, and the West Indies. In his book, *Birth After Cesarean: The Medical Facts*, he wrote, "These reports document thousands upon thousands of successful VBACs. In contrast, I was unable to find even a single medical report published anywhere in the world that came out in favor of routine repeat cesarean section."[14]

Clinical leaders, corporate employers, public interest groups and birth advocates endorsed the option of laboring for a VBAC. Large-scale efforts were made to change physician behavior and reimbursement rates (since a higher fee was paid for a cesarean than a normal delivery) and educate women about the safety and desirability of VBACs. Hospitals began to offer VBAC classes, and education videos were produced. Clinicians spent office time giving information to mothers to make an informed decision about their choice for birth.[15,16] Many mothers and birth advocacy groups began focusing on unnecessary repeat cesareans and pushed for women's right to labor for a VBAC.[17]

As more research became available the ACOG advised that women with one previous low vertical scar and women expected to have a big baby (more than 4000 g or 8 lb. 13 oz.) can also labor for a VBAC: "The evidence regarding the relative safety of vaginal delivery after cesarean birth is compelling. Women should be counseled and encouraged to undertake a trial of labor."[18] The following update stated that the "benefits of a trial of labor outweighed the risks."[19]

In 1995 twenty-eight health care organizations across the United States and Canada with very different populations collaborated to reduce cesarean section rates in their communities. The effort was a part of the Boston-based Institute for Healthcare Improvement's Breakthrough Series, a fast-track approach to making improvements in complicated health care systems. Encouraging women to plan a VBAC, implementing effective strategies to reduce routine repeat operations, and educating maternity care professionals about safe care for VBAC were key measures of the collaborative.[20] Luella Kein, M.D., past president of the American College of Obstetricians and Gynecologists, stated, "Reducing cesarean section rates is not easy. It will require a major change in attitude for patients, for obstetricians, for nurses, for hospitals, and for families... We need to close the gap between what we know to be an appropriate cesarean rate and what is actually done in practice. We could get a health bargain for women and a financial bargain for our health care system."[21]

FORCED CESAREANS—THE ACOG DRAFTS CONTROVERSIAL VBAC GUIDELINES

The VBAC rate in the United States climbed slowly but steadily till one in four women who had a prior cesarean labored for a VBAC. The national rate in 1995 had reached 27.5 percent. Then in 1999, the ACOG published more restrictive guidelines for VBAC, it seemed, to reduce the odds for medical malpractice suits that resulted from a uterine rupture. The guidelines stated that some third-party payers and managed care organizations "mandated" that all women with a prior cesarean delivery needed "to undergo trials of labor." Consequently physicians felt "pressured" to do so in "unsuitable" situations sometimes with patients who preferred to have a repeat operation. The ACOG stated that the increase in VBACs was paralled with an increase in reports of uterine rupture and other complications that led to malpractice suits.[22]

Instead of all prior guidelines since 1982 which recommended that anesthesia and a physician capable of performing an emergency cesarean delivery be "readily available" in active labor, the 1999 issue stated "*immediately available throughout active labor* [italics added]." Each hospital was to determine for itself how to interpret the words "immediately available." Many facilities interpreted "immediately available" to mean in-house availability. Large tertiary care centers have 24-hour in-house availability for any obstetric emergency including a cesarean section, but most U.S. hospitals do not.

Facilities that supported VBAC but did not have 24-hour emergency services would be open to the risk of medical-legal liability. The ACOG president cautioned in an article, "Nurse midwives and family practice physicians may be more receptive to the natural birth philosophy but must accept significant medical-legal liability risks if they offer patients trial of labor and VBAC and cannot provide immediate, appropriate surgical intervention in the case of maternal or fetal deterioration."[23] The ACOG presented no evidence-based references to substantiate the change in policy. The impact of this policy had a devastating effect on the health of women with a prior cesarean.

MALPRACTICE LIABILITY AND CONFLICT OF INTEREST WITH VBAC

Following the publication of the controversial guidelines some malpractice insurance companies restricted coverage for care providers who wanted to support VBAC. In late 2003 Northwest Physicians Mutual Insurance Company in Oregon began to require verification that the hospital where physicians and midwives practiced had a physician capable of performing a cesarean who was in the hospital or on campus throughout active labor. Physicians who had privileges at two separate hospitals (a common occurrence), or had multiple patients in labor at more than one hospital, could not meet those requirements. They asked their patients to sign a contract acknowledging that the physicians could not guarantee the patients could labor for a VBAC. In Southern states physicians covered by the ProAssurance professional liability company were required to sign a statement stating that they would follow the ACOG recommendations. The Utah Medical Insurance Association designed its own guidelines: physicians needed to be within 5 minutes of the operating room throughout a patient's labor, could not use prostaglandin agents, and could not support VBAC for twins. An advisor for the insurance association stated that VBAC was a high-risk obstetric procedure and a "huge area of litigation and loss around the country."[24]

In 2005 in the state of Oklahoma very few women had access to medical care if they wanted to labor for a VBAC. The Physicians Liability Insurance Company (PLICO), the state's largest provider of malpractice insurance whose board of directors at the time was composed entirely of doctors, made a decision not to cover any VBACs at all. Physicians who supported VBAC found themselves without medical liability coverage. The company was at the time a nonprofit subsidiary of the Oklahoma State Medical Association.[25]

Across the country women who wanted to plan a VBAC found themselves shut out of medical facilities, their physicians and midwives no longer able to support their choice of birth within their institutions. A 2001 survey of Utah's rural, suburban, and urban physicians practicing obstetrics found that 45 percent of all physicians reported a decline in VBAC practices in the preceding 12 months.[26]

Because women's choice of providers and hospitals is often dictated by their health insurance, for thousands of women the only alternative was a forced repeat cesarean section or to labor at home and arrive at the hospital ready to give birth. Facilities that no longer provided medical care for women who wanted a VBAC decided that it was too costly and sometimes impossible for lack of available staff to comply with the ACOG's revised recommendations. In fact one study that looked at staffing availability for hospital anesthesiologists in the state of Ohio determined that even if all hospitals that provided maternity care could afford to comply with the ACOG's new guidelines there were not enough anesthesiologists to meet the need.[27]

The International Cesarean Awareness Network (ICAN), a volunteer birth activist organization whose mission is to reduce cesareans and support VBAC, took the initiative to look into the impact of denial of service for VBACs—an issue that was virtually ignored by policy makers and the media. By November of 2004 the ICAN had documented the names of over 300 U.S. hospitals that no longer provided care for women who wanted to plan a VBAC. The organization viewed the denial of medical care for a planned VBAC as a civil rights issue.[28] From the many phone calls that the ICAN received from pregnant women looking for VBAC-friendly providers it was evident that the controversial guidelines put expectant mothers in a difficult situation. Some women would have to drive hundreds of miles to avoid a repeat surgery. Other mothers who did not want to submit to a forced cesarean looked for home birth midwives for support or chose to labor at home without medical assistance at all.[29]

Here is what some mothers wrote to a VBAC support Web site:

> I found out at my first prenatal appointment that the hospital I plan to deliver at has changed policies regarding VBAC. I want a VBAC. I feel so scared. I don't want this pregnancy to end so I don't have to deal with the issue. I have dreamed of going into labor and 'hiding' until delivery is imminent, then chance the 40 minute drive to the hospital and delivering on the roadside. Please help me.
>   P.S. All the hospitals in this area have the same policy.

> My hospital no longer allows VBACs. I investigated what would happen if I walked in ready to deliver, what they'd do, etc. I was told that if I came in at 8+ cm, they'd let me deliver vaginally—anything less and they'd either ship me off to another hospital or push to section me then and there.

This is from a certified nurse midwife:

> I live in W. Small hospital. No in house [*sic*] anesthesia. Nor VBAC unless the woman comes in advanced labor, then she labors in the OR (operating room). Documented in our practice guidelines that we don't do VBACs.

THE VERMONT/NEW HAMPSHIRE VBAC PROJECT

For maternity care providers in New Hampshire and Vermont, two states with cesarean rates among the lowest in the country, and VBAC rates among the highest, the ACOG's guidelines resulted in a sharp rise in cesareans and drop in VBACs in both states. In 1999 the VBAC rate in northern New England was 39.9 percent; by early 2002 it had decreased to 20.1 percent. In 2002 the two states would spend over $1.3 million extra to provide care for women who had a repeat cesarean rather than a VBAC. Based on a general risk of uterine rupture of 0.5 percent an estimated $7.5 million would be spent to prevent one fetal injury from a uterine rupture. Substantially more children would require intensive care services due to respiratory complications, some of them severe.

When maternity care providers in both states were polled 98 percent wanted to offer VBAC as an option to their patients. In response to the severely restricted choices for women the obstetric departments at Dartmouth Hitchcock Medical Center and Fletcher Allen Health Care collaborated to increase the availability of safe care for VBACs. In 2002 the Vermont/New

Hampshire VBAC Project had been created. Based on a review of the literature, the project found that the ACOG's "immediately available" recommendations actually applied to high-risk patients, not to low- or medium-risk patients. With careful planning and evidence-based guidelines providers and hospitals could safely care for women who wanted a VBAC.

The Network made regional recommendations for VBAC care based on women's risk status (low, medium, high) while ensuring patient and provider safety. The specific type of provider and resources required were matched to the patient's risk. The collaborative feels that "VBAC can be safely performed in community hospitals without excessive use of resources when patients are stratified by their risk."[30] The Network developed evidence-based documents for hospitals and health care providers and a pamphlet to help women make an informed decision about a repeat cesarean or a VBAC. They are available on their Web site. Although the project continues under the Northern New England Perinatal Quality Improvement Network (NNEPQIN) care providers have been severely restricted by the requirements imposed by malpractice insurance providers.[31,32] The Vermont/New Hampshire VBAC Project is an example of how collaborative care by dedicated providers in different communities can provide women with a safe option to a routine repeat cesarean section.

LITTLE EVIDENCE TO SUPPORT THE NEED FOR "IMMEDIATELY AVAILABLE" SURGICAL TEAM

By 2005 the VBAC rate had decreased to less than 8 percent.[33]

A study conducted in California showed that complying with the ACOG's controversial guidelines did not make VBAC any safer for mothers or their infants. The VBAC rate in California fell from 24 percent before the controversial guidelines to 13.5 percent after the guidelines were implemented. Researchers who examined births to women with a prior cesarean between 1996 and 2002 found no significant difference in maternal deaths for women who planned a VBAC with those who had an elective repeat operation. For normal weight babies there was no difference in neonatal mortality between women who had a routine repeat operation and women who labored for a VBAC. Of the women who labored for a VBAC in rural hospitals 79.5 percent had a normal birth, and in urban settings 83.3 percent had a safe VBAC. Neonatal mortality was not higher in rural hospitals.[34]

The American Academy of Family Physicians guidelines for a trial of labor after a cesarean (TOLAC) state that VBAC should not be restricted only to facilities with available surgical teams present throughout labor, since there is no evidence that these additional resources result in improved outcomes."[35] The Society of Obstetricians and Gynaecologists of Canada agrees that an approximate time frame of 30 minutes should be considered adequate in the set up of an urgent laparotomy (surgical incision in the abdominal cavity).[36]

Similarly, guidelines in Britain do not take extraordinary measures specifically for women who want to labor for a VBAC.[37] However, obstetric medical associations in Britain, Canada, Australia, New Zealand, and the United States agree that women who plan a VBAC should labor in a facility that can provide an emergency cesarean.

ROUTINE REPEAT CESAREANS ARE COST EFFECTIVE

At a time when reimbursement for professional health services is at a standstill or in some cases the fees have been reduced, VBAC is not likely to make financial sense for some institutions or provider groups. To comply with current recommendations it is obvious that very few institutions can afford to have a trauma-level team assembled at all times when a woman wants to labor for a VBAC. Nor can an independent physician with a private practice afford to sit by the bedside waiting for a woman to give birth. The financial downside of supporting VBAC was clearly stated in the controversial 1999 ACOG guidelines:

> It is often stated that the cost of VBAC is less than that of repeat cesarean delivery. However, for a true analysis of all the costs one has to include the costs to the hospital, the method of reimbursement... and medical malpractice payments. Higher costs may be incurred by a hospital if a woman has a prolonged labor or has significant complications, or if the newborn is admitted to a neonatal intensive care unit. Furthermore, 20–49% of women will fail the trial of labor, which will incur surgical costs. Increased time or attendance for a woman undergoing a trial of labor results in increased costs to the physician. The difficulty in assessing the cost-benefit of VBAC is that the costs are not all incurred by one entity.[38]

Since their first controversial VBAC guidelines publication in 1999 no entity has yet challenged the ethical, moral, legal, financial, and more importantly the health impact of forced repeat cesareans that ultimately benefit private medical associations and segments of the health care industry.

PLANNED OUT-OF-HOSPITAL VBAC

Some mothers consider the probability of scar separation to be low and choose to have a home VBAC rather than submitting to a forced repeat operation. To date there are no substantive reports on the safety of a home VBAC. But more mothers seem to be choosing this option because hundreds of hospitals have chosen to deny them care. Some mothers evaluate the risk for scar rupture as extremely low, knowing that their chances of having a normal birth will be much higher without medical interventions. They may feel securer, safer, and more supported in their own environment. Others will feel strongly that it's a risk they do not want to take.

Giving birth in a birth center increases the odds for a normal birth. However some mothers who plan a VBAC in a birth center will develop complications during pregnancy or just before labor and will need to be transferred to a hospital to continue their labor. There is evidence for laboring for a VBAC in a freestanding birth center. A study of women who gave birth at forty-one freestanding birth centers with midwifery care showed that overall 80.9 percent who had no prior vaginal births and 94.4 percent of mothers who did have a prior vaginal birth avoided another cesarean and had a VBAC and three out of four mothers gave birth at the birth center. However, there were an unexpected number of complications, and the authors of the study recommended, "Despite a high rate of vaginal births and few uterine ruptures among women attempting VBACs in birth centers, a cesarean-scarred uterus was associated with increases in complications that require hospital management. Therefore, birth centers should refer women who have undergone previous cesarean deliveries to hospitals for delivery. Hospitals should increase access to inhospital care provided by midwife/obstetrician teams during VBACs."[39] However, not all care providers or mothers who can't find supportive care for a hospital VBAC will agree with this conclusion. Many birth centers still support women who want to labor for a VBAC.

ESPECIALLY FOR MOTHERS

Making a Decision

Some mothers who have a cesarean know that when they become pregnant again they would want to plan a VBAC. Other mothers are sure they want a repeat operation. For some mothers the decision is sometimes difficult to make. Each woman is different and has the right to decide for herself, based on the best evidence, her prior birth experience, and what medical care and support is available to her, what feels best for her and her family.

What You Should Know about VBAC

VBAC is a safe alternative to a routine repeat cesarean. Many maternity care professional associations and birth advocacy groups support a woman's right to plan a VBAC. They include obstetric and gynecologist, family practitioners, and midwives. If you have a healthy pregnancy, have a low horizontal scar on the uterus, and go into labor on your own at term you have about a 70 percent to 75 percent chance that you and your baby will have a safe normal birth. With caregivers who support VBAC the rates are higher. Many hospitals and care providers no longer support women who want to plan a VBAC, not because it is not safe but of fear of a malpractice suit. Or because they feel it is too expensive to keep a full surgical team and anesthesia on standby in case a woman laboring for a VBAC needs a rapid cesarean as recommended by the American College of Obstetricians and Gynecologists.

Not all hospitals can provide an "immediate" cesarean, but most can provide one in 30 minutes or less. Hundreds of hospitals in the United States have decided for legal or economic reasons not to support women who want to labor for a VBAC. It can be extremely costly to have a full team on standby to perform a cesarean for all women who labor for a VBAC. It means that physicians, midwives, and anesthesiologist may not be able to care for other mothers. The American Association of Family Physicians (AAFP) and the Society of Obstetricians and Gynaecologists of Canada (SOGC) disagree with the "immediately available" recommendations. The AAFP states that health outcomes are not improved for mothers or babies when women labor in a facility that can perform an "immediate" cesarean. The SOGC state that when women labor for a VBAC, a time frame of 30 minutes is adequate. Often in emergencies a surgical team can begin a cesarean within a few minutes. The American College of Nurse Midwives (ACNM) strongly supports VBAC. The ACNM guidelines for VBAC state that midwives are qualified to care for women who want to plan a VBAC if appropriate arrangements for medical consultation and emergency care are in place.

Who Can Safely Plan a VBAC?

Women with one or two low horizontal uterine scars or a low vertical scar (depending on prior operative records); women who have had one vaginal birth or not; women who had a cesarean for a "big" baby, "failure to progress," a breech, or nonreassuring fetal heart tones (fetal distress); some women expecting twins or a "big" baby; women who go past their due date or go into labor before their due date and the baby is expected to be of normal weight; women who will labor for a VBAC 24 months after their prior cesarean delivery; and women who may want an epidural for pain relief can all plan VBACs.

Your risk for a uterine rupture is lower if you had one or two prior cesareans, if your labor is not induced, especially with prostaglandins, if your prior cesarean uterine incision was closed with two layers of sutures rather than one and you labor 24 months after your cesarean birth.

Factors That Increase Your Chances for a VBAC

Your chances for a VBAC increase if you have had one prior cesarean; you go into labor on your own; your labor is not augmented with oxytocin or prostaglandin; and you have had a prior vaginal birth and your baby is expected to weigh less than 9 lb. If you are in active labor when you arrive at a hospital labor and delivery unit your odds are more favorable.

The VBAC rate is higher for women who have midwifery care. If you are well prepared, have learned about strategies to enhance the progress of labor, and have resolved most of the emotional issues you may have had with your prior cesarean you are more likely to give birth without another cesarean section. If you think you may want an epidural for labor try to wait until you are in active labor. An epidural may slow your labor or the pushing phase and often caregivers don't feel comfortable if labor takes "too long." However studies show that an epidural will not reduce your chance for a VBAC.

You may want to have additional emotional support in labor, a professional doula or a friend or relative experienced with birth. An experienced doula can help you find comfortable positions to help your labor to progress, provide comfort and reduce your pain without medication, and support you with the kind of birth you want.

What Are the Risks of VBAC?

The main safety concern with VBAC is fear of the prior cesarean scar giving way during labor. The likelihood of a scar giving way in labor is about 2 to 7 per 1,000. This risk is not any higher than any other unpredictable emergency that can occur in any other labor, such as placental abruption (placenta separating from the wall of the uterus before the baby is born), nonreassuring fetal heart rate, and a prolapsed umbilical cord. The risk of laboring for a VBAC with one prior cesarean with a low horizontal scar is the same for women who give birth for the first time. The risk for infection is higher for mothers who labor but then have cesarean deliveries. If you have not had a normal birth before your prior cesarean or if you have had two prior low horizontal cesarean scars the risks are slightly higher. It may be possible for women with one low vertical scar to labor for a VBAC if the scar remains low in the bottom part of the uterus at term. Very rarely a low uterine scar may resemble an inverted T. The majority of maternity care professional associations recommend that women with a classical (vertical) scar on the body of the uterus have a repeat cesarean. The risk of the scar separating with a vertical scar is 4 to 9 percent. If you labor you may end up with a cesarean delivery for other reasons not related to the separation of the uterine scar.

What Care Does the Mother and Baby Need if the Scar Separates during Labor?

When the uterine scar gives way medical intervention with a rapid cesarean is necessary. The mother is at risk for hemorrhage and damage to the uterus or bladder. The baby is at serious risk for lack of oxygen. If the scar separates fully the baby may slide outside of the uterus and into the lower abdominal cavity. With a rapid cesarean, mothers and babies usually have favorable outcomes, although sometimes serious complications can arise. For every 10,000 women who labor for a VBAC with a low horizontal scar five to ten babies are likely to be seriously harmed or die. With proper care maternal death from laboring for a VBAC is extremely rare and occurs in less than 1 in 100,000 women who labor for a VBAC.

What Is the Mother Likely to Feel if the Uterine Scar Separates?

It is different for every mother. Sometimes the labor slows down, or the mother feels pain between contractions. Sometimes a mother may have heavy vaginal bleeding. There may be some tenderness or sharp pain at the site of the previous scar. If the mother has begun to push, the baby may slide back up in the birth canal. A uterine rupture cannot be diagnosed or anticipated until it actually happens. The most consistent sign of a rupture is an abnormal fetal heart rate. That is why continuous fetal monitoring is often recommended when laboring for a VBAC.

Where Is It Safe to Labor for a VBAC?

Thousands of VBACs have taken place in a hospital. So we have much information about the safety of laboring for a VBAC in a hospital. However, hundreds of hospitals in the United States have decided they will no longer care for women who want a VBAC. Some women are choosing to have a VBAC at home rather than being forced to have a repeat cesarean when no medical reason exists. Although many women have chosen to have a VBAC at home to date there is not enough information about the health outcomes of home VBACs. So it's difficult to make recommendations on home VBACs. Many caregivers support women who want a home VBAC and have established a relationship with a local medical facility and medical backup in case of complications.

If you would need to be transferred quickly to a hospital for care think about what needs to be in place: How far is the nearest medical facility? Who will go with you? How will you get there? How will you be cared for until you arrive? When you arrive will the medical staff be ready to care for you? Will there be an obstetrician available? Will there be an operating room available if you need surgery? Will there be appropriate emergency care for your newborn if needed? Obstetric professional societies do not recommend laboring for a VBAC at home.

Women who labor for a VBAC in a birth center and do not develop complications are more likely to have a normal birth. However, if you need an emergency transfer timing is very important. Find out what emergency measures are available to you in the event that you develop complications in labor. The American Association of Birth Centers does not currently support laboring for a VBAC in a birth center. It's possible that some birth centers will no longer support VBAC. However, midwives who have hospital staff priviledges go to the hospital with their patients for labor and birth.

WHERE CAN YOU FIND OUT ABOUT VBAC–FRIENDLY PROVIDERS?

Although many hospitals have stopped providing care for women who want to plan a VBAC, there are resources you can access. At this time, in the United

States all Level III hospitals, those that have emergency obstetric services available at all times and a neonatal special care nursery, meet the current ACOG recommendations for VBAC. These are usually large hospitals affiliated with a medical school. Call the hospitals covered under your medical insurance plan; ask if they support VBAC. If they do ask for the names of three providers on their staff. You can also access childbirth education and doula organization Web sites. Find members' names in your city or state. They may be familiar with VBAC-friendly providers. Check also the Web sites of midwifery organizations, like Mothers Naturally (http://mothersnaturally.org) and myMidwife (http://www.mymidwife.org/), and the American Association of Family Practitioners (http://www.aafp.org) to find out about VBAC-friendly care providers. Visit www.Choicesinchildbirth.org or www.BirthNetwork.org. Contact the International Cesarean Awareness Network; they have local chapters across the United States and Canada.

For Women Planning a VBAC: Things to Think about before or during Your Pregnancy

If you are considering planning a VBAC thinking about and discussing these issues with your partner and care provider will help you make the decision that is best for you:

- What are the advantages you see for yourself and your family? What are the disadvantages?
- What information do you need to have before you can feel really comfortable about planning a VBAC?
- What does your care provider think about planning a VBAC? Do you feel comfortable asking questions? Are your concerns being addressed? Will your care provider or health care plan refer you to another professional who does support VBAC?
- Within your health care insurance plan, do you have access to an obstetrician, a family practitioner, or a midwife who supports VBAC? Do you have access to a hospital or birth center experienced with VBAC? What guidelines or protocols do they have in place?
- Have you considered having a doula (a professional who provides labor support) to assist you before and during labor and birth?
- What community resources are available to help you prepare for your VBAC?
- How do your partner, family, and friends feel about your planning a VBAC?
- How would you feel if you labored for a VBAC but gave birth by cesarean?

For Partners of Women Planning a VBAC: Things to Think About

Mothers who want to plan a VBAC need the support of their partners as well as their maternity care professionals. Knowing you are there to support and guide her and to provide an emotionally safe environment to give birth in will go a long way to help her have the kind of birth she desires. It helps to discuss differences in your points of view about planning a VBAC during the pregnancy, so that she can labor confidently and meet the challenges ahead. These are some questions that may help to prepare both of you for the birth:

- What advantages do you see for your partner, yourself, and your family if you plan a VBAC? What are the disadvantages?
- When you and your partner talk about planning a VBAC, what do you agree and disagree about?
- Can you think of ways of working through these issues and coming to a resolution both of you feel good about?
- How do your friends and relatives feel about planning a VBAC?
- Supporting a woman in labor is hard work. Are you worried you won't be able to give her what she needs? Are you worried that she may end up with another emergency cesarean?
- You feel strongly that a scheduled repeat cesarean is the safest and easiest way to go for your partner and your baby. Can you understand why your partner feels strongly about having a VBAC?
- What information or resources do you need to make you feel comfortable about going ahead with a VBAC?
- Have you considered accompanying your partner when she goes for prenatal visits? Making a list of those issues you need more information about?
- Would you consider accompanying her to a community VBAC support group?

MAKING THE DECISION THAT IS RIGHT FOR YOU

After asking questions, reading books, searching the Internet, or contacting support groups you may come to the conclusion that a VBAC is not your best choice. You may not have enough support from your caregivers or your partner or enough resources you need to give you the confidence to labor for a VBAC. You may decide a repeat cesarean with caregivers whom you trust is best. Or you may find that although initially you had planned to have a repeat operation, over time during your pregnancy you find other mothers who planned a safe VBAC and change your mind. You may also find that unlike in your last pregnancy your current caregivers are supportive and are willing to work together with you to give you the best chance to have a normal birth. What matters is that you feel you have been involved in making those decisions as much as you would have liked to. You received the information you needed, and you feel that you made the best decision for yourself and your family.

RESOURCES

VBAC Guidelines

American Academy of Family Physicians. Policy on Trial of Labor after Cesarean (TOLAC). November 2005. http://www.aafp.org/online/en/home/clinical/ clinicalrecs/tolac.html (last accessed May 20, 2008).

American College of Nurse Midwives. Vaginal Birth after Cesarean. Position Statement. 2000. http://www.midwife.org/siteFiles/position/VBAC_05.pdf (last accessed May 20, 2008).

Enkin, M., M. J. N. C. Keirse, J. Nielson, C. Crowther, L. Duley, E. Hodnett, and J. Hofmeyr. Chapter 38: Labor and Birth after Previous Cesarean. In *A Guide to Effective Care in Pregnancy and Childbirth* (New York: Oxford University Press, 2000). http://www.vbac.com/chapter38.html (last accessed May 20, 2008).

Northern New England Perinatal Quality Improvement Network. VBAC Documents, http://www.nnepqin.org/ViewPage?id=3.

Society of Obstetricians and Gynaecologists of Canada. Guidelines for Vaginal Birth after Previous Caesarean Birth. Clinical Practice Guidelines, Number 155, February 2005. http://www.sogc.org/guidelines/index_e.asp# Obstetrics.

Resources Especially for Mothers

American Association of Birth Centers, http://www.birthcenters.org (last accessed May 20, 2008).

American Association of Family Physicians. A Shared Patient–Physician Tool. http://www.aafp.org/online/en/home/clinical/patiented/counselingtools/tolac.html (last accessed May 20, 2008).

Childbirth Connection. VBAC or Repeat Cesarean? http://childbirthconnection.org/article.asp?ClickedLink=293&ck=10212&area=27 (last accessed May 20, 2008).

Goer, Henci. Vaginal Birth after Cesarean: The Facts, http://parenting.ivillage.com/pregnancy/plabor/0,,bgjt,00.html (last accessed May 20, 2008).

Northern New England Perinatal Quality Improvement Network. Birth Choices after Cesarean. http://vbac.com/pdfs/FinalEd.pdf (last accessed May 20, 2008).

Rights of Women Seeking VBAC, International Cesarean Awareness Network. http://www.ican-online.org/vbac/enforcing-and-promoting-rights-women-seeking-vaginal-birth-after-cesarean-vbac-primer (last accessed May 20, 2008).

VBAC, Society of Obstetritians and Gynecologists of Canada, http://www.sogc.org/health/pregnancy-vbac_e.aspx (last accessed May 21, 2008.)

VBAC.com. http://vbac.com.

The VBAC Pages, http://www.vbac.org.uk/.

12

ELECTRONIC FETAL MONITORING: MORE INFORMATION IS NOT ALWAYS BETTER

The evidence indicates that EFM is of little if any proven benefit to low-risk patients than regular auscultation, and that EFM is a costly and dangerous procedure. Thus, its diffusion and routine use demonstrates a failure of public and private policies.[1]

A nonreassuring fetal heart (fetal distress) is one of the four main reasons for performing a cesarean. When electronic fetal monitoring (EFM) is used routinely to measure the baby's heart rate the number of cesareans goes up, but health outcomes do not improve. Listening to fetal heart tones through auscultation (listening to a patient's heart in order to make a diagnosis) and developing the skills to diagnose fetal well-being were discovered in Europe in the early nineteenth century. By the end of the century, the Pinard fetal stethoscope began to be used in pregnancy and childbirth. Auscultation, or listening to the fetal heart rate at specific intervals using a fetoscope remained the only method of detecting fetal well-being until the 1960s. EFM was introduced in the labor and delivery wards in the 1960s but before any scientific evaluation to show it was more effective than the traditional method of intermittent auscultation or a handheld Doppler ultrasound monitor.

During labor and birth abnormal changes in the baby's heart rate are associated with a low level of oxygen (hypoxia). Oxygen deprivation if prolonged or acute can lead to short- or long-term complications, neurological disability, or death. The theory was that EFM would detect fetal hypoxia sooner and more accurately than intermittent auscultation. Therefore when a nonreassuring heart rate pattern (fetal distress) would be identified efforts could be made to deliver the baby as quickly as possible.

"Like other kinds of birth technology," writes Marsden Wagner, M.D., M.S., a former director of the World Health Organization Women's and Children's Health, "the electronic fetal monitor first proved to be valuable for specific complications during labour. The indications for use gradually broadened beyond the scientific justification. By the early 1970s, it was used routinely on every labouring woman in a number of hospitals in Europe and the Americas."[2]

In its 1981 consensus report on cesarean delivery, the U.S. National Institutes of Health identified fetal distress as ranking third along with breech presentation as a reason for the rise of cesarean birth rates. "While evidence is lacking that the actual incidence of fetal distress has changed," stated the report, "the diagnosis of fetal distress has been made more frequently during the past 10 years."[3] By 1984 solid evidence from several randomized controlled studies of approximately 17,000 women showed no improvement in maternal or perinatal health with the routine use of electronic fetal monitoring compared with auscultation. There was no evidence that fewer babies died and no evidence that EFM prevented brain damage. Studies found no difference in Apgar scores (screening tool for fetal well-being at birth), cord blood gases at birth (indicating lower levels of oxygen), the number of babies who needed intensive care at birth, or long-term neurological problems.[4]

In 1996 a U.S. health technology evaluation report on electronic fetal monitoring confirmed what was already known a decade before. EFM detected a higher number of abnormal fetal heart rate patterns compared to auscultation but failed to show better outcomes over auscultation. Many babies born by instrumental delivery or cesarean section due to "fetal distress" were found to be normal at birth. EFM prolonged the progress of labor, probably because women were restricted to bed, and it triggered a "cascade" of costly interventions, each increasing maternal and infant health risks. One of the driving forces behind the use of EFM technology as compared to intermittent auscultation was the fear of medical malpractice claims. What was occurring in the legal arena was affecting the standard of care more profoundly than the scientific literature.[5]

In 2007 a systematic review of electronic fetal monitoring for low-risk women by the Coalition for Improving Maternity Services (CIMS) Expert Work Group found that compared with intermittent auscultation, EFM did not lower the incidence of low Apgar scores, the number of admissions to newborn special care nurseries, the incidence of cerebral palsy, or perinatal deaths. Fetal blood sampling (FBS) is a method of evaluating fetal blood gases and is used to confirm EFM tracings that indicate abnormal fetal heart rate patterns. When compared with intermittent auscultation, electronic fetal monitoring even when combined with FBS did not reduce perinatal mortality. Routine monitoring however increased the number of instrumental deliveries and cesarean sections without improving health outcomes.[6]

ROUTINE ELECTRONIC FETAL MONITORING CAUSES HARM WITHOUT IMPROVING OUTCOMES

Continuous fetal monitoring is usually recommended for high-risk mothers, especially when the mother has high blood pressure, is expecting twins, is overdue, has had a prior cesarean and if labor is induced or the mother has epidural analgesia for labor. But four decades of evidence show that the routine use of EFM exposes mothers and babies to increased risks without improving outcomes. Yet electronic fetal monitoring is still widely accepted as a reliable and valid technology for low-risk women. In 2005 a survey of women's childbearing experiences found that 93 percent of U.S. women were monitored continuously by EFM.[7] Ultimately routine use of EFM also reduces choices for women in labor. EFM restricts movement, reduces the opportunity for human interaction with the nursing staff, and increases the need for other interventions. Women are limited from using nondrug methods of pain relief such as walking, using a variety of comfortable postions, warm bath, and shower. With an EFM telemetry unit a woman in labor can be monitored continuously while she is walking in or near her labor room, but not many hospitals have these units. The evidence is clear that intermittent auscultation with a fetoscope or Doppler device is a better and safer method of monitoring low-risk women in labor. Women who choose to use a warm bath or birthing pool in labor can be monitored with a waterproof handheld Doppler.

ESPECIALLY FOR MOTHERS

Monitoring Your Baby's Heart Rate

It is important to monitor your baby's heart rate during labor. If a baby's oxygen level is low it may cause a baby to have a slow heart rate, a lower flow of blood out of the heart, and lower blood pressure. Reduced oxygen can affect the baby's brain, gastrointestinal (GI) tract, lungs, heart, and kidneys.[8]

A nonreassuring heart rate (not within normal levels) may indicate that the baby may not be getting enough oxygen and needs to be born as quickly as possible. There are different safe and effective ways to monitor the baby's heart rate and consequently the baby's oxygen supply during labor. A baby's heartbeat can be monitored with an electronic fetal monitor, continuously or intermittently (only for a specific period of time), and by auscultation with a fetal stethoscope (a Pinard) or with a handheld Doppler device. With auscultation your caregiver listens to the baby's heart rate every 15 to 30 minutes in the first stage of labor and every 5 minutes in the second stage or the beginning of pushing. With auscultation you are free to move around and use a variety of positions. A Doppler can also be adapted for use in water.

When healthy women are monitored routinely with an electronic fetal monitor compared to intermittent auscultation their risk for a cesarean or an instrumental delivery (with forceps or vacuum extractor) is increased by 30 percent. Using continuous EFM for healthy women does not improve a baby's well-being. It does not lower the baby's risk of needing admission to a special care nursery, having cerebral palsy, or perinatal death.

Continuous fetal monitoring is recommended when the mother has health complications. Some hospitals require that women have a 20-minute electronic fetal heart rate strip when they arrive at the labor and delivery unit. Evidence shows that this test does not improve the health of your baby, but it is more likely that your care provider will want to use continuous electronic fetal monitoring during your labor.[9]

If you need continuous fetal monitoring talk to your care providers at the hospital about ways you can safely move around and change positions during labor and ways to push your baby out using an upright position or while lying sideways. This will reduce your chances of having an instrumental delivery or a cesarean for fetal distress.

RESOURCES

Care Practices for Normal Birth. Care Practice #4. No Routine Interventions, http://www.lamaze.org/ExpectantParents/PregnancyandBirthResources/ AboutNormalBirth/NoRoutineInterventions/tabid/244/Default.aspx (last accessed April 2008).

The Informed Choice Initiative. Fetal Heart Monitoring in Labour, http://www.infochoice.org (last accessed May 21, 2008).

NICE, Monitoring Your Baby's Heartbeat in Labor, http://www.nice.org.uk/guidance/index.jsp?action=download&o=28972 (last accessed May 21, 2008).

13

Breech Version: A Safe Alternative to a Planned Cesarean

The results are consistent and clear: ECV (external cephalic version) should be offered to all women with an uncomplicated breech presentation at term.[1]

Breech presentation is one of four most common indications for performing a cesarean section. It is also one of the most preventable. The number of cesareans performed for a breech presentation has increased considerably over the last five decades. In 2002 86.9 percent of all breech pregnancies in the United States were delivered by cesarean section. With a procedure called breech version or external cephalic version (ECV) done at about 37 weeks of pregnancy up to eighty-six of breech babies can begin labor in a head-down position, reducing the number of women who would otherwise have a planned cesarean section. ECV, manually rotating the baby to a head-down position has been shown to be safe and effective in several randomized controlled studies.[2] However, in 2004 ECV was performed for less than 1 percent of breech pregnancies. ECV was successful for 49 to 67 percent of mothers who had the procedure. For women who had a successful procedure the cesarean rate was 13 percent compared to 90 percent for the women who did not have the procedure.[3]

At 28 weeks about 80 percent of babies spontaneously position themselves in a head-down position (vertex presentation) in the pelvic inlet. At term (37 weeks to 42 weeks) about 3 to 4 percent will still be in a breech presentation, that is, with their head up and buttocks, feet, or knees positioned towards the cervix. There are variations of the breech position:

Frank Breech (Photo 13.1): The baby is positioned bottom down with the legs bent upwards or extended straight upwards towards the face. Babies in a frank breech position may be able to be born vaginally.

Complete Breech (Photo 13.2): The baby is positioned bottom down with legs bent at the knees and the hips.

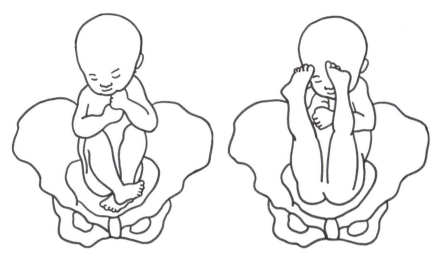

Photo 13.1. Complete Breech. *Source:* Illustration by Shanna dela Cruz.

Photo 13.2. Frank Breech. *Source:* Illustration by Shanna dela Cruz.

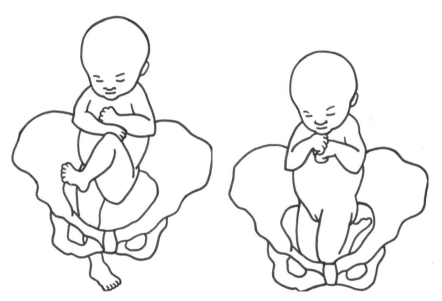

Photo 13.3. Footling Breech. *Source:* Illustration by Shanna dela Cruz.

Photo 13.4. Kneeling Breech. *Source:* Illustration by Shanna dela Cruz.

Footling Breech (Photo 13.3): With the bottom down, the baby may have one
or both legs positioned closest to the cervix. In this position one or both feet
would be the first part of the baby's body that would be born. A vaginal birth
for a baby in this position is more difficult and more likely to end up with
complications.

Incomplete or Kneeling Breech (Photo 13.4): One or both of the baby's knees
are closest to the cervix.

With both hands on the mother's abdomen and a technique called Leopold's
maneuver a physician or midwife can feel the position of the baby's head,
back, and bottom. Depending on the training and skills of health professionals
a number of breech presentations may not be detected with this method. At
times a breech is only diagnosed when the mother is already in labor, making
a cesarean the most likely option for birth.

Babies that are born preterm are often in a breech position; also with a twin
or in multiple pregnancies the baby is more likely to be breech. An excessive
level of amniotic fluid (hydramnios) or too little amniotic fluid (oligohydram-
nios) sometimes is the reason why a baby remains in a breech position at term.
A previous breech, a short umbilical cord, a uterus that is abnormal in shape
(for example, a bicornuate uterus), and fibroids also make it more likely that
the baby will be breech. With a breech, the placenta which usually attaches
itself to the top back wall of the uterus is more likely to attach itself towards
the bottom of the uterus (a condition known as low-lying placenta or placenta
previa) and partially or completely cover the cervix.[4]

HOW ARE BREECH BABIES DIFFERENT?

Most breech babies are born healthy. However, a baby in a breech position
is at higher risk for complications regardless of the method of birth. Breech
babies, whether born by cesarean or not, tend to have a higher incidence
of congenital birth defects, lower placental weight, and lower weight at birth
for same gestational age babies in a head-down position. Breech babies are
also more likely to be born preterm. Compared to babies in a vertex (head-
down) presentation, breech babies are also more likely to suffer from perinatal
complications and future handicaps and are also more likely to die soon after
birth. It is now known that poor outcomes of breech births are more likely to
be the result of preexisting conditions rather than whether or not a baby in a
breech position is born vaginally or by cesarean section.[5,6,7,8,9,10]

WHY ARE VAGINAL BREECH BIRTHS MORE DIFFICULT?

A breech birth presents unique challenges. With a vertex presentation both
the mother and the baby have an excellent chance for a normal uncomplicated
birth. Although most breech babies at term are born healthy, a breech poses
increased risks both for the mother and her baby. When baby's head comes

through the cervix first, it provides an effective wedge to dilate (stretch open) the cervix. With a breech the baby's buttocks or feet do not. With a vaginal breech birth (especially preterm) there is an increased risk that the umbilical cord may slip down between the baby's body and the mother's pelvic bones (cord prolapse), compromising the oxygen supply to the baby during labor or birth.

Depending on the gestational age of the baby and its position in relation to the mother's pelvis (frank or nonfrank breech presentation), the odds of a cord prolapse range from 1 to 20 percent. In inexperienced hands, there may be difficulty bringing the baby's head (head entrapment) or arms (nuchal arm) safely through the birth canal. The baby then would be at risk for asphyxia (suffocation) and for injury to the brachial plexus (a network of nerves the base of the neck, which affect the shoulder girdle, forearm, arm and hand).[11]

A vaginal breech birth may require, as vertex presentations sometimes do, the use of forceps or a vacuum extractor (instrumental delivery) and an accompanying episiotomy. Complications may be higher for vaginal breech births when labor is prolonged, induced, or augmented with oxytocin or prostaglandins and also when it is a footling breech and when a clinician is inexperienced and unskilled.[12]

EXTERNAL CEPHALIC VERSION (ECV) REDUCES THE ODDS FOR CESAREAN BY 30 TO 80 PERCENT

External cephalic version reduces the odds that a baby will be in a breech position at birth, and it also reduces the odds for a cesarean delivery.[13] When performed at term (37 to 42 weeks) the success rate of ECV is 30 to 80 percent. With ECV at term, 95 percent of babies will remain in a head-down position.[14]

With a breech version the physician's or midwife's hands try to rotate the baby from a breech presentation to a vertex presentation (head-down). It is done by gently disengaging the part of the baby that may have entered the pelvis, applying external pressure to the mother's abdomen, and gently guiding the baby into a forward or backward somersault while guiding the baby's head towards the pelvis. This skill is taught in midwifery programs and some obstetric residency programs, and there is evidence that breech versions were done by the ancient Greeks in the fourth century BC; they continue to be done in nonclinical settings as well. ECV is an effective method of reducing the odds for a cesarean for a frank, complete, or footling breech.[15]

Medical societies in the United States, Britain, Canada, Australia, and New Zealand and the International Federation of Gynecology and Obstetrics (FIGO) recommend that a woman with an uncomplicated breech at term should be offered the option of having an external version (ECV). All women between 37 and 42 weeks of pregnancy should be given information on the benefits and risks of ECV and the choice to undergo the procedure.[16]

An external version done very early in the third trimester from 32 to 34 weeks is not as effective and is not likely to lower the odds for a cesarean section.[17]

How Safe Is ECV?

External version is a relatively safe and successful procedure for most women when performed by experienced caregivers. Complications from ECV are rare.[18] Babies who have gone through the procedure are not at increased risk for admission to a special care nursery or perinatal death.

ECVs are more successful with an experienced care provider. Other factors such as the position of the baby, the level of amniotic fluid, and whether or not it's the mother's first pregnancy also play a role. To increase the odds of success for ECV sometimes tocolytic agents to prevent contractions are given to relax the uterine muscles. Epidural anesthesia and exposing the baby to noise stimulus (acoustic stimulation) close to the mother's abdomen have also been tried.[19] ECV can be attempted a second time if it is not initially successful.

For women who had a prior cesarean, two small studies found that ECV was safe and successful about 80 percent of the time. Breech versions have also been done in early labor, while the amniotic membranes were still intact. This option can be helpful for women who go into labor with an undiagnosed breech and a breech that has not yet fully engaged in the pelvis.[20]

To reduce the risk of complications ECV is usually attempted only with an uncomplicated single breech (frank, complete, or footling). ECV can also help to manipulate a baby from a transverse (side-lying) position to a vertex (head-down) position. ECV is done when the amniotic sac is still intact and there is a sufficient amount of amniotic fluid surrounding the baby; the baby's head should not be hyperextended (stargazer). With ECVs the baby's heart rate is monitored, and the procedure is done using ultrasound to visualize the baby's movements and the umbilical cord. The procedure is usually done in a hospital or physician's office with easy access to a cesarean should it become necessary. However, evidence shows that the risk of needing a cesarean is extremely low, and women no longer need to be routinely prepared for a possible surgery.[21] Breech versions are also performed by skilled practioners outside of a clinical setting (Photo 13.5).

An external version is not for women who have a heart problem, severe pregnancy-induced hypertension (high blood pressure that developed during the pregnancy) or who may have experienced hemorrhaging in pregnancy. ECV is not recommended for women with a uterus that is not shaped normally, who may have had uterine surgery other than a cesarean, or who may have a condition that prevents them from having tocolytic drugs. There is a difference of opinion when it comes to women who have diabetes and hypertension, are obese, or may be carrying a baby with congenital problems.[22,23,24]

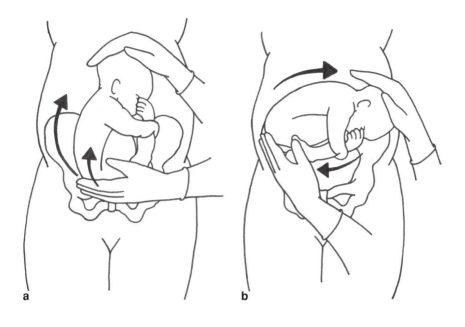

a

b

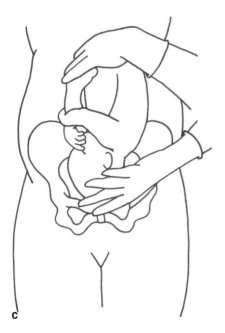

c

Photo 13.5. Movements for an external version: (a) moving the baby out of the pelvis; (b) baby being turned forward; and (c) baby turned to a vertex position (head down). *Source*: Illustration by Shanna dela Cruz.

Other Options for Turning a Breech

The Breech Tilt

It is possible that maternal posture may influence fetal position. Many postural techniques have been used outside of a clinical environment to turn a breech. With a breech tilt (in which the mother's head is positioned lower than her hips) gravity may encourage the baby to move toward the fundus (the top of the uterus), flex her chin, and turn her head towards the cervix to a vertex presentation. Although current evidence shows that by elevating her hips using either the knee-chest or flat-on-the-back position a woman is not more likely to have a vertex presentation at term, many women are willing to try these positions, and they are not harmful.[25]

Moxibustion

Moxibustion is a form of traditional medicine known to have been used more than 3,000 years ago. A stick or cone of an herb known as mugwort (*AiYe* in traditional Chinese) is ignited and placed on an acupuncture point of the body to stimulate the blood and life enerergy (qi) of the body. Commonly used to treat colds or inflammations the technique also stimulates fetal movements in pregnant women. Moxibustion is known for its ability to turn a breech into a normal head-down position. Fetal activity is encouraged by stimulating the acupressure point BL 67 found on the outside of the little toe. Moxibustion is usually used in combination with acupuncture. Although this technique can be taught by a qualified provider to the woman and her partner to be done at home, it is not a treatment option that is easily found in Western countries. Although evidence shows that moxibustion is effective and appears to be safe some researchers say that more studies are needed before it can be widely recommended.[26,27]

What Is the Safest Way for a Term Breech to Be Born?

When a breech version is not successful or the mother chooses not to have a breech version the safest way for a term breech to be born is still controversial. Having a vaginal breech birth or scheduling a cesarean are two options that the mother needs to consider carefully. Care providers who consider cesarean section to be the safest alternative for a term breech have argued that outcomes of breech studies in the past were biased or inconclusive. They could not be considered definitive enough to make clear recommendations about the safest method for breech births. Despite the fact that a randomized controlled trial (considered the gold standard) for term breech was conducted in twenty-six countries and included 2,088 frank or complete breech (called the International Term Breech Trial)[28] the debate has not yet been put to rest. The Term Breech Trial compared full-term breech babies born by scheduled cesarean with full-term breech babies born by planned vaginal birth. Initially the researchers concluded that babies were less likely to die with a scheduled cesarean. With time some critics found that the methods used to conduct the trial were scientifically unsound and the results highly controversial if not invalid.[29] A recommendation for routine cesarean section for all term breech was also questioned by maternity care professionals skilled in vaginal breech births.[30,31] By recommending cesarean section for all term breech babies the study did not consider the long-term health outcomes from a surgical birth for mothers.[32] Others have disagreed and found that a planned cesarean delivery for a full-term breech is safer for the baby.[33]

A 2-year follow-up by the researchers of the Term Breech Trial found that a planned cesarean for breech did not lower the risk of death or neurological development delays.

Performing a cesarean for a breech delivery is not altogether risk-free or necessarily less traumatic or damaging for the infant. It requires the skill to maneuver the fetus gently through a small incision in a thick muscular uterine wall. There may be difficulty in bringing out the baby's head through a relatively small incision in the uterine wall. For the baby, there is the potential for brachial plexus injury (paralysis of the arm from traction on the shoulder, temporary or long-term) or for small fractures of the lower limbs, if the practitioner is unskilled or specific maneuvers to deliver the breech are forceful or uncontrolled. A cesarean will expose a breech baby to the risks of surgery and complications from anesthesia. For mothers, there are the short-term and long-term risks associated with surgery and anesthesia: a uterine scar which will put her in a high-risk category in a subsequent pregnancy and the additional risk of placental problems and most likely a repeat cesarean in the next pregnancy.[34]

With experienced and skilled practitioners newborn outcomes with a planned vaginal breech birth are similar compared to those of breech births by elective cesarean section.[35] In countries such as France and Belgium where breech vaginal births are common, birth practitioners are skilled, and strict guidelines are followed before and during labor, neonatal complications for planned vaginal birth for a term breech are not significantly different than for term breech babies delivered by cesarean sections.[36]

Although vaginal breech delivery is a part of obstetrics and gynecology residence training, in the United States it is a quickly vanishing skill.[37] And as the evidence shows safe outcomes from a vaginal breech birth are dependent on the skill of the practitioner. Many women with a breech go into labor before term or at term regardless of whether or not a cesarean has been scheduled. So it is still important for clinicians to acquire the skills for facilitating the delivery of a vaginal breech.[38,39,40]

With regard to a full-term breech the Royal College of Obstetricians and Gynaecologists in the United Kingdom recommends that women be given accurate and comprehensive information about the benefits and risks of both a planned cesarean and a vaginal birth for themselves and their babies as well as the availability of caregivers skilled in term vaginal breech births.[41]

ESPECIALLY FOR MOTHERS

Ask your care provider to tell you if your baby is in a breech position or not by the 36th week of your pregnancy. This will give you time to plan for a breech version if you choose to have one. If your baby is breech here are your options:

Try the Breech Tilt; It Is the Least Invasive Approach

Although this option of turning a breech has not been studied enough to recommend its use, the breech tilt is an option that you can try for yourself and one that is not harmful. Start doing the breech tilt between 32 and 35 weeks of pregnancy, before your baby becomes engaged in your pelvis. Try this position on a flat and firm surface when your stomach is not full and when your baby is active. You will need one or two small pillows. Begin by lying flat on your back, knees drawn up and both feet flat on the floor. A rug or yoga mat would be more comfortable. Take some slow deep breaths to help you relax. Listen to soothing music if you wish. Place one or two pillows under your hips, so that your hips are about 12 inches or more above the floor. Your head and shoulders should be flat on the floor. Taking slow deep breaths, try to relax any tension you may be feeling, especially in your belly. Imagine your baby in slow motion trying to move downwards towards your pelvis. A source of music placed below your belly button may attract your baby towards the sound. Try to maintain this position for about 10 to 15 minutes three times a day. If you feel lightheaded or uncomfortable, stop. You may want to try it at another time. If you find that your baby has turned to a head-down position, stop the exercise, and try to take walks. This may help your baby to position himself in the pelvis.[42]

You May Want to Consider Moxibustion

The advantage of moxibustion is its effectiveness to turn a breech. Health insurance programs that cover alternative medicine treatments such as acupuncture usually cover moxubstion. There are disadvantages to moxibustion. The burning of mugwort sticks creates a pungent smell that may irritate some women who have respiratory problems. Some practioners use smokeles moxa sticks. There has also been the occasional report of external burns if the moxa stick is held too close. It may be difficult to find a licensed and qualified practitioner in your community. Acupuncture is included in the curriculum of a traditional Chinese medicine degree program. In the United States acupuncture practitioners are usually licensed under the state's acupuncture association or licensing board.[43]

Ask Your Care Provider about an External Cephalic Version (ECV)

Before doing an ECV most caregivers will do an ultrasound exam to see the position of the baby in your womb, locate the umbilical cord and placenta, and determine the amount of amniotic fluid that surrounds your baby. Ultrasound is often used during the procedure also. An electronic fetal heart monitor will measure your baby's heart rate before and during the procedure. To make sure your baby's heart rate has stabilized monitoring usually continues for about 30 minutes after. It is normal for the baby's heart rate to increase while it is being moved. If your baby does not tolerate the procedure it will be stopped.

Your caregiver may offer you a drug (such as terbutaline) to relax your uterine muscles, reduce contractions, and facilitate the breech version. Tocolytic drugs have side effects for both the mother and baby. You should discuss these with your caregiver.

You may be offered the option of having epidural anesthesia. Ask your caregiver about the benefits and risks of an epidural for this procedure. If you have Rh negative blood you will be offered Rh immune globulin to prevent incompatibility should your blood and your baby's come into contact during the version. This happens in about 4.1 percent of external versions.

To facilitate the movements of his hands over your abdomen, your caregiver will rub a lubricant on your belly. With both hands on your abdomen, your caregiver will place one hand on the baby's head and the other on the baby's bottom. He will lift the baby's bottom with one hand and gently push the head down with the other, backward or forward. If the procedure is successful you will likely go home. It is possible that you may want to have this procedure again if the baby was not able to be moved into a head-down position. Usually women find this procedure uncomfortable and sometimes painful. After the procedure, your caregiver will give you information about possible complications that may develop such as vaginal bleeding, going into labor, or the rupturing of your membranes. The probability of these complications is rare.[44]

If you have had a prior cesarean and have a low transverse scar on your uterus (bikini incision) and plan to have a VBAC you may want to ask your caregiver about the option of an external version. Although external versions have been safely tried under research conditions with women who have had one prior cesarean with a low horizontal uterine scar there is not enough information at this time to recommend or to contraindicate a version for women with a prior cesarean. ECV has been tried to turn a second twin from a breech to a vertex position, but it is still a controversial issue.

With a successful ECV about 96 percent of babies will remain in a vertex position.

If Your Breech Persists, Ask about a Vaginal Birth

If your baby persists in a breech position, find an experienced and skilled care provider to support you with a vaginal breech birth. Your provider should discuss with you and provide you with written information about the risks and benefits of a vaginal breech birth and real-time access to emergency medical services should they become necessary.

Although most breech babies are born healthy an experienced and skilled caregiver is important in planning a vaginal breech birth. Serious long-term injury and death of a breech when the mother labors are often the results of unskilled care providers or a lengthy response time in providing emergency medical services when complications arise. It is often difficult to find a care provider to support a vaginal breech birth, because they are not skilled, they cannot rely on a rapid response for emergency services, or their malpractice insurance providers exclude vaginal breech birth in their coverage.

You should be screened when you are close to your due date to identify what position your breech baby is in and where the placenta and umbilical cord are located. A baby in footling or kneeling breech position is considered unsafe for a vaginal birth. So is a baby with a hyperextended neck (chin tilting backwards, star gazer) and a large baby.

You Can Schedule a Cesarean Section

Most care providers are skilled at performing a cesarean section much more than at assisting in a vaginal breech birth. With regard to your health you should be given information regarding the benefits and risks of the operation, including how a cesarean would impact any future pregnancies. There is still controversy about whether or not scheduling a cesarean lowers the risk for babies when compared to a vaginal breech birth. If you choose a planned cesarean consider the recovery time you will need after the surgery and the support and resources available to you.

By understanding the benefits and risks of your options, finding out about the services and support that are available to you in your community, and discussing them with your caregiver, you will make the best decision that meets your needs.

RESOURCES

American Association of Family Physicians. What Can I Do If My Baby Is Breech? http://familydoctor.org/online/famdocen/home/women/pregnancy/labor/310.html (last accessed May 21, 2008).

Robertson, A. If Your Baby Is Breech. http://www.birthinternational.com/articles/andrea13.html.

Royal College of Obstetricians and Gynecologists. A Breech Baby at the End of Pregnancy. http://www.rcog.org.uk/index.asp?pageID=2310 (last accessed May 21, 2008).

14

ELECTIVE INDUCTION OF LABOR: A RISK FACTOR FOR CESAREAN DELIVERY

The increasing induction rates in the United States partly explains the rising C-section rate, which, in turn, is partly responsible for the rising rate of maternal mortality.[1]

An induction of labor is a complex and painful process that often requires additional medical interventions to keep the mother and baby safe from subsequent potential complications. Confining the laboring mother to bed, using continuous fetal monitoring, an epidural for pain, and the use of an IV are standard with an induction. Induction of labor is a risk factor for several complications for both mother and baby, including a higher risk for a cesarean section. Inducing labor with pitocin when the cervix is unripe (long and closed) sometimes causes the mother to labor for long hours with little progress. Cesarean section after a failed induction with pitocin is not uncommon.

There are several medical indications for inducing labor: when the mother or the baby's health would benefit more than continuing the pregnancy. In the case of diabetes, preeclampsia (high blood pressure), or a uterine infection. When an in utero baby is not growing at a normal rate (is small for gestational age), or the pregnancy is postterm (longer than 42 weeks), and when the bag of waters breaks prematurely (PROM, premature rupture of the membranes) before 37 weeks.

But elective inductions for no medical reason have been on the rise in the United States and in other countries. Increasingly labors are being induced for psychosocial reasons and for the physician's or hospital's convenience. A national survey of U.S. women who gave birth in 2005 showed that 21 percent tried to self-induce labor because they were tired of being pregnant and wanted to avoid a medical induction and to control the timing of their birth or because their caregiver was concerned about the size of the baby. More than four out of ten mothers (41 percent) reported that their caregiver tried to induce their labor.[2] In 2005 22.3 percent of all U.S. births were induced—a 50 percent increase since 1990. One out of four term births and one out of seven preterm births were induced.[3]

Elective induction rates vary widely among hospitals (12 to 55 percent) and among individual physicians (3 to 76 percent).[4] For some women an elective induction can almost double the risk for a cesarean, depending on the individual physician's practice style and medical specialty.[5] According to the WHO appropriate induction rates in any geographic region should not exceed 10 percent.[6]

RISKS OF ELECTIVE INDUCTION FOR THE MOTHER

There are several induction agents and differing guidelines for the appropriate timing, method, and dosing regimen, for ripening the cervix and inducing labor. Although oxytocin has been used for several decades, physicians are still debating what initial dosage is appropriate, at what intervals it should be increased, and for how long induction can safely continue."[7]

The risks associated with an elective induction (induction for no medical reason) may outweigh the perceived benefits of the procedure. Compared to women who go into labor on their own women whose labor is induced for no medical reason are at risk for several complications. Because contractions generated by an induction agent tend to be stronger and more frequent than with a normal labor, women are more likely to need pain medication including epidurals. Elective inductions increase the risk for cesarean delivery for both first time mothers and women who have given birth before. The risk for cesarean is higher for women aged 25 years or older and when the cervix is not ripe (not likely to dilate when labor is induced). Mothers who had a prior cesarean are at increased risk for uterine rupture. With an elective induction mothers are more likely to suffer from postpartum fever and need a longer hospitalization.[8]

Inductions also increase the risk for third degree perineal tears. A third degree tear is a partial or incomplete tear of the anal sphincter muscles. An induction increases the risk for third degree tears up to two percent.[9] With an oxytocin induction mothers are more likely to suffer from water intoxication,[10] a condition in which water enters the body faster than it can be removed. This condition causes an electrolyte imbalance which causes cells to swell. With water intoxication women often have difficulty initiating breast-feeding.

Amniotic fluid embolism is one of the leading causes of maternal mortality in developed countries. It is thought to result from the simultaneous tear in the fetal membranes and uterine vessels, which can cause the amniotic fluid to pass into the mother's venous circulation and eventually to her lungs. Artificially strong uterine contractions may increase this risk. A study that looked at three million hospital births found that medical induction of labor nearly doubled the risk of amniotic fluid embolism. Although the risk for amniotic embolism was low (about 6 per 100,000 for single births and 14.8 per 100,000 for women with a multiple birth) for 13 percent of the mothers who had single fetus the condition was fatal.[11]

RISKS OF ELECTIVE INDUCTION FOR THE BABY

Elective induction also impacts newborns. All induction agents increase the risk for stronger than normal contractions (uterine hyper stimulation) and affect the baby's oxygen supply and consequently its heart rate (causing fetal distress). Newborns are more likely to experience shoulder dystocia (a life-threatening complication of second stage) when labor is induced. At birth they are more likely to need resuscitation, treatment in an intensive care unit, and neonatal phototherapy to treat jaundice.[12]

Elective inductions are a risk factor for preterm birth and low birth weight (less than 2,500 g). The March of Dimes has identified increasing elective inductions and elective cesarean deliveries as two of the reasons for the increase. With elective inductions and cesareans babies are more likely to be born preterm.[13] According to the Centers for Disease Control (CDC) the number of infants delivered preterm (less than 37 completed weeks) has been increasing since the mid-1980s. In 2004 one out of every eight births in the United States was preterm. Preterm infants have a higher mortality rate compared to those born between 37 and 41 weeks of gestation. In 2004 36.5 percent of all infant deaths in the United States were from preterm-related causes. The CDC suggested that increases in cesarean deliveries and induction of labor for preterm infants were related to the increase in preterm-related infant deaths.[14]

REDUCING ELECTIVE INDUCTIONS REDUCES HEALTH RISKS

One U.S. health care system with hospitals in Utah and Idaho concerned about the rising elective induction rates and increase in related neonatal complications initiated evidence-based guidelines in 1999 to reduce induction rates. Some physicians within the system induced labor for nonmedical reasons or before pregnancy reached full term. When labor was induced before 39 weeks, babies were two to three times more likely to be admitted to intensive care units. Labor was also often induced with an unripe cervix. The Bishop score is a fifteen-point scoring system that evaluates whether or not the cervix is ripe, that is, favorable for induction. It measures five factors: cervical dilation, effacement, consistency, position in vagina, and station of fetal head. The guidelines developed by Intermountain Health Care set a minimum score of eight for first-time mothers and a score of ten for mothers who had given birth before as a requirement for inducing labor.

With an unripe cervix first-time mothers whose labor was induced took almost twice as long to give birth and were six times more likely to give birth by cesarean. Women who had given birth before were more than three times as likely to need a cesarean. After guidelines were implemented, the induction rate for pregnancies of less than 39 weeks was reduced from 27 to 5 percent. Physicians reduced their induction rate with an unripe cervix from 15 to 6 percent. An important component of the initiative was the development of a comprehensive patient education pamphlet which discussed the risks of elective inductions and safe guidelines for appropriate induction of labor.[15]

INDUCTION FOR A "BIG" BABY

Care providers sometimes suggest inducing labor before term to prevent an anticipated "big" baby (over 8lbs 13oz or 4,000 g). However, evidence shows that inducing labor for this reason in nondiabetic mothers does not reduce cesareans or instrumental deliveries; nor does it improve outcomes for mothers or babies. Induction may actually increase the risk of a cesarean section.[16] Only three out of ten pregnant women who are told they are carrying a big (macrosomic) baby actually give birth to a big baby. Inducing labor for a big baby almost doubles the odds for a cesarean. And the outcome is not any better.

INDUCTION FOR POSTTERM PREGNANCY

With a normal pregnancy labor can begin anytime between 38 and 42 weeks.

With an incorrect estimate of the due date and an elective induction the baby can be born preterm or can be of low birth weight. There is a 2-week margin of error in calculating due dates.[17] By having an ultrasound before 20 weeks the due date can be estimated more accurately, especially for women who do not have a 28-day menstrual cycle or for women who become pregnant after stopping to take a contraceptive pill.[18] Many women know exactly when they became pregnant.

For women who do not want to be induced by the end of the 41st week, the Royal College of Obstetricians and Gynaecologists of Britain recommends a "wait and see" (expectant management) approach during which the baby is assessed twice weekly by electronic fetal monitoring, and the mother is given a single ultrasound to determine the level of amniotic fluids.[19]

PRELABOR RUPTURE OF THE MEMBRANES (PROM): INDUCE OR WAIT?

For about 20 percent of mothers the bag of waters will break before the due date. When more than 37 weeks pregnant nine out of ten mothers whose water breaks will go into labor on their own within 24 hours. Some care providers recommend an induction as soon as the bag of waters is broken and there are no contractions. Waiting for contractions to begin on their own may be safe for women past their 37th week. Waiting exposes women to a slight risk for infection, so discussing symptoms of infection to watch out for with your care provider is important. So is the color or odor of the amniotic fluid. Avoiding an induction as soon as the bag of waters breaks reduces the risk for a cesarean.[20]

AMNIOTOMY (BREAKING THE BAG OF WATERS) DOES NOT REDUCE CESAREANS

Some care providers recommend an amniotomy (breaking the bag of waters) early in labor to reduce the length of labor and reduce the risk for cesarean section. An amniotomy shortens labor by about 1 to 2 hours and may reduce the need for oxytocin. But it can also increase the risk of infection for both mother and baby. It is more likely to affect the baby's heart rate in a negative way and increase the risk of the baby's umbilical cord slipping through the cervix before the baby (cord prolapse) making a cesarean delivery more likely. Breaking the bag of waters does not have any benefits for the baby. It also tends to increase the risk of a cesarean delivery.[21]

PROSTAGLANDIN E2 OR PGE2 (TRADE NAMES PREPIDIL, CERVIDIL)

Prostaglandin is a common agent available as a gel or a removable tampon in the United States and as a tablet in the United Kingdom. By ripening the cervix before an oxytocin induction women are more likely to give birth within twelve to 24 hours. They are also less likely to have an epidural or an instrumental delivery (with forceps or vacuum extractor). However, there is an increased risk that the uterus will contract more often and more strongly than normal (uterine hyper stimulation).[22] Some studies show that using a cervical ripening agent does not decrease the risk for a cesarean and may in fact increase the rate for a surgical delivery.[23]

PROSTAGLANDIN E1 OR MISOPROSTOL (CYTOTEC)

Another ripening agent commonly used off label is misoprostol or prostaglandin E1. Its trade name is Cytotec. The drug originally developed to treat people with ulcers is not approved by the FDA for induction of labor. Although studies have shown that this product is effective for ripening the cervix and may reduce the risk for a cesarean delivery[24] it does have serious side effects including hyper stimulation of the uterus, hemorrhage, placental problems, uterine rupture, amniotic fluid embolism, hysterectomy, and death of the mother and/or the baby. The excessive contractions caused by it reduce the available oxygen to the baby.

Although the manufacturer of the drug (Searle) had sent a letter to all U.S. physicians warning of the dangers of using the drug off label at any time during pregnancy or childbirth,[25] the American College of Obstetricians and Gynecologists petitioned the FDA to continue to allow its use for induction of labor.[26] The FDA has not yet banned the use of misoprostol for induction but has issued an FDA Alert which is posted on their Web site: "This Patient Information Sheet is for pregnant women who may receive misoprostol to soften their cervix or induce contractions to begin labor. Misoprostol is sometimes used to decrease blood loss after delivery of a baby. These uses are not approved by the FDA. No company has sent the FDA scientific proof that misoprostol is safe and effective for these uses. There can be rare but serious side effects, including a torn uterus (womb), when misoprostol is used for labor and delivery."[27]

Cytotec is commonly used in countries in which abortion is illegal because of its ability to stimulate contractions. Researchers and consumer advocacy groups have called for a ban on the use of Cytotec because of reported dangerous and deadly effects on some women and their infants.[28, 29, 30] Cytotec is especially dangerous for women laboring for a VBAC. Essentially, the use of cytotec in pregnant women is an uncontrolled medical experiment in which women have not consented to participate.

MECHANICAL METHODS OF INDUCTION MAY REDUCE THE RISK FOR A CESAREAN

Sometimes a Foley catheter (commonly used to empty the bladder) or natural (lamineria) or synthetic dilators can be inserted into the cervix to stimulate labor. These devices increase the production of prostaglandin, stretch the cervix and do not have the potential for excessive contractions. They can also be removed at any time. However, oxytocin is also more likely to be needed. Compared to induction with oxytocin because of an unripe cervix, these mechanical methods reduce the risk for a cesarean delivery.[31]

STRIPPING OR SWEEPING THE MEMBRANES

Sweeping the amniotic membranes is a less invasive alternative to stimulating labor. This method also releases prostaglandins locally. It can be done during a cervical exam, is generally safe, and does not increase the risk of infection when there are no complications. Sweeping the membranes can reduce the need for oxytocin or prostaglandins which can hyperstimulate uterine contractions (causing too many or too strong contractions). The procedure may be uncomfortable, cause some bleeding, and initially cause irregular contractions. However, it may inadvertently also break the bag of waters, putting a time limit on how long a woman can labor before a cesarean or an instrumental delivery is recommended.[32]

NIPPLE STIMULATION

Nipple stimulation has been found to be effective in inducing labor in low-risk women with a favorable cervix and does not increase the risk for hyperstimulating the uterus. Women are 30 percent more likely to go into labor within 72 hours when using nipple stimulation as opposed to waiting for contractions to begin on their own. However there is no difference in the cesarean section rate.[33]

Especially for Mothers

An induced labor can be long and very painful. When labor is artificially started the risk for other related complications for you and your baby increase. So does the risk for a cesarean section. All forms of induction have the potential to over stimulate contractions. There are medical reasons that make induction the safer option for you or your baby, when continuing the pregnancy would put you or your baby at risk. But inductions for nonmedical reasons have increased by 50 percent in the last 15 years, and they are affecting the health of mothers and babies. If there are no medical indications for inducing labor Lamaze International recommends you allow your body to go into labor spontaneously, when your baby is ready to be born. The natural rhythm of contractions produced by the mother's own oxytocin allows her the freedom to move around, change positions, or try taking a bath or shower to reduce stress and pain. Avoiding an induction will reduce the risk for other complications.[34, 35] Henci Goer, author of *The Thinking Woman's Guide to a Better Birth* makes the following suggestions to avoid the complications associated with an induction:

- If your labor needs to be induced you are more likely to have a vaginal birth when your cervix is ripe.
- Your risk for infection is reduced if your bag of waters remains intact. This will cushion the baby, facilitate movement through the pelvis, and reduce the risk for a cord prolapse.
- Ask your care provider to use a low dose oxytocin infusion at half-hour intervals to reduce your risk for contractions that are too strong and too close together. Your baby is less likely to be affected by a reduced amount of oxygen.
- If your labor has a consistent pattern of contractions after 4 cm or more, your body may continue to labor on its own if your turn off the oxytocin.
- Consider waiting for starting an epidural till you are in active labor—4 cm or more.
- If you have had a prior cesarean, inducing labor may increase your risk for a uterine rupture.

There are less invasive methods to artificially soften the cervix and begin labor. Try to find out more about stripping the amniotic membranes, using a Foley catheter or laminaria, and nipple stimulation. Induction rates vary among care providers and hospitals. Try to find a provider and hospital with low induction rates. This will reduce your risk for other complications and a cesarean.

Resources

Goer, H. Elective Induction of Labor. http://hencigoer.com/articles/elective_induction.

Intermountain Healthcare. Elective Labor Induction—When Is It Okay?, http://intermountainhealthcare.org/xp/public/managehealth/patiented/mombaby/.

Lamaze International. Care Practice #1: Labor Begins on Its Own, http://www.lamaze.org/ChildbirthEducators/ResourcesforEducators/CarePractice Papers/LaborBeginsOnItsOwn/tabid/487/Default.aspx (last accessed 7/3/07).

Lamaze International. Tips for Avoiding Labor Induction, http://www.lamaze.org/ExpectantParents/PregnancyandBirthResources/MoreTipsand Tools/InductionTips/tabid/255/Default.aspx.

NICE. About Induction of Labor—Information for Pregnant Women, Their Partners and Their Families, http://guidance.nice.org.uk/CGD/publicinfo/pdf/English.

SOGC. Bringing Baby Safely into the World. Inducing Labour, http://www.rogc.org/pub_ed/bringingbay/induceLab_e.shtml.

Wagner, Marsden. Cytotec Induction and Off-Label Use. *Midwifery Today* 67 (Fall 2003), http://www.midwiferytoday.com/articles/cytotec.asp.

PART IV

REDUCING THE RISKS FOR CESAREAN

15

ESPECIALLY FOR MOTHERS: COPING WITH THE PAIN OF LABOR

NONDRUG OPTIONS FOR PAIN RELIEF

Every woman who has ever given birth has needed some form of pain relief, a way to reduce her pain, to make her more comfortable and to make her feel safe and supported. Praise and encouragement from experienced women around her to give her the strength to endure, to complete her journey. Different cultures have their own unique traditions to reduce pain and support women in labor. In the United States women have fewer options for pain relief than women in many other industrialized countries. Providing drugs is one method of coping with the pain of labor and birth. But it's not the only one. How satisfied women are with their birth experience is, interestingly enough, not based on how much or how little pain they experience, or what medical interventions they have, but on the quality of their relationship with the people that care for them during childbirth. The level of support they have and their involvement in making labor and birth decisions. These things are more important to women than the level of childbirth pain.

There are many alternative methods of pain relief. Each culture and tradition has rich resources and knowledge to draw from. Every woman is different and can choose what best meets her needs at different times during her labor and birth. These nondrug methods can reduce the need for multiple doses of medication and their effects on the progress of labor and on the baby.

With any of these methods you are still alert and can maintain control over your labor. You can choose to begin or stop them at any time, and you can use them in whatever place of birth you choose. Together with continuous emotional support and the freedom to move and change positions, these options can help to reduce your pain and provide a sense of well-being. Many of these pain relief options are used in home births and birth centers. Some hospitals welcome and support mothers who choose these methods, and many labor and delivery nurses are learning to provide some of these pain-relieving methods. The following methods of pain relief have been studied and found safe and effective in reducing pain:

Cognitive Strategies

Visualization, breathing techniques, and conscious relaxation of tense body muscles are effective strategies that are taught in childbirth classes. Chanting phrases, affirmations (positive messages), prayers, or mantras and listening to music or peaceful environmental sounds can also be relaxing.

Warm Water Baths (Hydrotherapy)

Women who labor in water have less pain and are less likely to need drugs and oxytocin to stimulate labor contractions. Warm water reduces blood pressure and muscle tension and eases the pain of contractions. Women who use warm baths tend to have shorter labors if they enter the bath after active labor has begun (Photo 15.1). Women who make use of hydrotherapy are also less likely to experience fetal malpresentation (baby in an occiput posterior presentation or deep occiput transverse position). Being immersed in water is most effective if the water is at body temperature (98–100°F) and reaches up to the shoulder level and the laboring mother stays in the water for no longer than 1 to $1\frac{1}{2}$ hours at a time (Photo 15.2). Water that is too hot raises the mother's body temperature and increases the baby's heart rate. Portable water tubs are available in most birth centers or can be rented for home use. Some hospitals also have tubs in their labor and delivery units. Sitting or standing up under a warm shower can also reduce muscle tension and ease pain.

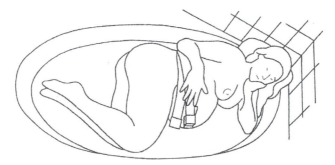

Photo 15.1. A mother laboring in a tub. *Source*: Illustrations by Shanna dela Cruz, copyright Ruth S. Ancheta (1994, 1999, and 2005). Reproduced by permission from Simkin, P. and Ancheta, R. (2000, 2005). *The Labor Progress Handbook: Early Interventions to Prevent and Treat Dystocia.* Oxford: Blackwell Publishing.

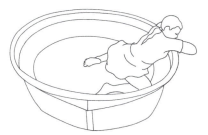

Photo 15.2. A mother laboring in a birthing pool. *Source*: Illustrations by Shanna dela Cruz, copyright Ruth S. Ancheta (1994, 1999, and 2005). Reproduced by permission from Simkin, P. and Ancheta, R. (2000, 2005). *The Labor Progress Handbook: Early Interventions to Prevent and Treat Dystocia*. Oxford: Blackwell Publishing.

Touch, Massage, and Acupressure

Massage and touch therapy are proven to reduce pain and anxiety and help women to cope better with labor pain. They also improve newborn outcomes. Simple touches such as holding a mother's hand, wiping her brow, and stroking and massaging her shoulders, feet, or back improve her comfort level and emotional state. There are specially trained pregnancy massage therapists who assist mothers during labor. Not all mothers feel comfortable with touch or massage, and some mothers will find it helpful for some parts of labor and not for others.

Hypnosis

Women who use hypnosis tend to use less pain medication, are less likely to need oxytocin to augment their labor, and have shorter lengths of labor and fewer operative deliveries. Hypnosis can help to reduce stress and anxiety and promote a positive response to the pain of labor. Women who have used hypnosis have expressed a sense of calm and control over their birth.

Hot and Cold Treatment

Using hot wet towels or face cloths across a woman's lower abdomen, lower back, or other tense muscle areas can lessen muscle spasms, provide comfort, and lessen pain. Rice-filled packs or cloth packs filled with synthetic beads can be heated in a microwave and used for comfort and pain relief. A cold compress or frozen gel pack can ease muscle spasm in the lower back and a cold towel can be refreshing to cool the mother's forehead or back of the neck.

Creating Your Own Birth Environment

Laboring at home or in a birth center gives women a sense of privacy, a familiar environment, and familiar birth attendants with whom she has developed a relationship. Often in a hospital the birth attendants are unfamiliar and the environment is noisier and less private. Hospital routines are likely to increase a woman's level of stress. It may help to create a personal environment by reducing the lighting, closing the labor room door, adjusting the room temperature, and bringing in familiar and relaxing music.

Any of these alternative methods of reducing pain and stress can be used for part of the time during labor, or a combination of them may meet your needs for all of labor and birth. They have no known negative side effects.

USING DRUGS FOR PAIN RELIEF

Analgesics

The drugs used to relieve pain in labor, or in general, are called analgesics. Analgesics whether given as an injection, by IV, or by mouth enter the mother's blood stream and are transferred to her baby. For a drug to be effective it is prescribed based on the mother's body weight, that is, an adult dose. Given that the baby's weight is a fraction of the mother's, and it's drug filtering system still immature, the drug's dosage will have a more powerful effect on the baby. Often, analgesics are given in early labor so that there is time for the drug to wear off.

Drugs circulate back from the baby through the placenta, and the mother filters it through her own system. It is difficult to assess how much of any drug will still be in the baby's system once it is born or to what extent it will affect the baby. The lower the dose and the longer the span between the time the medication was given and the time the baby is born, the more mature the baby is the less of an impact the drug has. Analgesics can slow down fetal heart rate and breathing and sedate the baby. At birth babies may have trouble breast-feeding and staying alert. Some drugs can be found in the baby's blood stream days after the birth.

Drugs commonly available for pain during labor include narcotics like morphine, Demerol, fentanyl, nubaine, and Stadol. Barbiturates such as Nembutal and Seconal are given for relaxation or sedation. Tranquilizers such as Vistaril, Phenergan, Versed, and Valium are used to reduce nausea and vomiting, side effects of the narcotics. Analgesics raise the threshhold for pain but do not eliminate the pain altogether. Often contractions slow down a while right after the mother has analgesics. Mothers may experience dizziness, nausea, restlessness, a drop in blood pressure, low heart rate, and respiratory depression.

EPIDURAL FOR PAIN RELIEF

Epidural analgesia is a way of providing pain relief for labor by inserting medication into the epidural space located near the spine through a thin plastic tube. The medication numbs the nerves of the uterus and the birth canal. The mother feels the numbing effect from the waist area down to the thighs and sometimes to the toes. The lighter the dose of anesthetic the easier it is for the mother to move her legs and change positions in bed. An epidural can be given continuously by infusion, or the medication can be increased when the last dose wears off. Women can also self-administer a predetermined dose of the drugs. This is called patient-controlled analgesia.

With a combined spinal-epidural (CSE) medication is first injected into the spinal fluid by puncturing the dura mater, the sheath surrounding the spinal cord, and then administering additional medication into the epidural space. With CSE pain relief is faster, and movement is easier. Although the CSE is known as a walking epidural, most mothers do not walk during labor, and a staff person is usually needed to accompany the mother while she is out of bed.

Epidural analgesia is an effective method of pain relief. Unlike systemic drugs that are given through an IV or by injection, an epidural does not make you drowsy. It can be helpful if you have been in labor a long time and are very tired and need to rest. Sometimes it can relax you enough to make your labor progress. It is helpful that when you are ready to push, you do so when you feel the urge to. Pushing forcefully and holding your breath for a long time is more likely to reduce the oxygen to the baby and affect its heart rate. It is also helpful if you push in an upright or side lying position. With an epidural you will need more time to push your baby out.

What Are the Advantages of Using an Epidural?

An epidural allows the mother to stay alert throughout labor and delivery. The pain of contractions is effectively reduced in about 10 to 20 minutes. An epidural can provide a rest period when labor is long. The baby is less medicated compared to using systemic drugs, but the drugs and anesthetic used do cross the placenta.

What Are the Disadvantages of an Epidural?

A woman's ability to move around, walk, or change positions will be limited. An IV, bladder catheter, and continuous electronic fetal monitoring are necessary with an epidural. The medication in the epidural may cause an erratic heart rate for the baby. Drugs can cause various degrees of maternal, fetal, and neonatal toxicity. The epidural sometimes does not fully relieve the pain.

Studies show that use of epidural analgesia may have the following results:

- Labor tends to take longer.
- Pitocin is needed to stimulate contractions.
- Mothers may experience low blood pressure.
- An epidural may cause maternal fever when used for long hours.
- Mothers sometimes experience headache, nausea, vomiting, or itching when epidural narcotics are used.
- There is an increased incidence of hemorrhage after the birth.

- Higher likelihood of needing forceps, a vacuum extractor, or a cesarean.
- The baby may have difficulty in positioning itself favorably for the birth (mal-positioning).
- Newborns and mothers are more likely to be screened and treated for infection.
- Initiating breastfeeding may be more difficult.

RESOURCES

ACNM, Pain during Childbirth, http://www.midwife.org/share_with_women.cfm (last accessed May 23, 2008).

American Academy of Family Physicians. Labor Pain: What to Expect and Ways to Relieve Pain, http://www.aafp.org/afp/20030915/1121ph.html (last accessed May 22, 2008).

American Psychological Association, Hypnosis, http://www.apa.org/divisions/div30/forms/hypnosis_brochure.pdf.

Childbirth Connection, Labor Pain, http://childbirthconnection.org/article.asp?ck=10191.

Goer, H. Epidurals for Labor Pain. http://parenting.ivillage.com/pregnancy/plabor/0,8jzw-p,00.htm (last accessed May 22, 2008).

Hypnobirthing, http://www.hypnobirthing.com/ (last accessed May 22, 2008).

MIDIRS, Infochoice.org, Non-Epidural Strategies for Pain Relief during Labor, The Use of Epidural Analgesia for Women in Labour, http://infochoice.org/ic/ic.nsf/TheLeaflets?openform (last accessed May 22, 2008).

MIDIRS, Infochoice.org, The Use of Water during Childbirth, http://www.infochoice.org/ (last accessed May 22, 2008).

Waterbirth International, http://www.waterbirthinternational.org (last accessed May 22, 2008).

16

LABOR SUPPORT BY WOMEN FOR WOMEN

> I have worked with doulas frequently over the last ten years or so and have found them to be a great benefit to my patients. In fact, I like the concept so much that I hired a doula for my practice to be with any of my patients who wanted one during the labor and delivery process. There is no doubt in my mind that the presence of a doula helps lower the use of epidurals and pain medicine during labor, and it improves the labor and delivery process for patients as well.[1]

Isolating healthy childbearing women from their family members and their social network when they go into labor, restricting their freedom of movement to the confines of their beds and instructing them to lie down on their backs when they are about to give birth are harmful birth practices initiated in the twentieth century, when all childbirth including for healthy, low-risk women was moved from home to the hospital. While advances in medicine, surgical procedures, and technology proved to be invaluable for women whose pregnancies and births were complicated by a medical or "abnormal" condition best cared for in a hospital, the rationale for the wholesale movement of all childbearing women to medical institutions and their treatment as at-risk patients has increasingly come under scrutiny.[2] A highly valuable component of childbirth that was eliminated from institutionalized maternity care was the personal emotional and physical support and encouragement that women had from trusted female relatives, friends, and birth attendants. Research conducted in several countries under highly varied hospital environments has shown that not only is that kind of nonmedical one-to-one support highly valued by women but is also extremely effective in improving health outcomes for mothers and their babies and reducing the odds for cesarean section.[3]

Women who give birth at home with professional midwives or in a free-standing birth center benefit from extremely low rates of medical complications and cesarean rates that result from a model of care that values and provides continuous one-to-one emotional, informational, and physical support. Having examined the impact of hospital birth practices on women in labor researchers from the Cochrane Pregnancy and Childbirth Group state that concerns "about the consequent dehumanization of women's birth experiences have led to calls for a return to continuous support by women for women during labour."[4]

In a hospital setting a similar model of continuous nonmedical support provided throughout labor and birth by a trained labor support professional (doula) or a lay female labor companion experienced with childbirth can enhance the process of labor and reduce the need for pain medication, medical interventions, and cesareans. Mothers are also highly appreciative of that support. These benefits have been observed across continents whether fathers were present during labor and birth or not.[5]

WHAT ARE THE SKILLS OF A PROFESSIONALLY TRAINED LABOR ASSISTANT?

Women trained as professional labor assistants or doulas bring specific knowledge, sensitivity, and skills to help enhance the progress of labor and reduce the emotional stress and physical pain of childbirth. Wherever women provide continuous support during childbirth, they share a few common elements. Labor companions do not leave the mother alone. They provide emotional support, reassurance, and praise for the mother's efforts. Their knowledge of the physiology of labor, specific breathing, and relaxation techniques, familiarity with hospital protocols and procedures, and understanding of the psychological factors that can impact the progress of labor are valuable skills and attributes that mothers appreciate. Doulas can provide comforting touch and massage and suggest a warm bath or shower when needed. They help the mother to interpret and cope with the increasing level of pain that is normal in labor. They advocate for the mother's individual needs and help her to communicate her wishes to her medical staff. Doulas provide a comfortable and emotionally safe environment, based on the mother's preference, where she can labor freely and give birth.

They can help the mother to maintain control over her labor, involving her in all decisions regarding her care. They help the fathers or partners to assist and participate at their own comfort level (Photo 16.1). Their individualized

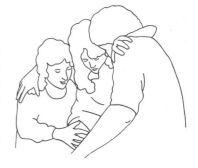

Photo 16.1. A doula and father supporting a mother in labor. *Source*: Illustrations by Shanna dela Cruz, copyright Ruth S. Ancheta (1994, 1999, and 2005). Reproduced by permission from Simkin, P. and Ancheta, R. (2000, 2005). *The Labor Progress Handbook: Early Interventions to Prevent and Treat Dystocia*. Oxford: Blackwell Publishing.

care and attention create a protective and nurturing environment that offsets the effects of the unfamiliar, intimidating, and often hurried institutional routines. After the birth they can enhance mother–infant attachment, help the mother to understand her newborn's behavior, and assist with the initiation of breast-feeding. In the days after birth doulas help the mother to integrate and process her birth experience.

Neonatologist Marshall H. Klaus, pediatrician John H. Kennell and psychotherapist Phyllis H. Klaus, the coauthors of *The Doula Book*, write, "Perhaps the most important insight needed by a doula-in-training is that every woman comes to labor with a different set of life experiences, needs, coping mechanisms, and responses. Each comes with a particular set of birth histories, information, worries, and histories. She approaches birth with her individual expectations and varied abilities to deal with pain or other difficult situations. The father, partner, close relative, or friend who accompanies the mother also comes with past life experiences and concerns. For this reason the doula must be adaptable, resourceful, and often creative to meet the different needs of each woman and the person accompanying her at birth."[6]

Continuous Support during Childbirth Improves Outcomes and Reduces the Risk of Cesareans

Many studies have compared maternal and infant outcomes when continuous support in childbirth was provided by a professionally trained labor assistant with outcomes from comparable clinical care provided to a similar group of mothers without continuous labor support and found several physical and psychosocial benefits. A review of five studies found that with continuous support women were less likely to request and use pain medication in labor. They were less likely to have an instrumental delivery (with forceps or vacuum extractor) and less likely to have postpartum pain. Newborns were less likely to need admission to a neonatal intensive care unit (NICU). When compared to continuous labor support provided to mothers by nurses employed by the hospital, women who were supported by a nonmedical trained or experienced woman had less need for oxytocin during labor, less need for pain medication, and fewer cesareans.[7]

The most recent review of fifteen randomized controlled trials (best available evidence) of continuous support in childbirth provided by a trained or experienced woman included 12,791 women in eleven countries. They were from different social backgrounds and varying hospital settings. Reviewers found that women who had the support were 41 percent less likely to have an instrumental delivery, 28 percent less likely to use any pain medication, and 26 percent less likely to give birth by cesarean section.[8]

Women were also more likely to feel in control of their birth. Women who received continuous labor support from midwives, student midwives, and nurses had a more positive overall experience than women who did not have that support. In some studies supported women had a shorter first stage of labor and less perineal trauma. Mothers tended to be less depressed at 6 weeks postpartum, had less difficulty with mothering, and were more likely to be breast-feeding 4 to 6 weeks after their birth.

This review also found that health outcomes were most beneficial and medical interventions rate most reduced when mothers had a labor companion but no loved one present at their birth, when labor support began in early labor, when epidurals were not easily available, when electronic fetal monitoring was not used routinely, and when labor support was provided by a woman who was not a hospital employee.

The researchers speculated that institutional routines, unfamiliar staff, the lack of privacy, and other conditions may have an adverse effect on labor progress and women's feelings of competence and self-confidence because women are uniquely vulnerable during labor. Consequently these negative feelings may affect their early adjustment to parenting and establishment of breast-feeding and increase their potential for depression. The effects of continuous labor support may safeguard them from those adverse effects.

Another viewpoint expressed by the researchers was the possibility that labor progressed with fewer complications because of specific skills that trained professionals bring to labor: encouraging women to remain upright and use gravity effectively, recommending specific positions to solve specific situations in labor, and using relaxation techniques to reduce the level of stress hormones (epinephrine). A high level of stress hormones can interfere with the pattern of contractions and reduce blood flow to the placenta and consequently to the baby. Reducing the need for pain medication including epidurals may in turn reduce the number of related medical interventions (the cascade of interventions) such as the use of continuous electronic fetal monitors, intravenous drips, and artificial oxytocin to counteract the slowing of labor by epidurals. Epidurals increase the need for other drugs to counteract hypotension and infections from catheters required to empty the bladder anesthetized by the epidural. Epidurals also increase the risk for instrumental deliveries due to the malpositioning of the baby. The authors of this Cochrane systematic review recommend that continuous support during labor should be the norm rather than the exception and that all women should be allowed and encouraged to have support people of their choice with them throughout labor and birth.[9]

Ginger Breedlove, Ph.D., C.N.M., A.R.N.P., F.A.C.N.M., coauthor of *The Community-Based Doula: Supporting Families Before, During, and After Childbirth* says,

> As more and more childbearing families are faced with the challenges of medical recommendation related to primary cesarean or repeat cesarean without trial of labor, doulas have continued to provide an alternative advocacy role assisting families in the decision-making process thereby leading to enhancement in informed consent. As a Nurse Midwife practitioner for over 25 years I have

observed hundreds of births with the presence of a multi-disciplinary team, including the active work of doulas in the hospital and in birthing centers. In this era of time constraints facing OB L&D nurses who have lesser time dedicated to bedside labor support, the doula and labor companions for the mother are integral for women who choose to labor without an epidural or with limited use of narcotics.[10]

ESPECIALLY FOR MOTHERS

In addition to medical care providers, when giving birth most mothers appreciate and come to depend on the emotional support, understanding, and experience of other women knowledgeable about childbirth. When giving birth at home or at a birth center this kind of support is complementary to the medical care that women receive. In the hospital medical care providers have more than one laboring mother to care for and have hospital duties to fulfill. In addition to having your partner with you at the birth, you may want to consider having an experienced female labor companion (a relative, friend, or doula) who you feel comfortable with and can trust to meet your nonmedical needs. If you think you would like to have an epidural for pain relief you may still benefit from the emotional support and guidance that a companion can provide throughout labor and after the birth.

Research shows that having a woman experienced in childbirth with you throughout labor and birth may help you have a shorter labor, make you feel more in control of your labor, and reduce your need for pain medication and for having an instrumental delivery (with forceps or vacuum extractor) or a cesarean section. You are also less likely to feel depressed and have an easier time initiating and maintaining breast-feeding for 6 weeks after the birth and more likely to feel less anxious about being a mother.

Talk to your partner about this option to find out if this arrangement can work for you. Some fathers and partners feel less anxious in the unfamiliar hospital environment and by not having to assume full responsibility for meeting the mother's needs during labor. They often can learn from your labor support companion many ways to help you have a more comfortable and satisfying birth. In some cultures it is the norm for fathers not to be closely involved in childbirth, so a female companion may be very helpful to you.

How Do I Select a Qualified Doula?

If you prefer to have a trained labor support assistant instead of a relative or close friend, you will benefit from taking the time to find out more about their training and the services they provide. Doulas can receive training and certification from several local, national, and international organizations. Training programs usually require prior knowledge of childbirth, selected reading material, and a 2- or 3-day seminar that includes hands-on practice of skills including relaxation and breathing techniques, positioning and movements to reduce pain and enhance the progress of labor, massage, and other comfort measures.

Doulas who are also certified have completed additional requirements that include attending several births, evaluations from medical care providers and parents, additional education, observation of a series of childbirth classes, and writing an exam or an essay that reflects a knowledge of the fundamental concepts of labor support.

How Do I Pay for a Doula's Services?

Many doulas have their own private or group practice. Fees for doula services in the United States vary from $250 to $1,500. Fees usually include two prenatal visits, continuous support throughout the entire labor, no matter how long it lasts, and one or two postpartum visits. However, some doulas provide free services, while they are still in training. Over a hundred U.S. hospitals provide doula services as part of their maternity care package by having doulas on staff or contracting with a doula service. With a hospital doula service, parents may or may not have the opportunity to meet their doulas before labor begins. Doulas assist mothers in home births as well as in birth centers. Many community maternity centers also employ doulas for their clients.

Parents in the United States may have a flex spending account in which a percentage of their wages is placed in a pretax account that can be used for uncovered medical expenses. Hospitals and individual physicians who directly employ doulas may also bill for doula services. Although the care that doulas provide is nonmedical, it does have medical and financial benefits. Some insurance companies reimburse parents for doula services. Medicaid funds are sometimes allocated for doula services by some county agencies, and private foundations have also provided grants to cover the cost of doula care.

What Questions Should I Ask a Prospective Doula?

Parents who are thinking about having a doula at their baby's birth may want to begin interviewing doulas about 2 months before the baby is due. You may want to have a phone interview before personally meeting her. To help you feel comfortable with the doula DONA International suggests that you ask these important questions:

- What training have you had?
- Tell me (us) about your experience with birth, personally as a doula?
- What is your philosophy about childbirth and supporting women and their partners through labor?
- May we call you with questions or concerns before and after the birth?
- When do you join women in labor? Do you come to our home or meet us at the hospital? The birth center?

- Do you meet me (us) after the birth to review the labor and answer questions?
- Do you work with one or more backup doulas when you are not available? Can we meet them?
- What is your fee? How do you expect payment to be made?

Parents need to feel comfortable and reassured with the doula they hire. Several doula training and certifying organizations require doulas to meet strict professional and ethical standards. By taking the time to interview a doula and find out about her professional training and the special services that she can provide you will be more satisfied with your birth experience.

A LETTER FROM A FIRST TIME MOTHER TO HER DOULA

Dear Ellie,

It has been three months since my daughter's birth. I have been blessed and delighted with motherhood. I enjoy her tremendously, and therefore I have neglected the rest of the world. I have been meaning to write and let you know how wonderful it was for my daughter and me that you were our doula. We are so glad we chose you to be with us for such a precious, intimate, soul-piercing moment—the birth of my daughter. I wanted to take the time to thank you for your care and concern about my well-being during labor. Starting with your massages, they were soothing and invigorating. I loved your rocking me. It produced in me a sense of calmness. You seemed to have known when to talk to me to keep me focused on my daughter's birth. You facilitated communication between my doctor and my nurses. At times I was out of it emotionally and physically that medical explanations had little meaning to me. You clarified, explained, asked questions and kept my interest at heart. You made a "dysfunctional labor," as my doctor labeled it, functional. My doctor spoke highly of you, and so did my family. My husband was so happy that you were there because it allowed him to relax and enjoy the process. He told me he trusted you implicitly.

Your hospital visit after the birth was deeply appreciated. I was feeling so overwhelmed and helpless by the ordeal of a cesarean, trying to breast-feed, changing diapers, answering phone calls, and trying to be graceful to my visitors. Your tips on organization and breast-feeding proved successful. Ellie, there was a sincere, loving level of care that you incorporated within your professional knowledge that made it easier for me to learn the techniques.

Your home visit was a delight. You helped me to give my newborn daughter her first bath and walked me gently through it, allowing me to lose the fear of hurting her. Yes, God danced the day she was born, and all the beings of this universe welcomed her to her home. I am bursting with pride, joy, and love for my daughter. Lastly, I must thank you for the list of reading material you recently sent me. Ellie, I couldn't have endured 28 hours of labor without your loving care and support. I am so happy you were there. We all thank you. Thank you for writing what took place when I gave birth to my daughter. I shall keep that account for her.

Love, M.

RESOURCES

For information about training and certification requirements for professional labor assistants or doulas and where to find one visit these Web sites:

Association of Labor Assistants and Childbirth Educators, http://www.alace.org.
Childbirth and Postpartum Professional Association, http://www.cappa.org.
DONA International, http://www.dona.org.
International Childbirth Education Association, http://www.icea.org.

17

GIVING BIRTH WITH MIDWIVES:
EXCELLENT OUTCOMES WITH
FEWER CESAREANS

Midwives believe that women's bodies are designed to give birth and know how to labor better than we understand, and that many of our attempts to control or improve the process end up disrupting it in ways that have unintended, often harmful consequences. Thus midwives endeavor to support and protect the normal process, because, as they have also learned, fear, discouragement, and seemingly harmless hospital routines and medical interventions can rob labor of its power.[1]

DEFINING THE PROFESSIONAL MIDWIFE

The word midwife has been used for centuries to describe a woman who is "with women" at birth. A midwife was traditionally an older female in the family or the community who gained her knowledge from experience rather than formal training. Traditional midwives still attend to women in developing countries. A professional midwife is a highly trained maternity care provider who works collaboratively with physicians and other maternity care professionals. Midwifery care is the best model of care for the majority of healthy pregnant women. Midwives are the primary caregivers for low-risk childbearing women in most industrialized countries. Midwifery care has been proven to reduce the rate of medical interventions in labor and birth that may cause harm when used routinely. Midwifery care also reduces the need for a cesarean section. Midwives meet more than women's medical needs. They also address the emotional, psychological, and cultural concerns of women in their childbearing year.

In *all* industrialized countries in the world except the United States professional midwives attend the majority of births. In Canada the profession of midwifery is rapidly gaining ground. Some provinces and territories have already passed legislation establishing midwifery care as an integral part of the health care service, and others are in the process of doing so. The model of care provided by midwives is based on the concept that pregnancy and childbirth are normal life events that should be carefully monitored but not interfered with unless necessary. Midwives look to maximize health outcomes using a minimum number of medical interventions.

In *Midwifery and Childbirth in America*, Judith Pence Rooks writes, "[E]xperience has taught midwives that when essentially healthy women labor in a secure environment; receive physical and emotional support; eat, drink, rest, move, and position themselves as they want; and when little is done to add to their discomfort and they are respected and encouraged and *expected to give birth successfully* [italics in original], most of them do."[2] Current evidence shows that this woman-centered, hands-on, low-tech approach to caring for low-risk women has produced excellent health outcomes.

The educational training, apprenticeship, and licensure requirements for the practice of midwifery vary from country to country. In the United States the legal standing and scope of practice of midwives vary from state to state. Regardless of the specific credential they hold or the professional philosophy of childbirth that they may have, the majority of midwives agree on the essential elements and scope of practice of their profession. In July 2005 the International Confederation of Midwives agreed upon the following:

> The midwife is recognized as a responsible and accountable professional who works in partnership with women to give the necessary support, care and advice during pregnancy, labour and the postpartum period, to conduct births on the midwife's own responsibility and to provide care for the newborn and the infant. This care includes preventive measures, the promotion of normal birth, the detection of complications in mother and child, the accessing of medical or other appropriate assistance and the carrying out of emergency measures. The midwife has an important task in health counseling and education, not only for the woman, but also within the family and community. This work should involve antenatal education and preparation for parenthood and may extend to women's health, sexual or reproductive health and childcare. A midwife may practice in any setting including in the home, the community, hospitals, clinics or health units.[3]

The philosophical foundation of midwifery care is based on protecting, supporting, and enhancing the normal process of birth. In contrast, the foundation of the biomedical model of care is the diagnosis and treatment of disease in which the focus is on the "abnormal" or pathological aspects of childbearing and birth. The biomedical model of care, obstetrics being one specialty, is risk-focused and tends to view all normal pregnancies and births as potentially becoming "abnormal" and all women needing medical interventions such as the routine use of electronic fetal monitoring and IV fluids (IV lines) "just in case." The model of care provided by midwives, which is based on their education and training in midwifery, is based on the concept that pregnancy and childbirth are normal life events; they should be carefully monitored but not interfered with unless necessary. Midwives look to maximize health outcomes using a minimum number of medical interventions. This model of care can be learned and practiced by all maternity care professionals.

WHAT IS THE EVIDENCE THAT MIDWIFERY CARE PROVIDES EXCELLENT OUTCOMES WITH FEWER INTERVENTIONS AND LOWER CESAREAN RATES?

The Mother-Friendly Childbirth Initiative (MFCI), an internationally supported consensus document of the Coalition for Improving Maternity Services (CIMS), promotes evidence-based, woman-centered maternity care. The Initiative advocates for all birthing mothers to have access to professional midwifery care. A systematic review of the evidence by the Coalition's Expert Work Group supports the excellent health outcomes provided by professional midwives. The CIMS Expert Work group found that compared with care provided by physicians for similar populations, maternity care provided by midwives results in the same or better maternal and perinatal health benefits. These are their findings:[4]

Compared to Care Given by Physicians, Women Cared for by Midwives Have Fewer Cesareans and More VBACs

Care provided by midwives avoids medical interventions and birth practices that are risk factors that lead to cesarean surgery. Avoiding the first cesarean scar has a significant beneficial impact on all future pregnancies.

Childbearing Women Attended by Midwives Are More Likely to Give Birth on Their Own without the Use of Forceps or Vacuum Extractors (Instrumental Deliveries)

Midwives are more likely to encourage the mother to walk, move around, and take comfortable positions during labor and birth. They are also more likely to give her time to push the baby out and to support her in using easier and more effective positions to give birth. This approach helps labor to progress and reduces the need for a cesarean. When a woman gives birth on her back with her legs in stirrups, she is pushing against gravity; labor takes longer; the tissues of her perineum (pelvic floor muscle) are pulled tight; it is more painful; she is more likely to tear; and her baby is at increased risk of abnormal heart rate patterns. She is also more likely to have an episiotomy and an instrumental delivery.

Both episiotomy and instrumental delivery are associated with third and fourth degree tears of the perineum, injuries to the sphincter muscle, and urinary and fetal incontinence. Women are more likely to experience pain with intercourse, hemorrhoids, infection, and additional pain for weeks and sometimes months after the birth. Many women experience psychological trauma and poor social functioning in the weeks after an assisted birth.[5] Midwifery care reduces the need for an episiotomy and instrumental assisted birth. Giving birth without these instruments reduces unintended harms to the mother and her newborn.

Women Cared for by Midwives Are Less Likely to Experience Hypertension during Pregnancy and during Labor

Hypertension is the most common complication of pregnancy and develops in about 5 to 10 percent of women. Hypertension is a medical condition that often requires a cesarean section for the safety of the mother and her baby. Pregnant women will develop complications including preeclampsia (a condition of pregnancy identified with high level of protein in the urine, swelling in the hands, legs, and feet and high blood pressure), liver failure, kidney failure, cerebral hemorrhage, abruptio placentae (a condition in which placenta detaches prematurely from the uterine wall), and a condition known as disseminated intravascular coagulation (DIC). DIC interferes with normal blood clotting. It is a life-threatening condition that may lead to thrombosis (excessive clotting) or hemorrhage throughout the body.[6] Women cared for by midwives are less likely to need a cesarean section due to hypertension.

Midwives Are Less Likely to Intervene in the Normal Progress of Labor than Physicians: They Artificially Induce and Augment Labor Less Often

Women whose labors are induced are more likely to need a cesarean section. Elective inductions (with no medical indication) are associated with an increase in the use of analgesia, epidurals, intrapartum fever, shoulder dystocia, instrumental delivery and increased cesareans for both first time and experienced mothers. Babies born by elective induction are more likely to suffer from nonreassuring fetal heart rate (fetal distress) and jaundice. They are also more likely to be of low birth weight and to require resuscitation at birth and admission to a neonatal intensive care unit (NICU).

Midwives Are Less Likely to Perform an Amniotomy (Breaking the Bag of Waters)

With an amniotomy the baby's umbilical cord is more likely to prolapse (come down ahead of the baby's head) and lead to fetal distress. Keeping the bag of waters intact until it breaks on its own also minimizes the risk for infection. Breaking the bag of waters early in labor may increase the odds for maternal and neonatal infection, nonreassuring fetal heart rate (fetal distress), and cesarean delivery.

Midwives Are More Likely to Monitor the Baby's Heart Rate by Auscultation (Listening to the Heart Rate with a Fetoscope or a Doppler Device) and Use the Electronic Fetal Monitor Intermittently (at Specified Intervals) Rather Than Continuously

Compared to the intermittent use of electronic fetal monitoring (EFM), routine use of electronic fetal monitoring increases the risk for an instrumental delivery and cesarean section without improving health outcomes.[7] In 2005 virtually all U.S. mothers (94 percent) had electronic fetal monitoring.[8] More than a decade ago the U.S. Preventive Services Task Force recommended against using electronic fetal monitoring for low-risk women in labor. Their evaluation found that physicians' fear of medical malpractice claims was affecting the standard of care more profoundly than the scientific literature.[9]

Midwives Encourage and Support Freedom of Movement for Labor and Birth

The connective tissue between the pelvic bones is very flexible during pregnancy as are all connective tissues in a pregnant woman's body. Walking and positions such as kneeling, squatting, and sitting upright during labor widen the diameters of the pelvis giving the baby more room to move downward and enhance the progress of labor. Lying flat on the back compresses the aorta that brings blood to the placenta, reducing the amount of oxygen available to the baby. Being upright, changing positions, and walking during labor according to women's needs is less painful. Being upright allows women to take advantage of gravity, align the baby, and facilitate the baby's movements through the mother's pelvis. Contractions are also more efficient. Women who walk during labor are less likely to have an instrumental delivery or a cesarean section. Women who choose to deliver in positions other than on their backs also have a shorter second stage, are less likely to need pain medication, and their babies have fewer abnormal heart rate patterns.[10]

Midwives Are More Likely to Allow Women in Labor to Eat and Drink and Receive the Nourishment They Need to Sustain the Energy They Need to Labor and Give Birth

Contrary to the commonly held belief that digestion slows down or stops during labor, research shows that calories consumed in labor are digested. When women in labor are denied oral fluids and food they experience a higher level of stress. The rational for not allowing women to eat or drink in labor is based on the belief that they may die from pulmonary aspiration of stomach contents during an unplanned cesarean section with general anesthesia. In the United States these odds are less than one in a million.[11]

Denying women nourishment during labor may lead to inefficient uterine contractions, slow progress in labor, and a diagnosis of dystocia (failure to progress). Midwives say that eating and drinking in labor allows women to feel normal and healthy rather than intimidated and apprehensive by authoritarian rules that deny them nourishment.[12]

Women Attended by Midwives Have Less Need for Pain Medication in Labor, Including Epidural Analgesia: Rather, Midwives Encourage the Use of Nonpharmacological Options for Pain Relief, Including Hydrotherapy and Massage.

Epidurals are associated with a higher risk of cesarean section for fetal distress and dystocia (nonprogressive labor).[13] Epidural analgesia in labor increases the risk for several complications, including hypotension (low blood pressure), intrapartum fever, longer first and second stages of labor, and an instrumental delivery. An epidural can slow labor and increase the need of oxytocin to activate labor again. Epidural analgesia may make it more difficult for a mother to give birth on her own. Babies are more likely to be in an occiput posterior (OP) position—an abnormal position that makes it difficult for the baby to move easily through the pelvic outlet. A cesarean section or assisted delivery is much more likely to be performed with a baby in the OP position.[14] Women cared for by midwives are encouraged to use nondrug methods of pain relief. Physical comfort, continuous emotional support, touch and massage, breathing techniques, freedom of movement, and immersion in warm water and intradermal water blocks for relief of back pain are all options that can help reduce the level and perception of pain.[15]

Midwife-Assisted Women Have a Lower Incident of Shoulder Dystocia Compared to Similar Women Being Cared for by Physicians

Shoulder dystocia, is a serious, potentially life threatening complication of second stage labor (the pushing phase). It requires specific maneuvers to deliver the baby's shoulders after the head has been born and when gentle traction is not successful. The safe delivery of a baby with shoulder dystocia requires excellent skills and a rapid response.[16] Physicians will often perform a cesarean rather than risk complications they anticipate would develop from trying to deliver a large baby with wide shoulders vaginally.

Midwifery Care Is Associated with Better Health Outcomes for Babies

Babies are less likely to be born preterm or have low birth weight. In a midwife's care babies are less likely to suffer from fetal distress (abnormal fetal heart tones) and birth trauma during labor and birth. They are also less likely to require resuscitation or special care in the neonatal intensive care unit (NICU). Midwives also have comparable or a fewer number of perinatal deaths (at 3 months).

Premature birth and low birth weight are currently a public health issue in the United States. The rate of premature birth increased almost 31 percent between 1981 (9.4 percent) and 2003 (12.3 percent) and is currently the highest ever in the country's history. Since 1996 steps taken to improve premature birth, low birth weight, and infant mortality have been slow.[17] The March of Dimes, a nonprofit organization devoted to preventing birth defects and premature birth is concerned that the increasing number of elective cesareans and medically induced labors have contributed to the rise in the number of late preterm births—babies born between 34 and 36 weeks of gestation. Compared to full-term babies, late preterm babies are more likely to have problems with maintaining their temperature, breathing, and feeding. They are also more likely to develop jaundice.[18]

With Midwifery Care Babies Are More Likely to Remain with Their Mothers throughout the Hospital Stay and Be Exclusively Breastfed up to 2 to 4 Months

The American Academy of Pediatrics, the U.S. Department of Health and Human Services, and other national and international maternal and child health organizations acknowledge breastfeeding as the most advantageous form of infant feeding. Babies that are breastfed have nutritional, immunological, and developmental advantages compared to babies that are fed milk substitutes.[19] Research shows that the mother's birth experience, the newborn's experience, and maternity birth practices have a strong influence on breastfeeding initiation and later infant feeding.[20] With a cesarean birth, mothers are less likely to initiate and maintain breastfeeding without skilled assistance and special support.

Care by Professional Midwives Reduces Costs When Compared with Physicians Working with Similar Populations

Pregnancy, childbirth, and newborn care are the second and third most expensive conditions treated in U.S. hospitals following coronary atherosclerosis (hardening of the arteries). The total national hospital bill for maternity care in 2004 was $41 billion, and for newborn care it was $34 billion. Midwives have lower rates of several childbirth-related procedures, The number of episiotomy, amniotomy, inductions, instrumental deliveries, and cesarean section and the use of electronic fetal monitoring, IV fluids, pain medications, and epidurals are lower for low-risk women cared for by midwives compared with a similar group of women cared for by physicians. Breastfeeding rates are higher and admissions to newborn intensive care units are lower with midwifery care.

Women Who Are Cared for by Midwives Are Very Satisfied with the Care They Receive

Women value the personalized care, education, and counseling that professional midwives provide. They also value the opportunity that midwives give them to participate fully in making all the decisions with regard to their care.

The model of care provided by midwives seems to be the most appropriate for low-risk women, and the "medical management model of care" is best applied and essential when during pregnancy and childbirth women are inherently at risk for or develop medical complications or diseases outside the health norms. The internationally recognized and respected researchers of *A Guide to Effective Care for Pregnancy and Childbirth* state,

It is inherently unwise, and perhaps unsafe, for women with normal pregnancies to be cared for by obstetric specialists, even if the required personnel were available. Because of time constraints, obstetricians caring for women with both normal and abnormal pregnancies have to make an impossible choice: to neglect the normal pregnancies in order to concentrate their care on those with pathology, or to spend most of their time supervising biologically normal processes. Midwives and general practitioners, on the other hand, are primarily oriented to the care of women with normal pregnancies, and are likely to have more detailed knowledge of the particular circumstances of individual women. The care that they can give to the majority of women, whose pregnancies are not affected by any major illness or serious complications, will often be more responsive to their needs than that given by specialist obstetricians.[21]

OPTIONS FOR MIDWIFERY CARE IN THE UNITED STATES

Although there is unquestionable evidence that midwifery care for low-risk pregnant women results in healthier mothers and babies access, to midwives and reimbursement for their services varies considerably in the United States. In 2005 11.2 percent of all vaginal births were attended by midwives. Although the 2005 rate was more than double the 1991 rate of 5.7 percent it is only a small fraction of births attended by professional midwives in other industrialized countries.[22]

In countries that provide health care through a national health care system midwives are required to meet professional requirements of one nationally established standard. In the United States, midwives learn their skills and obtain licensure in several ways. There are three national certification processes for midwifery that lead to a certification as a certified nurse midwife (CNM), certified midwife (CM), and certified professional midwife (CPM). In some states home birth midwives are licensed to practice without having met nationally recognized credentials. In those states, midwives are known as licensed midwives (LM) or registered midwives (RM). Nationally certified midwives must meet competency requirements and pass nationally accredited examinations.

CNMs and CMs

The certified nurse midwife (CNM) and the certified midwife (CM) credentials are both national credentials administered by the American College of Nurse-Midwives. Both require an undergraduate college degree and in most cases lead to a master's degree. CNMs are required to have a nursing background, whereas CMs are not; both CNMs and CMs undertake extensive inhospital midwifery training, and both must pass the ACNM written examination. CNMs and CMs practice primarily in hospitals, but they also work in birth centers, clinics, and the uniformed services and attend home births. Their practices generally include family planning and gynecologic services. CNMs are licensed in all fifty states, but the scope of their practice varies according to each state.

Despite the fact that midwives are trained to be licensed independent practitioners for midwifery care, five states still require that CNMs work under the
supervision of a physician. In July 2007 Pennsylvania became the last state to
grant prescriptive authority to CNMs. All states reimburse CNMs for care provided to women covered by Medicaid, and in thirty-three states private health
insurers are mandated by law to reimburse for CNM services.

Certified Professional Midwives

The certified professional midwife (CPM) credential was created by the
North American Registry of Midwives (NARM), the leading certification agency
for direct-entry midwifery in the United States. The CPM credential is accredited by the National Commission on Certifying Agencies (NCCA). Ten
direct-entry midwifery schools are accredited by the midwifery Education Accreditation Council (MEAC), which is recognized as an accrediting body for
midwifery schools by the CPMs attend births outside of a hospital setting.

This professional midwifery program includes apprenticeship, long-distance
learning, and university-based as well as institution-based programs. The CPM
credential values extensive and varied clinical experience as part of the learning process. Most states that license direct-entry midwives for out-of-hospital
practice require NARM certification, and all require that the applicant pass
NARM's written examination. As of 2007, direct-entry midwives were licensed
for out-of-hospital practice in twenty-two states. The NARM is a sister organization of the Midwives Alliance of North America (MANA), a professional
association which supports a nonmedicalized approach to birth and is inclusive
to all midwifery educational backgrounds and practice styles.[23]

The NARM recognizes that each midwife is an individual with specific practice protocols that reflect her own style and philosophy, level of experience,
and legal status and that practice guidelines may vary with each midwife.
However, CPMs are encouraged to practice according to the Midwives Model
of Care. This model is based on the fact that pregnancy and birth are normal
life events and includes monitoring the physical, psychological, and social well-
being of the mother throughout the childbearing cycle; providing the mother
with individualized education, counseling, and prenatal care, continuous hands-
on assistance during labor and delivery, and postpartum support; minimizing
technological interventions; and identifying and referring women who require
obstetrical attention. The application of this model has been proven to reduce
the incidence of birth injury, trauma, and cesarean section.[24] There are approximately 1,100 certified professional midwives (CPMs) in the United States.

THE "ETHIC OF CARING"

In their book, *Mainstreaming Midwives*, Davis-Floyd and Johnson have identified and refined common unifying elements of the unique and invaluable care
that all midwives provide to mothers and babies regardless of their educational credentials, legal status, or professional differences. They identify these

elements as comprising the "ethic of midwifery caring." These essential elements of the midwifery model of care are based on the concept of pregnancy and birth as normal life events and the unique relationship and interaction between midwives and the women they serve. This "ethic of caring" ultimately gives women a strong sense of autonomy and feeling of empowerment when they have given birth.

These elements are unique to the ethic of midwifery caring. Midwives seek opportunities to establish close connections with their patients. They build a personal dimension into the professional relationship. Regular prenatal visits provide the midwife with the opportunity to ask about her patient's family, job situation, social events, and the like. It also provides the woman the opportunity to get to know her midwife, since she also shares information about her personal and professional life. Midwives understand that a healthy pregnancy includes emotional well-being as well as physical well-being and take the time to address the issues that may be distressing to their clients. They also create a shared knowledge base with their clients, one that is based on the woman's personal and unique health condition rather than on preformulated risk factors.

Giving women concrete and particular information allows for medical decisions to be jointly made based on women's individual needs and circumstances. Their focus is on how well things are going rather than on how risky things can get. Feelings and intuitions are respected and are considered along with "rational knowledge." The quality of these interactions over the course of the pregnancy helps women to develop a sense of trust in themselves and in their midwives. Midwives are willing to be flexible and accommodate women's needs and requests within safety parameters.

This ethic of midwifery care, explain the authors, generates in women a sense of "embodied power." The mother's sense of intrinsic self-worth is enhanced, and over time during the pregnancy she develops a positive image of her pregnant body and her ability to cope with childbirth. The childbirth experience helps the mother to develop a strong sense of confidence in her ability to mother her child, and she learns to take more responsibility for making choices for her own as well as her family's health care.[25]

BARRIERS TO MIDWIFERY CARE: LIMITING CHOICES FOR CHILDBEARING FAMILIES

Despite the wealth of studies that demonstrate the excellence of midwifery care for low-risk women, the proportion being about 90 percent of expectant mothers in industrialized countries,[26] existing legal, political, and economic barriers to making midwifery care accessible to women are difficult to overcome. This is the case for both certified nurse midwives and certified professional midwives who practice outside of a hospital setting.

In 1998 the University of California, San Francisco, Center for Health Professions convened a Taskforce on Midwifery to explore the impact of market-driven changes in the delivery and financing of health care with regard to midwifery, issues facing their profession, and the role that midwives play in women's health care. As a result of their findings, the Taskforce made fourteen recommendations designed to benefit women and their families through increased access to midwives and the midwifery model of care. Their recommendations considered all three nationally recognized professional midwives: certified nurse midwives (CNMs), certified midwives (CMs), and certified professional midwives (CPMs). The two leading recommendations were that midwives should be recognized as independent and collaborative practitioners with the rights and responsibility that all independent professionals share and that every health care system should integrate midwifery into the continuum of care for women by contracting with or employing midwives and informing women of their options.[27]

Unlike in other industrialized countries where midwives and physicians work collaboratively, in the United States many licensed midwives continue to defend their right to practice in the face of strong opposition by state and national medical associations. Medical staff in some hospitals have used their power to deny hospital privileges to CNMs to prevent them from establishing practices in their area. They have restricted the midwives' ability to practice by requiring them to be employed by physicians, by requiring a physician to be present for all deliveries attended by CNMs, by arbitrarily requiring midwives to have a master's degree, and by requiring a physician to cosign nurse-midwives' entries on medical records. Some anesthesiologists have refused to give epidurals and some pediatricians have refused to examine babies for patients cared for by nurse-midwives. Physicians who support midwives and agree to provide backup have been threatened with the loss of their own jobs or hospital privileges. Despite the excellent track record of CNMs, some malpractice insurance companies have either denied them coverage or set exorbitant fees that have forced some independent practitioners and birth centers out of business.[28]

In July 2007 Pennsylvania became the last state to grant prescription authority to Certified Nurse Midwives.[29] In February 2008 a bill was introduced in the Oklahoma Senate (Bill 1638) to legally establish physician supervision of CNMs and other advanced practice nurses and to transfer their oversight from the Board of Nursing to the Board of Medical Licensure. CNMs are independent licensed practitioners who do not require physician supervison. Similarly, Oklahoma Senate Bill 1523 was introduced to establish physician ownership or direct operation of "retail health clinics" and legislate physician supervision for nonphysician practitioners.[30]

Despite the fact that the North American Registry of Midwives (NARM) is recognized by the NCCA as the certifying body for direct-entry midwives to earn the certified professional midwife (CPM) credential, many states still do not recognize or support the services CPMs provide. The legal status of direct-entry midwives and consequently access to midwifery care varies illogically from state to state. In some states direct-entry midwives are neither clearly legal nor illegal. The laws are silent, vague, or inconsistent. In some states, nonnurse midwifery is legal but not regulated. Some states do not require that midwives have a formal and extensive education but do license direct-entry midwives. Licensure or certification is optional in yet other states. The Department of Health and Social Services assumes responsibility for licensing direct-entry midwives in certain states.[31] The Midwives Alliance of North America (MANA) and the North American Registry of Midwives (NARM) Web sites post a current list of the legal status of direct-entry midwives state-by-state.

Susan Jenkins, an attorney in private practice and a birth policy activist, writes, "At a time when women are seeking out-of-hospital maternity care in increasing numbers, the expanded scope of medical and nursing practice acts in states without licensure has made direct-entry midwives the target of criminal prosecution, imprisonment and administrative proceedings. By contrast, in states with licensure, even licensed midwives are finding themselves in the precarious position of either following the guidelines of a flawed medical system or risking large fines, loss of licensure, and criminal prosecution and imprisonment."[32]

In 2008 the Birth Policy Coalition sponsored the The Big Push for Midwives national campaign to advocate for regulation and licensure of Certified Professional Midwives (CPMs) in all fifty states and the District of Columbia. The campaign is also fighting back against the attempts of the American Medical Association (AMA) Scope of Practice Partnership that effectively denies consumers access to legal midwifery care. As of 2008 forty states allowed CPMs to practice; of those, twenty-four license and regulate the profession. In the state of Missouri CPMs are still classified as felons. For 25 years vested interests have fought the passage of a bill to license CPMs in the state, despite the fact that they have met national standards and state regulations. In May 2008 the Missouri Senate passed a bill (HB2081) to provide legal access to out-of-hospital midwifery care and advocates were looking for the same from the Missouri House of Representatives.[33]

Regarding American midwives, Davis-Floyd and Johnson write, "Midwives do their best to provide women with birth options they would not otherwise enjoy and with lifetime health care based on notions of the normalcy of women's bodies and a sense of the importance of an ongoing relationship between the client and the practitioner. Legal or illegal, plain or professional, nurse- or direct-entry, American midwives remain dedicated to serving women and babies in woman-centered ways."[34]

ESPECIALLY FOR MOTHERS

Midwifery care and the excellent outcomes it provides is a choice that is being increasingly denied to women in the United States. Women who want to have access to midwifery care will have to take the initiative to guarantee their rights to access these services and to make sure that midwives are included as primary care providers entitled to reimbursement by health care insurance plans, Medicare and Medicaid.

If you are considering midwifery care, you may want to do the following:

- Ask your health insurance carrier if services provided by midwives are covered. If not, then why?
- Ask your employer to offer you a choice of health plans that cover midwifery services.
- Write to your state legislators and representatives in Congress about increasing safe access to professional midwifery care and decriminalizing the profession.
- Become involved in consumer advocate organizations that are working to legalize professional midwives and offer women choices for maternity care.

RESOURCES

ACNM. My Midwife, http://www.mymidwife.org.
American College of Nurse Midwives, http://www.midwife.org.
Birth Policy Coaltion, http://www.birthpolicy.org.
Citizens for Midwifery, http://www.cfm.org.
MANA. Mothers Naturally, http://mothersnaturally.org.
Midwives Association of North America, http://www.mana.org.
North American Registry of Midwie, http://www.narm.org.

18

OUT OF HOSPITAL BIRTH LOWERS THE ODDS FOR CESAREAN SECTION

> Birth is profoundly affected by the environment in which it takes place. Ideally, every laboring woman and the team that supports and facilitates her efforts to birth work together in an environment that is the most comfortable and safe for the birthing mother. For many women, families, and providers, that safe, comfortable place to birth is in the home or birth center.[1]

The safety of out-of-hospital birth is a controversial issue in some countries and respected as every woman's right in others. In many parts of the world women give birth at home out of necessity for lack of access to a maternity care facility or economic reasons or because their cultural traditions have always valued home birth as a social and spiritual life event. In countries where hospital births are the norm, some mothers prefer the privacy, comfort, freedom and control, and continuity of care that a home birth provides. Some families prefer to give birth in a birth center. Women who choose out-of-hospital birth and the care providers who support them view pregnancy and birth as a normal physiological process in which routine medical interventions are unnecessary. Should a medical complication develop, the use of interventions should be evidence-based. Current evidence supports the safety of both home birth and birth which takes place in birth centers. Without compromising the health and well-being of mothers and babies this low intervention model of care provided to women in out-of-hospital births substantially reduces the odds of needing a cesarean section.[2]

There is no evidence that hospital births are more or less safe for low-risk women who plan a home birth with a qualified professional and prearranged collaborative care and appropriate arrangement of transfer to a hospital if the need arises.[3,4] The World Health Organization recommends that healthy low-risk pregnant women should give birth where they feel safe with referral to a medical center and access to appropriate resources as necessary. This includes water births.[5]

In the Netherlands, midwives have practiced with legislative protection since the fifteenth century. Home birth is a culturally and legally supported choice that all women are entitled to. Pregnancy and childbirth are seen as normal and healthy events. Low-risk women with an anticipated normal birth are cared for by the "first line" of midwives and can choose to have their baby at home or at a maternity hotel, "kraamhotel." Since 1995 there has been a resurgence of home births in the Netherlands and one out of three women chooses home birth. Women with a high-risk pregnancy are referred to the "second line" or medical midwives who will care for them in a hospital setting supervised by a physician. Obstetrician-Gynecologists who practice in Holland are the primary caregivers only for pregnant women with serious medical complications. They are known as the "third line" of midwifery care.[6]

Mary Zwart, professional Dutch midwife and founder of the European Perinatal School gives us an insight into the process of establishing a successful collaborative model of care in the Netherlands: "The Kloostermanlist (named after a Dutch obstetrician) was the initial attempt at collaborative care between Dutch midwives and Dutch obstetricians. It was first published in 1985 and at first fully rejected by the physicians. Eventually collaboration between midwives, family physicians, obstetricians, perinatologists and pediatricians was achieved. Today known as the Vademecum, the risk selection list is collaboratively revised every 5 years, but it is the 'fist line' midwife that is still responsible for the referral to another level of care. This Dutch model of midwifery care and support for home birth with established collaborative care from all maternity care disciplines is responsible for the excellent maternal and perinatal outcomes of home births in the Netherlands."[7]

In Wales the government supports the training of midwives in home birth skills and encourages women with normal pregnancies to consider giving birth at home.[8] The U.K. Department of Health supports women's rights to choose their place of birth, and home is one of their options.[9] In New Zealand home birth is now a free service available to all women who choose one. In 2003 New Zealand midwives attended 72.6 percent of normal births.[10,11]

Australia has a public hospital system free to all birthing families who choose a hospital birth. However, the hospital system is highly medicalized, and Australian women who want to have a home birth must cover their own costs. Few private health insurance companies reimburse for the services of an independent midwife. Australia only recognizes registered midwives, who have been exclusively nurse-midwives until recently, when direct-entry midwives, trained in tertiary institutions, have entered the midwifery workforce. In most states existing legislation forbids unregistered midwives from attending home births. Currently in Australia there is a growing consumer movement advocating for the government to sponsor community-based midwifery, with the choice of home or hospital birth (as exists in the neighbouring New Zealand). Advocates have developed a National Maternity Action Plan that calls for choice of birthplace for pregnant women and continuity of care with a community-based midwife.[12]

Midwifery care and home birth in Canada is rapidly gaining public and legislative support. Home birth and midwifery care is publicly funded in some provinces and privately funded in others. The Canadian Association of Midwives works collaboratively with the Society of Obstetricians and Gynecologists of Canada to provide safe care for home birth and access to emergency services and hospitals when transport is needed.[13]

HOME BIRTH LOWERS THE ODDS FOR A CESAREAN

In 2005 99 percent of all women who gave birth in the United States did so in a hospital. Of the 1 percent of out-of-hospital births, 65.4 percent were home births.[14] Low-risk women who plan a home birth with a professional midwife or physician have similar health outcomes and in some cases better outcomes compared to similar women who have hospital births. They also have lower cesarean rates.[15] A Cochrane review of the safety of home births for low risk women found no strong evidence to favor either planned hospital or planned home birth. The shift from planned home birth to planned hospital birth for low-risk women, concluded the authors of the study, was not supported by good evidence. Moreover, hospital birth for these healthy women may increase unnecessary interventions and complications without any beneficial outcomes.[16]

One study is often cited as evidence that home birth is less safe than births occurring in a hospital.[17] However researchers repeatedly disqualify the study for these reasons: Some births were unattended (that is, no qualified health professional was assisting). Women were not low-risk, and preterm births, twins, and breech presentations were included. Some birth attendants were not qualified to attend births at all. And not all women actually planned to give birth outside the hospital.[18]

Home Birth Is Safe When Four Important Criteria Are Met

Planned home birth is as safe as planned hospital birth for similar groups of women when four important criteria are in place:

1. Pregnant women are low-risk.
2. Home is chosen as the intended place for birth.
3. The primary care provider is qualified according to professional licensing standards and trained to assist at home births.
4. A collaborative relationship with consulting physicians and a medical center exists with clear guidelines for continuity of care should a complication arise where the mother or baby would benefit from the transfer.

Based on a systematic review of 16 years of scientific studies the evidence shows that compared to low-risk women who plan a hospital birth, low-risk women who plan home births have similar or better outcomes with fewer medical interventions and fewer cesareans. In 2007, a systematic review conducted by the Coalition for Improving Maternity Services Expert Work Group compared the outcomes of low-risk women who planned home births with a similar group of low-risk women who planned to give birth in a hospital. The researchers found several health advantages from home births for both mothers and their infants. Overall, home births required less medical interventions but had similar or better outcomes and fewer cesareans. Women who gave birth at home had the same or lower rates of induction and augmentation of labor. They were less likely to need IV fluids, to have an amniotomy (intentional breaking of the bag of waters), or to have continuous electronic fetal monitoring. (Routine continuous electronic monitoring and amniotomy are associated with an increased risk for cesarean section.) At home women had more freedom of movement and more choice of positions for labor and birth. Ultimately the home birth group had fewer cesareans and more VBACs, less or similar incidents of maternal infection requiring antibiotics after birth, and less need for a blood transfusion.

Perinatal outcomes from the planned home births were similar to planned hospital births. Similar numbers of newborns were admitted to the intensive care unit, and similar or fewer numbers of newborns suffered from birth traumas. The number of babies who died in the first 28 days (perinatal mortality) was similar in the home birth and hospital birth groups. Overall 85 percent of women who fist gave birth in a hospital and went on to have a home birth preferred their experience of birth at home. Of women who planned to have other children 91 percent said they would have another home birth.[19]

There is a long-standing perception in the United States that women who choose to have a home birth with a nonnurse professional midwife put themselves and their babies at great risk. The argument has been that unlike some other countries, the United States does not have an integrated health care system with efficient emergency services in place to receive transfers from home births. The largest prospective study of home births in North America with professional midwives gives us an accurate picture of the safety of home birth when the four criteria of planned home birth are met.[20]

This landmark study published in the *British Medical Journal* included data on 5,418 low-risk pregnant women across the United States and Canada who planned to give birth at home with a direct-entry (certified professional) midwife. A total of 409 midwives participated in the study. The births took place in 2000 in areas of both countries where home birth is not well integrated into the health care system. The study authors followed the home births up to 6 weeks postpartum and compared the home birth outcomes with data from official birth certificates of low-risk hospital births which took place in the United States in that same year.

Medical intervention rates were consistently low, and so was the cesarean rate. The cesarean rate was 3.7 percent for the home birth group compared to 19 percent for the hospital births. The home birth group had a 9.6 percent rate for continuous electronic fetal monitoring compared to 84.3 percent for hospital births. Induction of labor was 9.6 percent compared to 21 percent for the hospital births. Augmentation of labor was twice as high in the hospital birth group, 18.9 percent versus 9.2 percent. The combined forceps and vacuum extraction rate was 1.6 percent for the home births compared to 7.4 percent. The epidural rate was 4.7 percent for the home birth group compared to 63 percent for all risk categories in the United States during 2000.

The need to transfer women to a hospital during or after birth was 12.1 percent. The majority of women were transferred during labor for failure to progress, pharmacological pain relief, or exhaustion. After the birth 1.2 percent of the mothers were transferred for maternal hemorrhage (0.6 percent) or a retained placenta (0.5 percent). No mothers died. and the intrapartum and neonatal mortality rate for this low-risk group was 1.7 deaths for 1,000 home births, the same as in other studies of low-risk home births and hospital births in North America. Home birth for a breech and twin pregnancies are controversial. Some midwives are skilled and experienced with these types of births; others "risk out" these clients and refer the mothers to other care providers. There were eighty planned breech home births in this study. Two of these infants died. There were no deaths among the thirteen sets of twins born at home. At 6 weeks postpartum 98.3 percent of babies and 98.4 percent of mothers were in good health, and 95.8 percent were breastfeeding, 89.7 percent exclusively.

Pregnancy and childbirth are significant life events with cultural and psychosocial implications for the mother and her family. Current evidence confirms that for normal pregnancies women who choose to give birth at home have lower risks of complications and lower cesarean rates when cared for by qualified professionals with access to medical consultants and prearranged transfer to a medical facility. National and state health services, employers, and health insurers should include planned home births and the qualified professionals who attend them in their maternity care reimbursement policies.

FREESTANDING BIRTH CENTERS

In countries with a national health care system that has birth centers, birth "hotels" or "home-from-home" birth centers operate under the supervision and licensing of the national department of health. In the United States some hospitals offer low-risk expectant mothers the choice of giving birth in their birth center as opposed to their labor and delivery units. Inhospital birth centers have in-house capabilities for emergency services if they become necessary. The safety of inhospital birth centers is acknowledged. However, the safety of giving birth in freestanding birth centers in the United States has sometimes been questioned. A freestanding birth center is a safe option for low-risk women considering an out-of-hospital birth. Current evidence supports the safety, excellent health outcomes, low-intervention rates, and lower cesarean rates associated with freestanding birth centers when compared with low-risk births in a hospital setting.[21]

Freestanding birth centers are independently run and staffed by qualified professionals. Care is provided by midwives and rarely by physicians. Birth centers have contractual agreements with family physicians, obstetricians, pediatricians and other professionals. They are integrated into the community health care system and have established protocols for transfer to hospitals in case of need. Birth centers provide prenatal care and care during labor and birth, as well as postpartum care and breastfeeding support for low-risk women, in a homelike setting. Some birth centers are also equipped for water births.

The birth center model of care is focused on wellness, safety, responsibility for self-care, and shared decision making. The staff helps to educate the mother and her family in each step of her pregnancy to enhance her self-confidence and ability to give birth. Expectant mothers are given the freedom to choose how they want to give birth. They can assume any position they wish for labor and birth. Family members and children are welcome to participate at the birth. Birth centers do not have routine procedures such as continuous fetal monitoring, episiotomy, and use of IVs. Each birth is individually considered. Mothers are free to move, eat, and drink as they wish during labor. The baby's heart rate is typically monitored by auscultation (handheld device) or a fetoscope. Mothers and newborns are not separated at birth; there are no newborn nurseries. Breastfeeding is highly encouraged, and bonding and breastfeeding follow naturally after the birth. All newborn exams are performed close to the parents. Birth centers provide continuity of care and support for early parenting by helping families identify appropriate resources in their community.

In case of complications, birth centers have plans for the transport of the mother and her baby to a hospital facility for additional care. According to the American Association of Birth Centers, about 12 percent of women need to be transferred during labor, but only about 2 percent of these are emergency transfers. In the United States many major health insurers and state Medicaid programs cover the cost of giving birth in a birth center.

The American Association of Birth Centers recommends and encourages freestanding birth centers to become licensed and accredited. Licensing and the regulation of birth centers vary with each state. To ensure the safety of childbearing women the American Public Health Association (APHA) Guidelines for Licensing and Regulating Birth Centers recommends that outside of the mother's home or a hospital, any professional office or facility that operates as a birth center for normal uncomplicated pregnancies should be licensed and accredited according to national safety standards.[22]

GIVING BIRTH IN A BIRTH CENTER LOWERS THE ODDS FOR CESAREAN SECTION

Birth centers are a safe place to give birth. They also serve the psychosocial needs of women and their families. In 2005 10,217 women gave birth in a freestanding birth center.[23] A systematic review of seven high quality studies by the Coalition for Improving Maternity Services Expert Work Group compared health outcomes of women who gave birth in a birth center with similar groups of women who gave birth in a hospital. They found that birth centers used fewer interventions, had lower cesarean rates and similar or better perinatal outcomes. These findings were similar despite the fact that the births took place in several different countries.

Both groups of women, those who intended to give birth in a birth center and those who planned a hospital birth, had similar antepartum (before labor) hospital admission rates. The women who gave birth in a birth center had fewer inductions of labor and fewer oxytocin augmentations of labor. They were less likely to have an amniotomy (artificial breaking of bag of waters). And they were also less likely to be monitored continuously by an electronic fetal monitor. They had fewer episodes of fetal heart rate abnormalities. These women were much more likely to walk during labor, eat, and drink and less likely to need intravenous fluids (IVs). Women who gave birth in a hospital used analgesia and epidurals more than the women in the birth center who were more likely to use nonpharmacological pain relief. The nonpharmacological methods of pain relief provided in the birth centers were highly effective, since the majority of women did not use analgesia or chose to have an epidural. In the birth centers more women had normal births (not requiring forceps or vacuum extraction). They also had fewer cesareans. Women in birth centers had similar rates of infection and use of antibiotics as the women who gave birth in the hospitals.

With regard to the health of the newborns, there were fewer incidents of fetal heart abnormality for babies born in birth centers. Fewer infants required an evaluation and treatment for infection. Epidurals used in labor raise the mother's body temperature, indicating she may have a fever. To rule out a neonatal infection newborns are tested for the possibility of infection also. The appearance of thick meconium (baby's first bowel movement in utero) in the amniotic fluid is a sign of fetal distress. Both groups of newborns had a similar rate of thick meconium. The infant low birth weight rates were similar. The same number of newborns needed to be admitted to an intensive care unit after birth, and a similar number were readmitted following complications.[24]

The Coalition for Improving Maternity Services Expert Work Group's review included the National Birth Center Study, the largest study of birth centers in the United States. It reported on 11,814 women who were admitted in labor at eighty-four birth centers in the United States in 1992. The women in the study received safe care with fewer interventions and fewer cesareans. Only 4.4 percent of the mothers needed a cesarean section. Of all the labors 90 percent were monitored by auscultation (handheld device) and 10 percent with electronic fetal monitoring. Only 20 percent needed IV fluids, and 41 percent had clear fluids or solid food during labor. Only 3 percent of mothers chose to have an epidural (and consequently were transferred to a hospital), and 13 percent chose to have systemic analgesics (for example, Nubain, Demerol, and Stadol). Half the mothers used either the shower or the tub to help with pain relief, and 35 percent chose to have a massage during labor. When giving birth, 89 percent of the mothers chose not to deliver on their backs. When congenital anomalies (inherent birth defects) were excluded the perinatal mortality rate was 0.7 per 1,000 live births. The overall perinatal mortality rate was 1.3 per 1,000 births, a significantly lower rate than the national average for U.S. births that same year.[25,26]

Research shows that the overwhelming majority of women who chose an out-of-hospital birth expressed great satisfaction with their care and said that if they would become pregnant again, they would choose to do the same.[27] It is the midwifery model of care that is practiced at home births and in birth centers that ensures low intervention rates, fewer complications, good outcomes, and lower cesarean rates.

DELEGITIMIZING OUT-OF-HOSPITAL BIRTH IN THE UNITED STATES

In the United States, despite clear evidence to support the safety of out-of-hospital birth with qualified midwives, some medical societies and state legislations are denying childbearing women the option to choose out-of-hospital birth. In the October 2006, the executive board of the ACOG (American College of obstetricians and Gynecologists) issued a statement of policy, "Out-of Hospital Births in the United States." In it the ACOG stated, "Studies comparing the safety and outcome of U.S. births in the hospital with those occurring in other settings are limited and have not been scientifically rigorous. The development of well-designed research studies of sufficient size, prepared in consultation with obstetric departments and approved by institutional review boards, might clarify the comparative safety of births in different settings. Until the results of such studies are convincing, ACOG strongly opposes out-of-hospital births. Although ACOG acknowledges a woman's right to make informed decisions regarding her delivery, ACOG does not support programs or individuals that advocate for or who provide out-of-hospital births." The ACOG also stated that hospitals and birth centers within a hospital complex were the safest place to give birth.[28]

The ACOG's policy statement on out-of-hospital birth was strongly refuted by several professional organizations and consumer advocates groups. In a letter to the ACOG issued by the American College of Nurse-Midwives (ACNM) and cosigned by eight other leading organizations in maternity care, the ACNM wrote, "The troubling nature of this statement places in jeopardy access to a valid, evidence-based system of care. Providers who support evidence-based care have an ethical responsibility to offer access to care at all levels and in all settings for these families."[29] The American Association of Birth Centers (AABC) also responded to this policy: "The statement does not appear to be evidence-based, and AABC has been unable to find a factual basis to support this sweeping pronouncement."[30]

Childbirth Connection (formerly the Maternity Center Association) of New York, a nationally recognized nonprofit maternity care advocacy group for improving the quality of maternity care and five other nationally influential health advocacy organizations also addressed their concerns. They anticipated that this policy would undermine women's legal entitlement to informed consent which the ACOG's own *Ethics in Obstetrics and Gynecology* supported. The groups also expressed concern that the medical association's position conflicted with currently established state, federal, and corporate policies that support women's choice for out-of-hospital births, the professionals and facilities that provide the services, and the regulatory and reimbursement policies related to out-of-hospital births that were already in place.[31]

In May 2007 in response to public and professional concerns, the American College of Obstetricians and Gynecologist issued another statement of policy, "Home Births in the United States." In this statement, the ACOG revised its position and acknowledged that freestanding birth centers that meet recognized accreditation standards are also a safe place to give birth. However, its position regarding home birth did not change. Nor did ACOG cite any study to support its position.[32,33] In February 2008 the organization once again reiterated its position against home births, this time blaming women for putting their babies at risk: "ACOG does not support programs that advocate for, or individuals who provide, home births.... Childbirth decisions should not be dictated or influenced by what's fashionable, trendy, or the latest cause célèbre."[34]

The Need to Support Out-of-Hospital Birth

Evidence shows that collaborating and consulting throughout the perinatal period with other maternity services results in safer outcomes for mothers and babies. Noncooperation from maternity care professionals can impact their transfer to a higher level of care when necessary and the quality of the care they receive.[35] Ultimately, professional associations and policy makers who do not support or encourage collaboration with legally qualified midwives who support out-of-hospital birth may be putting women and their infants' health and well-being at risk.

ESPECIALLY FOR MOTHERS

Some mothers feel safe giving birth in a hospital; others feel safe giving birth at home or in a birth center. Out-of-hospital birth is a safe option for low-risk women who are cared for by professionally recognized midwives and physicians. Out-of-hospital birth gives women more freedom to shape their birth environment, but it also requires them to take more responsibility for their own care. Women who choose to give birth at home or at a birth center are usually ready to take more responsibility for their care during pregnancy as well as for labor and birth. They are also willing to forgo an epidural for pain relief. If you are considering having an out-of-hospital birth find out if there is a hospital nearby that will care for you in case there is a need to transport you or your newborn for medical care. These are some questions you may want to ask your midwife for a home birth or your care providers at a freestanding birth center.

For a Home Birth—Questions to Ask Your Midwife or Physician

- How, when, and where did you receive your midwifery education?
- Are you certified or licensed? By whom, and till what date?
- How many births have you attended alone? And how many with a partner?
- What prenatal tests do you recommend? At which time in the pregnancy?
- What physician collaboration or backup do you have?
- If there is a complication, and you recommend a transfer during labor, will you accompany me to the hospital? Would you stay with me?
- What is the approximate rate of complications requiring transport in your practice?
- Do you carry oxygen to births? (The answer should be yes).
- Do you carry a vacuum extractor to births? (The answer should be no).
- Do you maintain statistics from your practice? May I see them?
- How many women are due within a month of my due date?
- Do you work with a partner? If so, what are his or her qualifications?
- What is your plan if another one of your clients is in labor at the same time as I am?
- Do you participate in a local professional association? Peer review?
- Do you use pharmaceutical products to induce labor? What about complimentary/alternative therapies?
- What do you use to treat postpartum hemorrhage?
- In what situations would you consider referring me to a physician or hospital during my prenatal care? During labor? After the birth?
- What emergency equipment would you bring to the birth?
- Is your certification in neonatal resuscitation up to date?
- Do you work with a pediatrician or family physician?
- What is your schedule for prenatal visits? How many home visits do you do make before the baby comes? How often?
- How often will you make postpartum visits?
- What do your fees include?
- May we contact your former clients?

For a Freestanding Birth Center—Questions to Ask

- Is the birth centered licensed? Is it accredited?
- What are the working hours? Is it always open?
- Which number can I call if I have questions? Which number does my family/ friends call when I am at the birth center?
- Do you have hydrotherapy tubs?
- Is there a playroom for children and/or a room for the family?
- Can my family stay with me during labor and birth?

- Do you provide translators?
- What arrangements are in place in case of complications?
- How quickly can I be transferred to a hospital if necessary?
- Do you accept my health insurance plan? Will I need to pay for any additional services?
- What classes do you offer for expectant parents?
- When would you consider me high-risk and no longer ineligible to give birth in your center?
- Do members of the birth center staff have privileges at the community hospital?
- Would the birth center staff come with me to the hospital and stay with me until the birth?

RESOURCES

American Association of Birth Centers, http://www.birthcenters.org (last accessed May 23, 2008).

Childbirth Connection, Choosing a Caregiver, http://www.childbirthconnection.org/article.asp?ck=10158 (last accessed May 23, 2008).

Goer, Henci. Is Home Birth Safe? http://parenting.ivillage.com/pregnancy/plabor/0,6rl1,00.html (last accessed May 23, 2008).

Home Birth, U.K., http://www.homebirth.org.uk/ (last accessed May 23, 2008).

Midwives Alliance of North America, http://www.mana.org (last accessed May 23, 2008).

19

Especially for Mothers: Reducing the Odds for a Cesarean—What To Do during Pregnancy

Every woman should have the opportunity to receive accurate and up-to-date information about the benefits and risks of all procedures, drugs, and tests suggested for use during pregnancy, birth, and the postpartum period, with the rights to informed consent and informed refusal.[1]

Today cesareans are increasingly being performed for reasons that are no longer strongly supported by evidence. Whether or not you will have a cesarean is dependent on many things other than your health or the health of your baby. Who you choose as your care provider, where you choose to give birth, and what tests of procedures you may have during pregnancy make a difference. By making informed choices you lower your odds for having a cesarean delivery. The chapter lists the important issues you may want to think about.

Explore Your Options for Care Providers

Evidence shows that for healthy, low-risk pregnant women, care provided by professional midwives reduces the risk for cesarean section when compared to care provided by physicians for a similar group of women.[2] Family physicians also have a lower rate of cesareans compared to obstetricians/ gynecologists. You may want to find out more about access to midwifery care and accredited birth centers in your community and coverage for midwifery services by your health care insurance provider.

Consider Your Place of Birth

If you are a healthy woman with an uncomplicated pregnancy you should know that having your baby at home (with a qualified professional and access to a medical facility) or at a freestanding birth center (with access to a medical facility) reduces the odds for complications that may lead to a cesarean section once labor has begun. Giving birth at home or at a birth center is safe for women with an uncomplicated pregnancy.[3]

HAVE AN EARLY ULTRASOUND TO DETERMINE YOUR "REAL" DUE DATE

Many women have labor induced because they have been told that their pregnancy has gone past their due date. Induction of labor for healthy women increases the risk for a cesarean. About 4 to 14 percent of women do not go into labor on their own by the end of the 42nd week. Calculating the due date by going back to the first day of the last menstrual period, as it is often done, may be an inaccurate form of measure. This method is based on a 28-day menstrual cycle. If a woman's cycle is other than 28 days or if she became pregnant while she was on oral contraceptives or soon after their use the date may be off by 3 days. Often women are induced because they don't go into spontaneous labor by their due date, increasing their risk of cesarean section. Evidence shows that calculating the due date based on an early ultrasound scan is a more accurate method of estimating the due date (when women are not sure of the date of conception) and would avoid induction for an otherwise post–due date pregnancy.[4]

AVOID A ROUTINE ULTRASOUND IN LATE PREGNANCY (AFTER 24 WEEKS OF GESTATION)

Some care providers recommend a late pregnancy ultrasound routinely, even for women with no medical risk factors. Research shows that routine late pregnancy screening does not improve health outcomes for mothers or babies when compared with women who do not have the screening. However, routine late pregnancy ultrasound screening can potentially increase the use of major interventions including a cesarean section.[5]

AVOID SCREENING FOR A "BIG" BABY (MACROSOMIA)

Sometimes a care provider recommends that a woman be screened—by X-ray, ultrasound, computerized tomography scanning, or magnetic resonance imaging (MRI)—to determine the weight of her baby at birth. Based on these measurements the care provider decides whether or not the baby is "too big" to be born vaginally. This is called pelvimetry. Pelvimetry is an inaccurate method of predicting the size of the baby and cannot predict whether or not the baby will move down through the mother's pelvis. An ultrasound screening has an error margin of 10 to 20 percent. Women who have pelvimetry are more likely to have a cesarean, but there is no evidence that the health outcomes of babies are improved. Medical experts state that pelvimetry should not be used to make decisions about a vaginal or a cesarean birth.[6]

You have a better chance of easing your labor with a big baby when you are free to move and change positions in labor and birth. Learn more about effective positions. Find out more about helping labor progress and discuss your options with your care provider. This will help you make an informed decision about the best way for you to have your baby.

RECONSIDER AN ELECTIVE CESAREAN FOR A "BIG" BABY

Given that the diagnosis of fetal macrosomia (big baby) is inexact, an elective caesarean section should not routinely be offered to women who are not also diabetic. Based on expert opinions a cesarean may be considered when the baby is expected to weigh more than 5000 g when diabetes is not a factor and more than 4500 g for women with diabetes.[7] There is a strong belief that "big" babies born vaginally are at high risk for shoulder dystocia. Shoulder dystocia is a complication that can occur in the pushing phase. When the baby's head is delivered but the shoulders remain stuck the baby's chest can become compressed reducing the oxygen supply to the heart and brain. Often those "big" babies are born within normal weight range. Experts state that almost of half of the cases of shoulder dytocia occur in infants weighting less than 4000 g.[8]

Shoulder dystocia can be resolved when care providers are skilled and experienced with specific manueuvers (like McRoberts' position or the Gaskin maneuver).[9] There is no evidence to suggest that a cesarean is safer for a big baby, but often a cesarean is recommended because many practioners are not experienced with shoulder dystocia.[10] Compared to care provided to a similar population midwives have a lower or equivalent rate of shoulder dystocia than physicians.[11]

RETHINK AN ELECTIVE CESAREAN FOR TWINS AT TERM

With a twin pregnancy the risks of life-threatening complications at the time of birth are greater. However, if the twins are ready to be born and the first twin is in a head-down position (cephalic presentation) there is no evidence that a cesarean section improves the health of the second twin. If the first twin is breech, there is currently not enough information about which is the best option, but most practitioners will recommend a cesarean. It is becoming increasingly difficult to find a care provider skilled and experienced with twin vaginal births. Should you decide a cesarean is the best option for you it's best not to schedule it before the 38th week of pregnancy because it increases the risk of breathing problems for the twins at birth.[12,13]

RECONSIDER AN ELECTIVE CESAREAN FOR SMALL FOR GESTATIONAL AGE BABY

Babies who do not grow to their potential in the womb are born smaller. They are known as small for gestational age. Those babies are at higher risk of neonatal morbidity and mortality. But, as yet, it is unknown whether or not a planned cesarean improves their health outcomes. Medical experts recommend that a woman should be given accurate information regarding both vaginal and cesarean births, so she can make an informed decision about how she wants to give birth.[14]

RECONSIDER AN ELECTIVE CESAREAN TO PREVENT PELVIC FLOOR DYSFUNCTION

Increasingly women are hearing that by having a cesarean and by bypassing labor they will be protected from experiencing urinary or anal incontinence. However, the evidence shows that a scheduled cesarean does not protect women from moderate to severe urinary incontinence and anal incontinence in the long term. In the short term an elective cesarean will reduce the odds for urinary incontinence in approximately 6 percent or less women at 1 year after childbirth and will protect about 3 percent of women from anal incontinence at 1 year.

There is no strong evidence that planning a cesarean instead of having a normal birth protects women from experiencing incontinence beyond the age of fifty. Severe symptoms of postpartum urinary incontinence are similar in the long run whether women have a planned cesarean or not. Much of the damage done to the pelvic floor can be linked to common birth practices, like women being instructed to push forcefully in second stage or to push when they don't feel the urge. With an instrumental delivery (with forceps or vacuum extractor) and an episiotomy women are more likely to suffer from damage to the pelvic floor.[15,16,17]

When a care provider pushes down on the mother's abdomen to hasten the birth of the baby (applying fundal pressure) there is increased risk for perineal tears that can extend into or through the anal muscle. Women are more likely to suffer from third and fourth degree perineal lacerations with an episiotomy and an instrumental delivery. This condition can have significant long-term effects.[18]

Compared with women who give birth on their own, women who have an instrumental delivery are more likely to have complications that include anal muscle tears, pain, sexual problems, bowel problems, and infection.[19]

Incontinence is associated with other issues not related to childbirth at all. These include smoking, hormone therapy, having had a hysterectomy, repeat urinary tract infections, excess weight, and some chronic diseases and medications. Women may want to consider these factors before scheduling a cesarean to prevent damage to the pelvic floor.[20]

IF YOU HAVE A SERIOUS INFECTION

Hepatitis B

If you have hepatitis B and you agreed to have your baby vaccinated and receive immunoglobulin at birth you can have a normal birth. A planned cesarean will not reduce the risk of transmitting the infection to the baby.[21]

Hepatitis C

If you are infected with hepatitis C a planned cesarean will not reduce the chances of transmitting the virus to your baby. However, it will increase the risks for complications for you and your baby.[22]

HIV

If you are HIV positive and become pregnant a planned cesarean delivery may reduce the risk of mother-to-child transmission of HIV.[23]

HIV and Hepatitis C

If you are infected with the HIV and also infected with the hepatitis C virus a planned cesarean may reduce the chance of transmission of both infections to the baby.[24]

Genital Herpes

Genital herpes is an infection of the areas surrounding the vagina, lips around the opening of the vagina, and the anus. It is caused by the herpes simplex virus (HSV). It is possible to acquire a genital herpes infection not and notice any other symptoms but have painful sores or watery blisters in these areas. The virus can also become active more than once. Aciclovir is the usual treatment for genital herpes, and mothers can use the medication during pregnancy. About 40 percent of women who are infected for the first time during pregnancy pass the infection to the baby during a vaginal birth.

If you acquire a primary (first time) genital herpes simplex virus (HSV) infection in the last trimester of your pregnancy having a planned cesarean will decrease the chance of infecting the baby. You should have the option of having a cesarean if you develop genital herpes for the first time in the last 6 weeks of your pregnancy. However, if you have had HSV before you ever became pregnant or earlier in the pregnancy but it was treated, you are likely to have passed your immunity on to the baby. It is uncertain at this time if a planned cesarean will reduce the risk of infecting the baby. Get as much information as you can, so you can make an informed decision about which way is best for you to give birth.[25]

Resources

American Academy of Family Physicians, http://familydoctor.org/online/famdocen/home/common/infections/hepatitis/032.html (last accessed May 23, 2008).

American Academy of Family Physicians, http://familydoctor.org/online/famdocen/home/common/infections/hepatitis/071.html (last accessed May 23, 2008).

American Academy of Familiy Physicians, http://familydoctor.org/online/famdocen/home/women/pregnancy/illness/093.html (last accessed May 23, 2008).

American Academy of Family Physicians, http://familydoctor.org/online/famdocen/home/women/pregnancy/illness/760.html (last accessed May 23, 2008).

American Association for Birth Centers, http://www.aabc.org (last accessed May 23, 2008).

American College of Nurse Midwives, http://www.midwife.org (last accessed May 23, 2008).

Childbirth Connection, for more information about preventing pelvic floor dysfunction, visit http://childbirthconnection.com/article.asp?ck=10206 (last accessed May 23, 2008).

Lamaze International, Lamaze Six Care Practices That Support Normal Birth; Care Practice #1 Labor Begins on Its Own, http://www.lamaze.org/Childbirth Educators/ResourcesforEducators/CarePracticePapers/LaborBeginsOnItsOwn/tabid/487/Default.aspx (last accessed May 23, 2008).

MIDIRS, Informed Choice, http://www.infochoice.org (last accessed May 23, 2008).

Midwives Alliance of North America, http://www.mana.org (last accessed May 23, 2008).

The Pink Kit, http://www.birthingbetter.com/ (last accessed May 23, 2008).

Royal College of Obstetricians and Gynaecologists. Genital Herpes in Pregnancy, http://www.rcog.org.uk/index.asp?PageID=1117 (last accessed May 23, 2008).

Simkin, Penny. Comfort in Labor, http://www.childbirthconnection.org/home.asp?Visitor=Woman (last accessed May 23, 2008).

U.S. Centers for Disease Control and Prevention, http://www.cdc.gov/ncidod/diseases/hepatitis/ (last accessed May 23, 2008).

U.S. Centers for Disease Control and Prevention, http://www.cdc.gov/hiv/topics/perinatal/ (last accessed May 23, 2008).

U.S. Centers for Disease Control and Prevention, http://www.cdc.gov/std/Herpes/STDFact-Herpes.htm (last accessed May 23, 2008).

U.S. National Instititutes of Health. HIV during Pregnancy, Labor and Delivery, and after Birth, http://aidsinfo.nih.gov/ContentFiles/Perinatal_FS_en.pdf (last accessed May 23, 2008).

20

ESPECIALLY FOR MOTHERS: REDUCING THE ODDS FOR A CESAREAN—WHAT TO DO DURING LABOR AND BIRTH

Procedures used during labour which are known to increase the likelihood of medical interventions should be avoided where possible. For example, continuous electronic monitoring during labour in low-risk women is associated with an increase in emergency caesarean section but no long-term health gain, and use of epidural anaesthetic in labour increases the need for forceps or ventouse (vacuum extractor). However, it is important that women's needs and wishes are respected and they should be able to make informed decisions about their care.[1]

ARRIVE AT THE HOSPITAL WHEN YOU ARE IN LABOR

Many healthy full-term pregnant women are admitted to the labor and delivery unit at the hospital before they are in active labor, when the membranes are intact, the cervix has not effaced, and contractions are irregular. There are usually no medical complications, no vaginal bleeding or signs of fetal distress. Once admitted there is a tendency to expect labor to progress according to an established timeline. Induction of labor, use of an IV, and continuous electronic fetal monitoring are more likely to be used. Women are more likely to be restricted to bed, and their ability to walk, move, and change positions will be limited. Healthy women at term who are admitted to the hospital labor and deliver unit only when they are in active labor are less likely to have their labor induced and to use pain medications. They are also more likely to feel more in control during labor.[2]

AVOID CONTINUOUS ELECTRONIC FETAL MONITORING IF YOU ARE LOW-RISK

Monitoring the baby's heart rate during labor is important. A nonreassuring heart rate may indicate that the baby may not be getting enough oxygen and needs to be born as quickly as possible. There are different safe and effective ways to monitor the baby's heart rate and consequently the baby's oxygen supply during labor. A baby's heartbeat can be monitored with an electronic fetal monitor (EFM), continuously or intermittently (only for a specific period of time) and by auscultation with a fetal stethoscope (Pinard) or with a handheld Doppler device. With auscultation your caregiver listens to the baby's heart rate every 15 to 30 minutes in the first stage of labor and every 5 minutes in the second stage or the beginning of pushing. You are free to move around and use a variety of positions. A Doppler device can also be adapted for use in water. Research shows that when healthy women are monitored routinely and continuously with an electronic fetal monitor compared to intermittent auscultation their risk for a cesarean or an instrumental delivery (with forceps or vacuum extractor) is increased by 30 percent. Using continuous EFM for healthy women does not improve a baby's well-being. It does not lower the baby's risk of cerebral palsy, perinatal death, or needing admission to a special care nursery. Continuous fetal monitoring is recommended in special situations when the mother has high blood pressure, is expecting twins, is overdue, or has had a prior cesarean. It is also advised when the baby seems smaller than expected (low birth weight) and when labor is induced.[3, 4]

AVOID THE ROUTINE USE OF INTRAVENOUS FLUIDS

IV fluids are needed if you labor is induced or augmented, if you have an epidural, if you need antibiotics, or if you become dehydrated. If there is no medical reason to have IV fluids you will have more freedom to move and change positions. You are also less likely to have fluid overload, which makes initiation of breast-feeding more difficult. Preventing women in labor from eating and drinking (fasting) increases the length of labor and the level of psychological distress. It also increases the level of ketones in their bodies.[5] Use of IVs also increases the risk for infection.

AVOID AN AMNIOTOMY (ARTIFICIAL RUPTURE OF THE BAG OF WATERS)

Some care providers recommend amniotomy early in labor to reduce the length of labor and reduce the risk of cesarean section. An amniotomy can shorten labor by about 1 to 2 hours and reduce the need for oxytocin (used to induce or augment labor). However, it can also increase the risk of infection for both mother and baby. It is more likely to affect the baby's heart rate in a negative way and increase the risk of the baby's umbilical cord slipping through the cervix before the baby, compromising the baby's oxygen supply. Breaking the bag of waters does not have any benefits for the baby. Evidence suggests that amniotomy alone tends to increase the risk of a cesarean delivery, not reduce it.[6, 7]

Read Chapter 10 which deals with helping your labor to progress.

To Reduce the Odds for a Cesarean in Second Stage (Pushing Phase) Take the Time You Need to Give Birth

Many care providers arbitrarily limit the mother's time for pushing the baby out (second stage labor) to 2 hours. It is a common concern that prolonging the second stage of labor may compromise the level of oxygen available to the baby. However, current evidence shows that for women whose labor begins on its own, if the mother's and the baby's vital signs are stable and birth is progressing, there is no reason to terminate labor with a cesarean or instrumental delivery.[8,9] You will likely be less fatigued, and your baby will be in a healthier condition if you push only when you feel the urge to do so. Forceful pushing can compromise the baby's heart rate and increase your risk for perineal tears. Pushing in an upright position helps your progress and is less painful.

Resources

ACNM, Am I in Labor?, http://www.midwife.org/share_with_women.cfm (last accessed May 23, 2008).

ACNM, When Does the Bag of Water Break?, http://www.midwife.org/share_with_women.cfm (last accessed May 23, 2008).

Lamaze International. Care Practice Papers, http://www.lamaze.org/Childbirth Educators/ResourcesforEducators/CarePracticePapers/tabid/90/Default.aspx (last accessed May 23, 2008).

PART V

CHANGING THE STATUS QUO

21

WHY NORMAL BIRTH MATTERS

As a responsible doctor, I can promise you the finest care and a pain-free birth. These days, women all across North America and Europe are having their babies with little or no pain. Why should you allow yourselves anything less? The latest methods of obstetrics—chloroform, ether, chloral, opium, the use of forceps— these things can make birthing the joyful experience it was meant to be. I can even administer Twilight Sleep if desired.[1]

These are the words of Dr. Thomas, a fictional character in Ami McKay's novel *The Birth House* set in the early years of World Word I. Twilight sleep was an amnesic state induced in women in childbirth. The drugs used were a combination of scopolamine and morphine. The drugs allowed for childbirth without pain, at least without the memory of pain, but they also completely detached the mother from her birth experience and depressed the newborn's baby's central nervous system. The promise of modern medicine and birth technology to improve on and perfect the inherent process of childbirth seems to have reached its limit; at least for now. It seems that in our endless search to appease the pain of childbirth and safeguard the mother's and her newborn's life we have come too far. We have forgotten to ask the mother what she wants; how she feels; how she is affected by the potent drugs and the needles, catheters, tubes, and wires that are keeping vigil over her and her unborn child; if all these interventions make it easier or harder for her to become a mother, to care for her newborn as she would like to; and if she is empowered or feels weakened or defeated by her experience of childbirth. With the scepter of potential mortality at each and every birth we have not stopped to ask ourselves why, when our use of birth technology and cesarean rate is at its highest ever, is the maternal and infant mortality rate also higher: why things are not getting better but worse. The evidence seems to tell us that in our efforts to improve on or preempt the process of birth we have in some ways caused harm.

There is a growing global movement to reduce unnecessary medical interventions in childbirth and to rehumanize birth. In Britain, the Maternity Care

Working Party (MCWP) an independent, multidisciplinary body of physicians, midwives, nurses, hospitals, and consumer advocate groups is raising awareness about the public health impact of the rising cesarean rates. They have signed a consensus statement, "Making Normal Birth a Reality," to share their views about why normal birth matters. The group serves in an advisory position to the All Party Group on Maternity—a group of members of parliament. The MCWP has voiced its concerns about the rising intervention rates, planned and unplanned cesareans, and instrumental births (with forceps and vacuum extractor). They recognize that these procedures significantly impact mothers and infants both physically and psychologically. They state, "We all want mothers and babies to come through birth healthy and well-prepared for the changes, demands, and emotional growth that follows."[2] They have recommended that inductions, continuous electronic fetal monitoring, and use of epidurals be reduced because of their established link to emergency (unplanned) cesareans, instrumental delivery, and no improvements in long-term health. That evidence-based information be shared with women, so they can plan for the kind of birth they want, and that women are offered a choice of place of birth and one-on-one midwifery support in active labor. They are encouraging childbirth classes that teach women about nondrug methods for coping with pain, freedom of movement and positioning in labor, and access to water births, massage, and aromatherapy. They are making these recommendations based on the best available scientific evidence. And because normal birth makes it easier for a new mother to breastfeed, to "get her family life to a good start," and ultimately to protect the mother's and baby's long-term health. Government policies will be implemented and funding will be available to educate and train birth professionals to support women in childbirth without technological interventions.

Several maternity care advocacy groups in Europe are aiming to make a "radical change" from "industrial" and "productivist" obstetrical care to normal birth with education and awareness campaigns. An example of this is the annual World Respected Childbirth Week. The campaign is also active in other countries including the Netherlands, the Czech Republic, and Argentina. The Alliance Francophone pour l'Accouchement Respecté (AFAR), a French language network of citizens and nonprofit societies involved in the support of, and providing information about, gentle childbirth and care of the newborn states that the "marketing of birth, in France, is obvious in the dismantling of small obstetrical units to the benefit of 'birth factories.' Fear of litigation has pushed professional attendants to shelter behind protocols imposing an increasing number of interventions, most of which are useless or detrimental to the natural process of birthing."[3]

In Latin America, where in some countries the cesarean rate in private hospitals can reach 90 percent, there is a social movement pushing back the worst of medical interventions: enemas, shaving, fasting, fundal pressure, episiotomy, strapping women's hands during vaginal births and cesareans. Medical anthropologist Robbie Davis-Floyd states, "Nothing is as certain to start a social movement as a pendulum swing this far on the wrong side of the scientific evidence."[4] In many Latin American countries professional organizations, grassroots activists, and nongovernmental organizations have taken the initiative and responsibility to humanize maternity care. The First International Congress on the Humanization of Birth was held in Fortaleza, Brazil, in November 2000. Government and nongovernmental organizations were invited to participate. Two thousands participants including physicians, midwives, health officials, doulas, lactation consultants, and childbirth educators attended it.

In the United States, as the Institute of Medicine concluded, there is a need for fundamental change in our health care delivery system. Given the intricate and tangled web of hundreds of stakeholders and no comprehensive national health office to jumpstart the process, that change will not be easy to make. It is however, possible to aspire to a model of maternity care that is evidence-based and mother-, baby-, and family-friendly; a model of care that respects women's right (a human right) to participate in all decisions regarding their care, to choose their own place of birth and caregiver, to give birth in a supportive and secure environment, and to make the choices that are best for themselves and their family; a model of care that optimizes physical and psychological health outcomes.

That model of care is the Mother-Friendly Childbirth Initiative (MFCI)—the first consensus declaration of a multidisciplinary group of professional organizations and individuals in North America to address the issues of childbirth. Ratified in 1996, the initiative is the bedrock of the Coalition for Improving Maternity Services (CIMS). The CIMS is a collaborative effort of numerous individuals and more than fifty organizations representing over 90,000 members. Its mission is to promote an evidence-based wellness model of care that improves outcomes and substantially reduces costs. The Mother-Friendly Childbirth Initiative has been adopted as a model of care by maternity care and breastfeeding organizations around the world. Several of the Ten Steps of the Mother-Friendly Childbirth Initiative that directly affect breastfeeding success are included in the World Health Organization's Guide to Infant and Young Child Feeding: A Tool for Assessing National Practices, Policies, and Programmes. The MFCI may inspire more childbearing women to advocate for their rights to fully participate in their care and all those who devote their professional lives to maternity care to swing the pendulum towards evidence-based mother-centered care.

THE MOTHER-FRIENDLY CHILDBIRTH INITIATIVE

The First Consensus Initiative of the Coalition for Improving Maternity Services (CIMS).

Mission, Preamble, and Principles

Mission

The Coalition for Improving Maternity Services (CIMS) is a coalition of individuals and national organizations with concern for the care and wellbeing of mothers, babies, and families. Our mission is to promote a wellness model of maternity care that will improve birth outcomes and substantially reduce costs. This evidence-based mother-, baby-, and family-friendly model focuses on prevention and wellness as the alternatives to high-cost screening, diagnosis, and treatment programs.

Preamble

Whereas

- In spite of spending far more money per capita on maternity and newborn care than any other country, the United States falls behind most industrialized countries in perinatal morbidity and mortality, and maternal mortality is four times greater for African-American women than for Euro-American women;
- Midwives attend the vast majority of births in those industrialized countries with the best perinatal outcomes, yet in the United States, midwives are the principal attendants at only a small percentage of births;
- Current maternity and newborn practices that contribute to high costs and inferior outcomes include the inappropriate application of technology and routine procedures that are not based on scientific evidence;
- Increased dependence on technology has diminished confidence in women's innate ability to give birth without intervention;
- The integrity of the mother–child relationship, which begins in pregnancy, is compromised by the obstetrical treatment of mother and baby as if they were separate units with conflicting needs;
- Although breastfeeding has been scientifically shown to provide optimum health, nutritional, and developmental benefits to newborns and their mothers, only a fraction of U.S. mothers are fully breastfeeding their babies by the age of six weeks;
- The current maternity care system in the United States does not provide equal access to health care resources for women from disadvantaged population groups, women without insurance, and women whose insurance dictates caregivers or place of birth;

Therefore,

We, the undersigned members of CIMS, hereby resolve to define and promote mother-friendly maternity services in accordance with the following principles:

Principles

We believe the philosophical cornerstones of mother-friendly care to be as follows:

Normalcy of the Birthing Process
- Birth is a normal, natural, and healthy process.
- Women and babies have the inherent wisdom necessary for birth.
- Babies are aware, sensitive human beings at the time of birth and should be acknowledged and treated as such.

- Breastfeeding provides the optimum nourishment for newborns and infants.
- Birth can safely take place in hospitals, birth centers, and homes.
- The midwifery model of care, which supports and protects the normal birth process, is the most appropriate for the majority of women during pregnancy and birth.

Empowerment
- A woman's confidence and ability to give birth and to care for her baby are enhanced or diminished by every person who gives her care and by the environment in which she gives birth.
- A mother and baby are distinct yet interdependent during pregnancy, birth, and infancy. Their interconnectedness is vital and must be respected.
- Pregnancy, birth, and the postpartum period are milestone events in the continuum of life. These experiences profoundly affect women, babies, fathers, and families and have important and long-lasting effects on society.

Autonomy. Every woman should have the opportunity to:
- Have a healthy and joyous birth experience for herself and her family, regardless of her age or circumstances;
- Give birth as she wishes in an environment in which she feels nurtured and secure, and her emotional well-being, privacy, and personal preferences are respected;
- Have access to the full range of options for pregnancy, birth, and nurturing her baby and to accurate information on all available birthing sites, caregivers, and practices;
- Receive accurate and up-to-date information about the benefits and risks of all procedures, drugs, and tests suggested for use during pregnancy, birth, and the postpartum period, with the rights to informed consent and informed refusal;
- Receive support for making informed choices about what is best for her and her baby based on her individual values and beliefs.

Do No Harm
- Interventions should not be applied routinely during pregnancy, birth, or the postpartum period. Many standard medical tests, procedures, technologies, and drugs carry risks to both mother and baby and should be avoided in the absence of specific scientific indications for their use.
- If complications arise during pregnancy, birth, or the postpartum period, medical treatments should be evidence-based.

Responsibility
- Each caregiver is responsible for the quality of care she or he provides.
- Maternity care practice should be based not on the needs of the caregiver or provider but solely on the needs of the mother and child.
- Each hospital and birth center is responsible for the periodic review and evaluation, according to current scientific evidence, of the effectiveness, risks, and rates of use of its medical procedures for mothers and babies.

- Society, through both its government and the public health establishment, is responsible for ensuring access to maternity services for all women, and for monitoring the quality of those services.
- Individuals are ultimately responsible for making informed choices about the health care they and their babies receive.

These following principles give rise to the following steps, which support, protect, and promote mother-friendly maternity services.

Ten Steps of the Mother-Friendly Childbirth Initiative for Mother-Friendly Hospitals, Birth Centers, and Home Birth Services

To receive CIMS designation as "mother-friendly," a hospital, birth center, or home birth service must carry out the above philosophical principles by fulfilling the Ten Steps of Mother-Friendly Care.

A mother-friendly hospital, birth center, or home birth service:

1. Offers all birthing mothers:
   - Unrestricted access to the birth companions of her choice, including fathers, partners, children, family members, and friends;
   - Unrestricted access to continuous emotional and physical support from a skilled woman—for example, a doula or labor-support professional;
   - Access to professional midwifery care.
2. Provides accurate descriptive and statistical information to the public about its practices and procedures for birth care, including measures of interventions and outcomes.
3. Provides culturally competent care—that is, care that is sensitive and responsive to the specific beliefs, values, and customs of the mother's ethnicity and religion.
4. Provides the birthing woman with the freedom to walk, move about, and assume the positions of her choice during labor and birth (unless restriction is specifically required to correct a complication) and discourages the use of the lithotomy (flat on back with legs elevated) position.
5. Has clearly defined policies and procedures for:
   - collaborating and consulting throughout the perinatal period with other maternity services, including communicating with the original caregiver when transfer from one birth site to another is necessary;
   - linking the mother and baby to appropriate community resources, including prenatal and post-discharge follow-up and breastfeeding support.
6. Does not routinely employ practices and procedures that are unsupported by scientific evidence, including but not limited to the following:
   - shaving;
   - enemas;
   - IVs (intravenous drip);
   - withholding nourishment or water;
   - early rupture of membranes; and

- electronic fetal monitoring; other interventions are limited as follows:
  - Has an induction rate of 10% or less;
  - Has an episiotomy rate of 20% or less, with a goal of 5% or less;
  - Has a total cesarean rate of 10% or less in community hospitals and 15% or less in tertiary care (high-risk) hospitals;
  - Has a VBAC (vaginal birth after cesarean) rate of 60% or more with a goal of 75% or more.
7. Educates staff in non-drug methods of pain relief and does not promote the use of analgesic or anesthetic drugs not specifically required to correct a complication.
8. Encourages all mothers and families, including those with sick or premature newborns or infants with congenital problems, to touch, hold, breastfeed, and care for their babies to the extent compatible with their conditions.
9. Discourages non-religious circumcision of the newborn.
10. Strives to achieve the WHO-UNICEF "Ten Steps of the Baby-Friendly Hospital Initiative" to promote successful breastfeeding:
    1. Have a written breastfeeding policy that is routinely communicated to all health care staff;
    2. Train all health care staff in skills necessary to implement this policy;
    3. Inform all pregnant women about the benefits and management of breastfeeding;
    4. Help mothers initiate breastfeeding within a half-hour of birth;
    5. Show mothers how to breastfeed and how to maintain lactation even if they should be separated from their infants;
    6. Give newborn infants no food or drink other than breast milk unless medically indicated;
    7. Practice rooming in: allow mothers and infants to remain together 24 hours a day;
    8. Encourage breastfeeding on demand;
    9. Give no artificial teat or pacifiers (also called dummies or soothers) to breastfeeding infants;
    10. Foster the establishment of breastfeeding support groups and refer mothers to them on discharge from hospitals or clinics.

Over the years, since the MFCI was ratified in 1996, the Coalition has learned that making change in a practice or an institution is a long and challenging process and that it may take years to meet the requirements for designation. In recent years the CIMS has encouraged and valued step-by-step implementation of the Mother-Friendly Childbirth Initiative. Maternity care professionals, each within their own scope of practice, continue to find ways to meet those challenges, so they can provide the kind of care that mothers and babies deserve.

22

RESOURCES: TRUTH AND TRANSPARENCY IN MATERNITY CARE

> Women can not make informed choices about their maternity care if they do not have access to the information that is most likely to influence their outcomes. They cannot decrease their exposure to injury from injudicious use of interventions without knowing where and with whom intervention rates are too high. Without transparency, our health care system gives women a false sense of choice.[1]

Before the introduction of the Internet, clear, easy to read evidence-based information on the benefits and risks of cesarean section and medical interventions associated with increased cesarean rates was not easily available to the public. Access was limited mostly to health professionals and parents who attended childbirth classes that provided evidence-based information. With increased access to this technology it became possible for maternity care advocates, researchers, professional associations, and birth advocacy groups to keep up with the latest evidence and educate consumers about their right to fully participate in their care. These advocacy groups and professional associations have played a key role in providing consumers and professionals with evidence-based information regarding cesarean sections and routine practices likely to increase the risk for the surgery. They have made childbearing women aware of the choices available to them. They have also provided a wide net for women and health professionals to communicate with each other worldwide on issues that are critical to the childbirth experience.

AMERICAN COLLEGE OF NURSE-MIDWIVES' REDUCE CAMPAIGN

The American College of Nurse-Midwives (ACNM) recognizes that the rising cesarean rate is driven by both the primary cesarean rate and the decline in the vaginal birth after cesarean (VBAC) rate without any corresponding improvement in maternal or neonatal health. It is the ACNM's position that primary elective cesarean section, major abdominal surgery in healthy women with no medical indication, as a substitute for vaginal birth is not supported by scientific evidence. The ACNM launched the REDUCE (Research and Education to Reduce Unnecessary Cesareans) campaign in 2005 to proactively address the steady rise in cesareans which the College views as preventable and unnecessary. The ACNM developed fact sheets and reports to assist media in accurately reporting on the short- and long-term complications associated with the surgery. The College is concerned that women are not aware of the serious risks associated with the surgery, and it has taken an active role in keeping the public informed about national developments in cesarean-related issues. Professionals and consumers interested in reducing cesareans can access educational materials, legislative action advice, and media packets to promote the issue on a national or community level. The ACNM encourages women to explore their options for care providers and methods of pain relief and avoid routine medical interventions. The professional association has identified the misinterpretation of scientific evidence and a lack of respect for the risks of cesarean surgery as two factors for the increase in cesarean delivery. The REDUCE campaign educational materials are available at no cost from their Web site, http://www.midwife.org.

BirthNetwork National

BirthNetwork National is a leading voice of consumers concerned about the barriers to evidence-based maternity care. Founded in 1999, BirthNetwork National is a nonprofit, volunteer-run organization that promotes awareness about birth options and strives to make those options available to women through its various programs and local chapter activities. Unlike many other activist organizations, BirthNetwork National does not advocate for a specific type of health care provider or encourage any one particular method of giving birth. Rather, its goal is to help mothers make their own personal and informed decisions about where, how, and with whom they want to give birth based on the full scientific evidence.

In addition to chapters working within communities to increase awareness about evidence-based maternity care and publishing a printed and online provider listing guide the organization has dedicated its large volunteer base to the work of the Transparency in Maternity Care Project. BirthNetwork leaders have rallied around the project as a "for consumers, by consumers" project that will change the way that women make decisions about their maternity care. BirthNetwork encourages women who want to make maternity care safer and more satisfying to become active with a local chapter, to start a chapter in their area, or to inquire about volunteer opportunities at the national level. Their Web site is http://www.birthnetwork.org.

Childbirth Connection

Childbirth Connection is a national not-for-profit organization that improves the quality of maternity care through research, education advocacy, and policy.

Founded in 1918 as Maternity Center Association (MCA), the young organization carried out a program that reduced maternal and infant deaths in New York City. During the twentieth century, the MCA played a central role in such core areas as maternity nursing, childbirth and parent education, nurse-midwifery education, and the freestanding birth center model of care. In 1999, the organization began its long-term national program to promote evidence-based maternity care and ensure that families receive safe, effective care that reflects best scientific evidence. Childbirth Connection works with childbearing women, health professionals, policy makers, and journalists through its highly regarded Web site (http://www.childbirthconnection.org), publications, media outreach, and other channels. The group has extensive resources for childbearing women and health professionals relating to cesarean section and vaginal birth. Childbirth Connection carried out the first and, to date, only systematic review to identify all harms that differ in likelihood between vaginal and cesarean births. Results are presented in a booklet, *What Every Pregnant Woman Needs to Know about Cesarean Section*, which helps women make informed decisions and has been endorsed by over thirty organizations and is available on their Web site. Childbirth Connection also helps the public understand cesarean trends and the drivers behind them, associated costs, best evidence about vaginal birth after cesarean versus repeat cesarean, and related topics. The organization actively advocates nationally for childbearing families and engages diverse stakeholders in improving the quality of maternity care, including the establishment of performance measures and incentives for appropriate use of cesarean section Their Web site is http://www.childbirthconnection.org.

CITIZENS FOR MIDWIFERY

Citizens for Midwifery (CfM) is a national, nonprofit, grassroots consumer advocacy organization founded by several mothers in 1996. The organization promotes the Midwives Model of Care, provides advocacy tools, educational material, and networks with other organizations to support legislative efforts that promote access to midwifery at a state level. In recent years CfM has provided support in various ways to midwifery and birth activist organizations around the country, including several states that have passed laws allowing midwives trained in the Midwives Model of Care© to attend births outside the hospital. Scientific evidence supports a noninterventionist, individualized, evidence-based model of care as being integral to reducing complications of childbirth and cesarean section. The goal of Citizens for Midwifery is to see that this evidence-based, respectful model of care is available to all childbearing women and universally recognized as the best kind of care for pregnancy and birth for all providers and settings. The CfM works to improve access to the Midwives Model of Care for women of all ages, ethnic backgrounds, races, religions, sexual orientations, abilities, and socioeconomic circumstances. Education and legislative information is posted at no cost on their Web site, http://www.Cfmidwifery.org.

COALITION FOR IMPROVING MATERNITY SERVICES

Established in 1996 the Coalition for Improving Maternity Services (CIMS) is a collaborative effort of numerous individuals and more than fifty organizations representing over 90,000 members. It's a volunteer, nonprofit organization. The CIMS' mission is to promote a wellness model of maternity care that will improve birth outcomes and substantially reduce costs. The CIMS Mother-Friendly Childbirth Initiative was the first evidence-based consensus document on labor and birth drafted by a multidisciplinary group of professional organizations and individuals in the history of North America. The consensus document gave rise to the evidence-based Ten Steps of Mother-Friendly Care, a model of maternity care that supports normal birth and reduces the risk of complications and cesarean section. The initiative has been recognized by national and international organizations including the World Health Organization and UNICEF. The CIMS conducts research, collaborates with maternity care organizations, holds annual forums, and disseminates all research findings at no cost. In 2005–2006 the CIMS Expert Work Group systematically reviewed 15 years of scientific studies and found that the mother-friendly model of maternity care is still strongly founded on scientific evidence and provides the best outcomes for mothers and babies.[2] In addition the CIMS Expert Work Group found strong evidence to support the valuable contributions of midwifery care and the safety of out-of-hospital birth. The research report, "Coalition for Improving Maternity Services Evidence-Basis for the Ten Steps of Mother-Friendly Care," was published as a supplement of the winter 2007 issue of *The Journal of Perinatal Education*. Thanks to a generous grant from the New Hampshire Charitable Foundation the findings of this research project and its publication in *The Journal of Perinatal Education* is available worldwide at no cost from the CIMS Web site, http://www.motherfriendly.org.

DONA INTERNATIONAL

DONA International, formerly Doulas of North America, was founded in 1992 by Dr. Marshall Klaus and Dr. John Kennell, expert researchers on maternal-infant attachment, and Phyllis Klaus, C.S.W., M.F.C.C., Penny Simkin, P.T., and Annie Kennedy, renowned experts in childbirth, newborn care, and the postpartum period. The word, "doula" was chosen by the founders to describe a woman who provides continuous emotional and physical support during labor and birth, and/or afterwards. There are birth doulas and postpartum doulas. Drs. Klaus and Kennell conducted research on continuous nonmedical emotional support during labor and found (as have numerous other studies) significantly improved health outcomes for the laboring women who received the support, when compared to women who received usual hospital care. These included reduced risks of cesarean section, fewer requests for pain medications, fewer forceps or vacuum extractor deliveries, and increased satisfaction with the birth experience among the supported women. DONA

International publishes evidence-based research and position papers on doula care, sponsors yearly educational forums, provides training and certification for the profession, and a directory of certified professional doulas. Graduates of DONA International trainings are educated to work within evidence-based standards of practice and a code of ethics. Research materials on doula care, including the most recent Cochrane reviews on the benefits of continuous support in labor, are available from their Web site, http://www.dona.org.

INTERNATIONAL CESAREAN AWARENESS NETWORK

The International Cesarean Awareness Network (ICAN) is a volunteer non-profit organization dedicated to preventing unnecessary cesareans through education, providing support for cesarean recovery, and promoting vaginal birth after cesarean. The organization was founded in 1982 as the Cesarean Prevention Movement by Esther Booth Zorn and has grown to nearly a hundred chapters. The organization's early efforts were focused on challenging the long-held belief "once a cesarean, always a cesarean" by providing education, advocacy, and support for women who had cesarean surgery. The ICAN works to ensure that women have easy access to accurate information about pregnancy and birth, so that they can make informed, evidence-based decisions about where and how they birth and understand their right to consent to or refuse interventions, including surgery. The ICAN has kept the excessive cesarean rate issue and the pervasive denial of medical care for VBAC up-front and center through media and advocacy efforts. The ICAN is the only organization currently tracking the number of hospitals that are banning VBAC. The ICAN's international volunteer base offers support in person and online, as well as through a toll-free telephone line. These support vehicles serve an essential role in providing a safe and supportive environment for women who had a difficult or traumatic cesarean or are pursuing a VBAC. The ICAN's Web site is http://www.ican-online.org.

INTERNATIONAL CHILDBIRTH EDUCATION ASSOCIATION

The International Childbirth Education Association (ICEA) is a nonprofit organization established in 1960. As a professional organization it provides training and continuing education programs, evidence-based educational resources, and professional certification programs for maternity care professionals. The ICEA is founded on freedom of choice based on knowledge of alternatives in family-centered maternity and newborn care. ICEA has historically been proactive in providing evidence-based information and advocacy support for reducing nonmedically indicated cesareans. In 1990–1991 ICEA and the Cesarean Options Committee mailed over 1,200 copies of the pamphlet *ICEA Review: Vaginal Birth after Cesarean Section* to hospitals and health agencies across the United States. The organization developed fact sheets and position statements on cesarean section and VBAC for both consumers and professionals. In 1980 the ICEA published the booklet *Unnecessary Cesareans—Ways to Avoid Them*, one of the first publications on cesarean prevention. In 2000 the organization published *The VBAC Source Book and Teaching Kit*. The ICEA's evidence-based position papers and statements on induction, epidural anesthesia, amniotomy, and other cesarean-related issues are available at a nominal fee from their Web site, http://www.icea.org.

LAMAZE INSTITUTE FOR NORMAL BIRTH

The Lamaze Institute for Normal Birth was launched to support initiatives that provide credible, relevant and useful information about normal birth to new and expectant parents and childbirth professionals. Forming the foundation of the Lamaze Institute for Normal Birth are the six care practices that support normal birth. These evidence-based practices, adapted from the World Health Organization, are: labor should begin on its own; laboring women should be free to move throughout labor; laboring women should have continuous support from others throughout labor; there should be no routine interventions during labor and birth; women should not give birth on their backs; and mothers and babies should not be separated after birth and should have unlimited opportunity for breast-feeding. The Lamaze Institute for Normal Birth supports community-based efforts to promote normal birth by providing grants and organizational resources to Birth Networks, grassroots organizations that provide pregnancy, birth, and parenting support and resources to families. The Institute also works closely with other organizations and individuals who support normal birth and conducts research and education to further the understanding of the benefits and physiology of normal birth to mother and baby. All materials are available from their Web site, http://www.lamaze.org.

TRANSPARENCY IN MATERNITY CARE PROJECT: THE BIRTH SURVEY

The Transparency in Maternity Care Project was founded and is run by a grassroots volunteer committee of the CIMS dedicated to ensuring public access to quality of care information specifically related to maternity care providers and institutions. The CIMS committee believes women should have access to information that will help them choose maternity care providers and institutions that are most compatible with their own philosophies and needs. At the heart of the project is an ongoing, online consumer survey, The Birth Survey, that asks women to provide feedback about their birth experience with a particular doctor or midwife and within a specific birth environment. Responses are made available online to other women in their communities who are deciding where and with whom to birth. Paired with this experiential data will be official statistics from state departments of health, listing obstetrical intervention rates at the facility level. The goal of the committee is to give women a mechanism that can be used to share information about maternity care practices in their community while at the same time providing practitioners and institutions feedback for quality of care improvement efforts. The Birth Survey was launched in New York State in 2007. Plans are in place to extend the project across the country. Its Web site is http://www.thebirthsurvey.com.

These national organizations have played a key role in keeping consumers, policy makers, and health professionals informed and updated on all issues related to the rising cesarean section rate and its impact on maternal and newborn health. They have spoken up where medical associations, public health services, and the media have maintained their silence. They have made it their goal to provide evidence-based information about birth practices, place of birth, and care providers that impact the rate of cesarean deliveries. Above all they are educating childbearing women about safe alternatives and offering them choices for childbirth that have been ignored or contested by the organized medical community.

GLOSSARY

Aciclovir. An antiviral agent used to treat herpes virus infections.

Amniotic fluid embolism. An obstetric emergency in which amniotic fluid, fetal cells, hair, or other debris enters the mother's blood stream through the placental bed of the uterus and triggers an allergic reaction. This reaction results in heart and lung collapse and blood clotting.

Antepartum. The time between conception and the onset of labor.

Apgar score. An index used to evaluate the condition of a newborn infant based on a rating of 0, 1, or 2 for each of the five characteristics of color, heart rate, response to stimulation of the sole of the foot, muscle tone, and respiration, with 10 being a perfect score.

Apnea. Transient cessation of breathing.

Asynclitic. The entry of the fetal head in the pelvic inlet in an oblique angle.

Atalectasis. Collapse of all or part of the lung.

Auscultation. The act of listening to sounds arising within organs as in the heart or the uterus during pregnancy.

Bacterial sepsis. Infection caused by bacteria accompanied by fever and a high white blood cell count.

Birth trauma. An injury or wound to living tissue of the infant.

Bladder catheter. A thin tubular medical device inserted in the bladder to withdraw urine.

Breech presentation. A fetus that presents buttocks or legs first at the cervix.

Bupivacaine. A local pain-numbing anesthetic.

Cardinal movements. Specific head and body position changes that the fetus makes to adjust and pass through the birth canal. They include descent, flexion, internal rotation, extension, restitution, external rotation, and expulsion.

Cerebral palsy. A disability resulting from damage to the brain before, during, or shortly after birth and outwardly manifested by muscular incoordination and speech disturbances.

Cervical dilation. The stretching or enlarging of the cervix.

Cervix. The narrow lower or outer end of the uterus.

Cesarean. The surgical incision of the walls of the abdomen and uterus for delivery of the baby.

Colostrum. The first secretions from the breast before the true milk comes in. It contains serum, white blood cells, and antibodies.

Complete breech. Breech with flexed thighs and knees.

Cord prolapse. Umbilical cord prolapse is an obstetric emergency during labor that endangers the life of the fetus. It occurs when the umbilical cord presents itself outside of the uterus while the fetus is still inside. It can happen when the water breaks.

Deep vein thrombosis. A blood clot that forms in a deep vein, most commonly in the deep veins of the lower leg.

Dehiscense. The thinned area of the uterus wall at the site of the prior cesarean incision. It occurs in about 1 percent to 2 percent of women. It's also called an incomplete or asymptomatic uterine rupture. It heals on its own.

Doula. A woman trained to provide continuous physical and emotional support in labor.

DSM. *Diagnostic and Statistical Manual of Mental Disorders.*

Dystocia. An abnormal or difficult childbirth or labor. It may be due to incoordinate uterine contractions, abnormal fetal lie or presentation, or cephalopelvic disproportion.

Ectopic pregnancy. The fertilized egg implants itself and grows outside the uterus, usually in one of the fallopian tubes.

Effacement. The thinning out and softening of the cervix during labor.

Electronic fetal monitoring. An electronic method for examining the condition of a baby in the uterus by noting any unusual changes in its heart rate.

Endometritis. Inflammation of the endometrium, the inner lining of the uterus.

Endorphins. Endogenous opioids produced by the pituitary gland and the hypothalamus. Endorphins work as "natural pain killers."

Epidural analgesia. A form of regional anesthesia/analgesia involving the injection of drugs through a catheter placed into the epidural space.

Episiotomy. A surgical incision through the perineum made to enlarge the vagina and assist childbirth.

External cephalic version (ECV). A process by which a breech baby can sometimes be turned from buttocks or foot-first to headfirst.

Fetal distress. The presence of signs in a pregnant woman—before or during childbirth—that the fetus is not well.

Fetal scalp blood sampling (FBS). A technique of sampling blood from the fetal scalp to assess the acid-base status during labor.

Footling breech. One or both feet come first, with the bottom at a higher position.

Frank breech. The baby's bottom comes first, and his or her legs are flexed at the hip and extended at the knees.

Freestanding birth center. A birth center not in a hospital or on hospital grounds.

Fundus. The top portion of the uterus, opposite the cervix.

Genital herpes. A viral infection caused by the herpes simplex virus.

Gestation. The number of weeks counted from the first day of the last menstrual period.

Gravida. Any pregnancy regardless of duration; also includes present pregnancy.

Hypoxia. A shortage of oxygen in the body.

Hysterectomy. The surgical removal of the uterus.

Induction of labor. Starting of labor contractions by artificial means.

Infant respiratory distress syndrome. A syndrome caused in premature infants by developmental insufficiency of surfactants and structural immaturity in the lungs.

Informed consent. The process of understanding the risks and benefits of treatment before making a voluntary decision to accept or reject a procedure, drug, or test. This is a right protected by law.

Informed refusal. The right of a patient to refuse any drug, test, or procedure for any reason. This is a right protected by law.

Instrumental delivery. Use of forceps or vacuum extractor to bring the baby out of the birth canal.

Intrapartun. The time between the onset of true labor until the birth of the infant and placenta.

Intraventricular hemorrhage. Bleeding in the brain of the infant.

Jaundice. Yellowish discoloration of the skin, conjunctiva (a clear covering over the sclera, or whites of the eyes), and mucous membranes caused by increased levels of bilirubin in the blood.

Lactation. The process of providing milk to the young; also the period of time that a mother lactates to feed her young.

Lactation specialist/consultant. A health care professional trained to help mothers with specific issues related to breastfeeding. The International Board of Lactation Consultant Examiners (IBLCE) is the internationally recognized certifying agency for lactation consultants.

Latch on at breastfeeding. Refers to the way the baby latches onto the breast. With a correct position the mother's nipples do not get sore and the baby can easily access the milk.

Late preterm birth. Babies born between 34 and 36 weeks of pregnancy.

Left occiput anterior (LOA). The fetal occiput (head) is directed towards the mother's left anterior side.

Lithotomy position. In it the patient lies with her legs in stirrups and her buttocks close to the lower edge of the table.

Low-segment uterine incision. A transverse (horizontal) incision in the uterus along the pubic hairline.

Low vertical uterine incision. A vertical uterine incision in the lower segment of the uterus.

Macrosomia. Also known as big baby syndrome, a fetus that weighs above 4,000 grams (8 lb. 13 oz.) in a diabetic woman or 4,500 grams (9 lb. 15 oz.) in a normal woman.

Meconium. The medical term for a newborn infant's first stools.

Morbidity. The incidence or prevalence of a disease.

Mortality. The death rate.

Multigravida. A pregnant woman who has been pregnant before.

Multipara. A woman who has had two or more births at more than 20 weeks gestation.

Necrotizing enterocolitis. The death of intestinal tissue; primarily affects premature infants or sick newborns.

Neonatal. Pertaining to the first 4 weeks (28 days) after birth.

Nosocomial infection. Hospital-acquired infection.

Occiput posterior presentation. The position of the fetus in cephalic (head-down) presentation in labor, with its occiput (back of the head) directed toward the right (ROP) or left (LOP) posterior quadrant of the maternal pelvis.

Occiput transverse position (deep). The position of the fetus during delivery in which the occiput (back of the head) turns but stops in the transverse diameter of the pelvis.

Opioid. Any synthetic narcotic that has opiate-like activities but is not derived from opium.

Oxytocin. A natural hormone secreted by the hypothalamus.

Partogram. A visual/graphical representation of related values or events over the course of labor. Measurements might include statistics such as cervical dilation, fetal heart rate, and other vital signs.

Patient-controlled analgesia. Self-administered, controlled dosage of pain relief.

Pelvic adhesion. Fibrous bands that form between tissues and organs, often as a result of injury during surgery. They may be thought of as internal scar tissues that have formed in the pelvic region.

Pelvic diameters. The three principal diameters of the pelvis—antero-posterior, transverse, and oblique.

Pelvimetry. The assessment of the female pelvis in relation to the birth of a baby.

Placenta accreta. A placenta that implants itself too deeply and firmly in the uterine wall to detach normally after birth.

Placenta increta. A placenta more deeply imbedded through the thickness of the uterine muscle.

Placenta percreta. A placenta more deeply imbedded through the thickness of the uterine muscle and sometimes an organ such as the bladder.

Placenta previa. Low-lying placenta that covers part or all of the inner opening of the cervix.

Placental abruption. Also known as abruptio placentae, a complication of pregnancy, in which the placental lining separates from the uterus of the mother. It is the most common cause of late pregnancy bleeding.

Planned (scheduled) primary cesarean. The first birth by cesarean scheduled before labor begins.

Postpartum. The time interval from the birth until the woman's body returns to a nonpregnant state.

Postterm labor. Labor that begins after 42 weeks gestation.

Post-traumatic stress disorder (PTSD). An anxiety disorder that can develop after exposure to a terrifying event or ordeal in which grave physical harm occurred or was threatened.

Preterm birth. A birth that occurs after 20 weeks gestation but before the completion of the 37th week gestation.

Primary cesarean. The first birth ever by cesarean.

Primigravida. A woman who is pregnant for the first time.

Primipara. A woman who has had one birth at more than 20 weeks gestation, regardless of whether or not it was a live birth.

Prostaglandin. One of a number of hormone-like substances that participate in a wide range of body functions such as the contraction and relaxation of smooth muscle.

Pulmonary aspiration. The diversion of the acidic stomach content to the trachea and the lungs.

Pulmonary embolism. Blood clot in the lungs.

Pulmonary hypertension. A condition resulting from constriction, or tightening, of the blood vessels that supply blood to the lungs.

Regional anesthesia. Refers to an epidural or spinal anesthesia or a combination of the two.

Respiratory distress syndrome (RDS). Also kown as hyaline membrane disease, a syndrome of respiratory difficulty in newborns caused by a deficiency of surfactant.

Right occiput anterior (ROA). The fetal occiput (back of the head) is directed towards the mother's right anterior side. It is the easiest position for birth.

Shoulder dystocia. A condition in which the baby's shoulder is wedged behind the mother's pubic bones.

Stillbirth. A baby born dead after 20 weeks gestation.

Sudden infant death syndrome (SIDS). The sudden, unexpected, and unexplained death of any infant or young child.

Surfactant. A wetting agent, a substance secreted by the cells lining the alveoli of the lungs to reduce surface tension. It prevents the alveolar walls from sticking together.

Systemic analgesics. Drugs for pain relief that are distributed throughout the body.

Term Birth. The normal duration of pregnancy, 38 to 42 weeks gestation.

Tocophobia. Fear of labor.

Tocolitic agent. An agent used to relax uterine muscles.

Trauma. An injury (as a wound) to living tissue.

Uterine rupture. Separation of the uterine wall.

Uterine scar. Site of the incision on the uterus from a prior cesarean section.

Vacuum extractor. An instrument used as an alternative for forceps; it has a suction cup that is placed on the baby's head. A vacuum is created using a pump, and the baby is pulled down the birth canal with the suction cup and the help of the mother's contractions.

Vertex presentation. Presentation in which the head of the baby appears first from the birth canal. Vertex refers to the baby's position as head-down.

NOTES

INTRODUCTION

1. Institute of Medicine, *Crossing the Quality Chasm: A New Health System for the 21st Century* (Washington, DC: National Academy Press, 2001), 1.

2. Ibid., 231.

3. Agency for Healthcare Research and Quality, *Priority Areas for National Action: Transforming Health Care Quality.* Summary of Institute of Medicine Report, January 2003, Agency for Healthcare Quality, http://www.ahrq.gov/qual/iompriorities.htm (last accessed May 15, 2008).

4. B. Hamilton, J. A. Martin, and S. J. Ventura, Preliminary data for 2006, National Vital Statistics Reports, 56(7), Health E-Stats. Hyattsville, MD: National Center for Health Statistics, 2007, Centers for Disease Control and Prevention, http://www.cdc.gov/nchs/products/pubs/pubd/hestats/prelim_births/prelim_births04.htm (last accessed May 15, 2008).

5. Office of Disease Prevention and Health Promotion, U.S. Department of Health and Human Services, Healthy People 2010, Maternal, Infant, and Child Health, 16–30. Washington, DC, Healthy People, http://www.healthypeople.gov/document/word/Volume2/16MICH.doc (last accessed May 15, 2008).

6. World Health Organization, WHO Consensus Conference on Appropriate Technology for Birth, Fortaleza, Brazil, April 22–26, 1985, in M. Wagner, *Pursuing the Birth Machine: The Search for Appropriate Birth Technology* (NSW, Australia: Ace Graphics:), 346.

7. Medical Leadership Council (MLC), *Coming to Term: Innovations in Safely Reducing Cesarean Rates* (Washington, DC: The Advisory Board Company, 1996).

8. Childbirth Connection, Why Is the Cesarean Rate Higher Than Ever, and Rising? Childbirth Connection, http://www.childbirthconnection.com (last accessed May 14, 2008).

9. F. Menacker, Trends in Cesarean Rates for First Births and Repeat Cesarean Rates for Low-Risk Women: United States, 1990–2003, *National Vital Statistics Reports* 54(4) (Hyattsville, MD: National Center for Health Statistics, 2005).

10. F. Menacker, E. Declercq, and M. F. MacDorman, Cesarean Delivery: Background, Trends, and Epidemiology, *Seminars in Perinatology* 30(5) (2006): 235–241.

11. J. Villar, E. Valladares, D. Wojdyla, et al., Caesarean Delivery Rates and Pregnancy Outcomes: The 2005 WHO Global Survey on Maternal and Perinatal Health in Latin America, *The Lancet*, May 23, 2006, DOI:10.1016/S0140-6736(06)68704-7.

12. World Health Organization, Women's Health, Western Pacific Region 2001, Korea, p. 286, World Health Organization Regional Office for the Western Pacific, http://www.wpro.who.int/internet/files/pub/360/283.pdf (last accessed May 15, 2008).

13. P. Hanvoravongchai, et al., Implications of Private Practice in Public Hospitals on the Cesarean Section Rate in Thailand, World Health Organization, http//www.who.int/hrh/en/HRDJ_4_1_02.pdf (last accessed May 16, 2008).

14. *Royal College of Midwives Journal*, Caesarean Conference Report: From Audit to Action, Royal College of Midwives Journal, http://www.midwives.co.uk/defaut.asp?chid=439&editorial-id=7089 (last accessed May 16, 2008).

15. Centers for Disease Control and Prevention, Morbidity and Mortality Weekly Report, Rates of Cesarean Delivery among Puerto Rican Women—Puerto Rico and the U.S. Mainland, 1992–2002, *Journal of the American Medical Association* 295(12) (2006): 1369–1371.

16. D. D. Lallo, C. A. Perucci, R. Bertollini, and S. Mallone, Cesarean Section Rates by Type of Maternity Unit and Level of Obstetric Care: An Area-Based Study in Central Italy, *Preventive Medicine* 25(2) (March 1996): 178–185, 8; IngentaConnect.com, http://ingentaconnect.com/content/ap/pm/1996/00000025/00000002/art/art00044 (last accessed May 15, 2008).

17. M. Wagner, *Pursuing the Birth Machine: The Search for Appropriate Birth Technology* (NSW, Australia: Ace Graphics, 1991).

18. M. Enkin, M. J. N. C. Keirse, J. Neilson, et al., *A Guide to Effective Care in Pregnancy and Childbirth*, third edition (Oxford: Oxford University Press, 2000).

19. M. Rosen and L. Thomas, *The Cesarean Myth: Choosing the Best Way to Have Your Baby* (New York: Penguin Books, 1989), ix.

20. M. Gabay and S. Wolfe, *Unnecessary Cesarean Sections: Curing a National Epidemic* (Washington, DC: Public Citizen's Health Research Group, 1994).

21. Institute for Healthcare Improvement, *Reducing Cesarean Section Rates While Maintaining Maternal and Infant Outcomes. Proceedings from a National Congress*, October 17–18, 1996, Orlando, FL.

22. Institute of Medicine, National Roundtable on Health Care Quality, Statement on Quality of Care, National Academies Press, 1998, 13, The National Academies Press, http://www.nap.edu/catalog/9439.html (last accessed May 15, 2008).

23. Childbirth Connection, What Every Pregnant Woman Needs to Know About Cesarean Section, Evidence Tables: Key Questions and Outcomes Examined, Childbirth Connection, http://www.childbirthconnection.org/pdf.asp?PDFDownload=ToCtablesA-F.

24. Australian and New Zealand Perinatal Societies, The Origins of Cerebral Palsy—A Consensus Statement, *Medical Journal of Australia* 162 (1995): 85–90; The Medical Journal of Australia, http://mja.com.au/public/isues/misc/mclann/mclann.html (last accessed May 14, 2008).

25. National Institute for Clinical Excellence, Caesarean Section: Clinical Guideline 13, April 2004, National Institute for Health and Clinical Excellence, http://www.nice.org.uk/page.aspx?o=cg013niceguideline (last accessed May 14, 2008).

26. Maternity Center Association, *What Every Pregnant Woman Needs to Know about Cesarean Section* (New York: MCA, July 2004).

27. M. Enkin, M. J. N. C. Keirse, J. Neilson, et al., *A Guide to Effective Care in Pregnancy and Childbirth*, 360.

28. B. L. Flamm and E. J. Quilligan, editors, *Cesarean Section: Guidelines for Appropriate Utilization* (New York: Springer-Verlag, 1995), 115–124.

29. Childbirth Connection, What Every Pregnant Woman Needs to Know About Cesarean Section.

30. M. R. DiMatteo, S. C. Morton, H. S. Lepper, T. M. Damush, et al., Cesarean Childbirth and Psychosocial Outcomes: A Meta-Analysis, *Health Psychology* 15(4) (1996): 303–314.

31. D. Bailham, and S. Joseph, Post-Traumatic Stress Following Childbirth; A Review of the Emerging Literature and Directions for Research and Practice, *Psychology, Health & Medicine* 8(2) (2003): 159–168.

32. March of Dimes, Cesarean Sections May Be Contributing to the Rise in Late Preterm Births, March of Dimes, http://www.marchofdimes.com/aboutus/15796_19306.asp (last accessed March 29, 2008).

33. World Alliance for Breastfeeding Action, Health Care Practices, World Alliance for Breastfeeding Action, http://www.waba.org.my/hcp.htm, May 15, 2008.

34. United States Breastfeeding Committee, Benefits of Breastfeeding, United States Breastfeeding Committee, http://www.usbreastfeeding.org/Issue-Papers/Benefits.pdf (last accessed May 15, 2008).

35. M. F. MacDorman, F. Menacker, and E. Declercq, Cesarean Birth in the United States: Epidemiology, Trends, and Outcomes, *Clinical Perinatology* 35 (2006): 293–307.

CHAPTER 1

1. B. W. Harrer, Jr., A Look Back at Women's Health and ACOG. A Look Forward to the Challenges of the Future, Obstetrics & Gynecology January 97(1) (2001): 1–4.

2. S. P. Chauhan, V. G. Berghella, M. Sanderson, et al., American College of Obstetricians and Gynecologists Practice Bulletins: An Overview, Obstetrics and Gynecology, 194 (2006): 1564–1575.

3. Physician Insurers Association of America, http://www.piaa.us (last accessed May 25, 2008).

4. S. P. Chauhan, V. B. Chauhan, B. D. Cowan, et al., Professional Liability Claims and Central Association of Obstetrics and Gynecologists Members: Myth versus Reality, American Journal of Obstetrics and Gynecology 192 (2005): 1820–1826.

5. Public Citizen Congress Watch, *Medical Malpractice Payout Trends 1991–2004*, (Public Citizen: Washington, DC, April 2005).

6. Health Affairs. Malpractice Premium Spike in Pennsylvania Did Not Decrease Physician Supply, Press Release, April 24, 2007, Health Affairs, http://www.healthaffairs.org/press/marapr0707.htm (last accessed September 13, 2007).

7. Birth Injury Info, For Parents and Lawyers: Electronic Fetal Monitoring, http://www.birthinjuryinfo.com (last accessed May 23, 2008).

8. Institute for Healthcare Improvement, Reducing Cesarean Rates While Maintaining Maternal and Infant Outcomes, National Congress, October 17–18, 1996, Orlando, FL.

9. M. MacDorman, W. M. Callaghan, T. J. Mathews, et al., Trends in Preterm-Related Infant Mortality by Race and Ethnicity: United States, 1999–2004, Centers for Disease Control, National Center for Health Statistics, http://www.cdc.gov/nchs/products/pubs/pubd/hestats/infantmort99-04/infantmort99-04.htm (last accessed May 16, 2008).

10. R. M. Silver, M. B. Landon, D. J. Rouse, et al., Maternal Morbidity Associated with Multiple Repeat Cesarean Deliveries, *Obstetrics & Gynecology* 107 (2006): 122–132.

11. C. Deneux-Tharaux, E. Caromona, M. H. Bouvier-Colle, and G. Bréart, Postpartum Maternal Mortality and Cesarean Delivery, *Obstetrics & Gynecology* 108(3) (2006): 541–548.

12. International Cesarean Awareness Network, VBAC Policies in US Hospitals, International Cesarean Awareness Network, http://ican-online.org/vbac-ban-info (last accessed May 16, 2008).

13. C. Merrill and C. Steiner, Hospitalizations Related to Childbirth, 2003 (HCUP), Statistical Brief #11, August 2006, Agency for Healthcare Research and Quality, http://www.hcup-us.ahrq.gov/reports/statbriefs/sb11.pdf (last accessed May 16, 2008).

14. R. M. Andrews and A. Elixhauser, The National Hospital Bill: Growth Trends and 2005 Update on the Most Expensive Conditions by Payer, HCUP Statistical Brief #42, December 2007, Agency for Healthcare Research and Quality, Rockville, MD, http://hcup-us.ahrq.gov/reports/statbriefs/sb42pdf (last accessed December 12, 2007).

15. K. Pollitz, M. Kofman, A. Salganicoff, et al., Maternity Care and Consumer-Driven Health Plans, Kaiser Family Foundation Report, June, 12, 2007, Kaiser Family Foundation, http://kff.org/womenshealth/upload/7636ES.pdf (last accessed May 16, 2008).

16. K. Levit, K. Ryan, A. Elixhauser, E. Stranges, et al., HCUP Facts and Figures; Statistics on Hospital-Based Care in the United States in 2005, Rockville, MD, Agency for Healthcare Research and Quality, 2007, http://www.hcup-us.nhrq.gov/reports.jsp (last accessed December 12, 2007).

17. K. Pollitz, M. Kofman, A. Salganicoff, et al., Maternity Care and Consumer-Driven Health Plans.

18. M. Sagady Leslie and S. Storton, The Coalition for Improving Maternity Services: Evidence Basis for the Ten Steps of Mother-Friendly Care. Step 1: Offers All Birthing Mothers Unrestricted Access to Birth, Companions, Labor Support, Professional Midwifery Care, Journal of Perinatal Education 16(1) (Suppl.) (Winter 2007): 10S–19S.

19. Childbirth Connection. Average Facility Labor and Birth Charge by Site, U.S. 2003–2005, Childbirth Connection, http://www.childbirthconnection.org/article.asp?ck=10463&ClickedLink=274&area=27 (last accessed May 14, 2008).

20. Office of Disease Prevention and Health Promotion, U.S. Department of Health and Human Services, Healthy People 2010, Maternal, Infant, and Child Health, 16–30, Washington, DC, Healthy People, http://www.healthypeople.gov/document/word/Volume2/16MICH.doc (last accessed May 15, 2008).

21. Women Deliver Global Conference, London, October 18–20, 2007, Why So High? USA Facts on Maternal Mortality: Women Deliver, http://womendeliver.org/publications/Why_So_High.htm (last accessed May 16, 2008).

22. L. A. Thompson, D. C. Goodman, and G. A. Little, Is More Neonatal Intensive Care Always Better? Insights from a Cross-National Comparison of Reproductive Care, *Pediatrics* 6 (109) (June 2002): 1036–1043

23. Save the Children, State of the World's Mothers, 2006, http://www.savethechildren.org/jump.jsp?path=/publications/mothers/2006/SOWM_2006_final.pdf (last accessed May 16, 2008).

24. M. F. MacDorman, E. Declercq, F. Menacker, et al., Infant and Neonatal Mortality for Primary Cesareans and Vaginal Births to Women with "No Indicated Risks," United States, 1998–2001 Birth Cohorts, *Birth* 33(3) (September 2006): 175–182.

25. Office of Disease Prevention and Health Promotion, U.S. Department of Health and Human Services, Healthy People 2010, Maternal, Infant, and Child Health, 16–30, Washington, DC, http://www.healthypeople.gov/document/word/Volume2/16MICH. doc (last accessed May 16, 2008).

26. Association for Health Care Journalists, http://www.healthjournalism.org/ resources-AHCJpubs.php (last accessed March 25, 2008).

27. United States Department of Health and Human Services, Agency for Research and Quality (AHRQ), National Healthcare Quality Report, 2003, http://www.ahrq.gov/ qual/nhqr03/nhqr03.htm (last accessed July 7, 2008).

28. National Committee for Quality Assurance, The State of Health Care Quality 2007, National Committee for Quality Assurance, Washington, DC, http://ncqa.org/ tabid/543/Default.aspx (last accessed May 16, 2008).

29. National Quality Forum, National Voluntary Consensus Standards for Perinatal Care Steering Committee, http://www.qualityforum.org/projects/ongoing/perinatal/ index.asp (last accessed March 23, 2008).

30. E. R. Declercq, C. Sakala, M. P. Corry, and S. Applebaum, Listening to Mothers II: Report of the Second National U.S. Survey of Women's Childbearing Experiences, New York: Childbirth Connection, October 2006.

CHAPTER 2

1. Coalition for Improving Maternity Services, The Mother-Friendly Childbirth Initiative, http://www.motherfriendly.org (last accessed May 16, 2008).

2. Institute of Medicine, *Crossing the Quality Chasm. A New Health System for the 21st Century* (Washington, DC: National Academy Press, 2001), 61–88.

3. M. A. Schuster et al., *The Quality of Health Care in the United States: A Review of Articles since 1987*, in Institute of Medicine, *Crossing the Quality Chasm. A New Health System for the 21st Century* (Washington, DC: National Academy Press, 2001), 231.

4. S. P. Chauhan et al., American College of Obstetricians and Gynecologists Practice Bulletins: An Overview, *American Journal of Obstetrics and Gynecology* 194 (2006): 1564–1575.

5. A. Coulter, J. Ellins, D. Swain et al., Picker Institute Europe, Assessing the Quality of Information to Support People in Making Decisions about Their Health and Healthcare, Oxford, November 2006, Picker Institute Europe, http://www.pickereurope.org (last accessed September 15, 2007).

6. Institute of Medicine, *Crossing the Quality Chasm*, 70.

7. FIGO, Ethical Issues in Obstetrics and Gynecology, November 2006, http://www.figo.org/docs/Ethics%20Guidelines%20-%20English%20version% 202006%20-2009.pdf (last accessed May 16, 2008).

8. H. Murkoff, A. Eisenber, and S. Hathaway, *What to Expect When You're Expecting*, third edition (New York: Workman Publishing, 2002), 299.

9. Institute of Medicine, Committee on Quality of Health Care in America. To Err Is Human: Building a Safer Health System, Report Brief, November 1999, Institute of Medicine, http://www.iom.edu/CMS/8089/5575/4117.aspx (last accessed May 17, 2008).

10. E. R. Declercq, C. Sakala, M.P. Corry, and S. Applebaum, Listening to Mothers II. Report of the Second National U.S. Survey of Women's Childbearing Experiences, New York: Childbirth Connection, October 2006.

11. National Institutes of Health, State-of-the-Science Conference Statement, Cesarean Delivery on Maternal Request, Final Statement, March 27–29, 2006, http://consensus.nih.gov/2006/2006CesareanSOS027main.htm (last accessed May 16, 2008).

12. American College of Obstetricians and Gynecologists, Surgery and Patient Choice, 2003, New ACOG Opinion Addresses Elective Cesarean Controversy, *ACOG News Release*, October 31, 2003, ACOG, http://www.acog.org/from_home/pubilcations/press_releasess/nr10-31-1.cfm (last accessed May 16, 2008).

13. R. L. Barbieri, It's Time to Target a New Cesarean Delivery Rate, *OBG Management* 6(9) September 2004, OBGManagement, http://obgmanagent.com/article_pages.asp?AID=3386&UID= (last accessed May 16, 2008).

14. Cindy Starr, Elective Cesarean Section: A New Dividing Line for Obs, *Contemporary OB/GYN*, June 2003, http://www.modernmedicine.com/modernmedicine/Cesarean+Section/Elective-cesarean-section-a-new-dividing-line-for-/ArticleStandard/Article/detail/114934 (last accessed May 16, 2008).

15. D. S. Cole, Highlights in Obstetrics, American College of Obstetricians and Gynecologists 51st Annual Clinical Meeting, 2003, Medscape.com, http://www.medscape.com/viewarticle/456324 (last accessed May 16, 2008).

16. D. S. Cole, Elective Primary Cesarean Delivery: What's the Big Deal? Highlights in Obstetrics from the 50th Annual Meeting of the American College of Obstetricians and Gynecologists, Los Angeles, CA, May 4–8, 2002, http://www.medscape.com/viewarticle/434586 (last accessed May 16, 2008).

17. F. D. Frigoletto, Jr., and C. Junge, High-Tech Birth: Do You Need a C-Section? *Newsweek*, April 25, 2007, Massachusetts General Hospital, Vincent Obstetrics and Gynecology Services, http://www.mgh.harvard.edu/vincent/news_April_25_05.htm (last accessed May 17, 2008).

18. Coalition for Improving Maternity Services, Evidence Basis for the Ten Steps of Mother-Friendly Care. Step 2. Provides Accurate, Descriptive, and Statistical Information About Birth Care Practices, *Journal of Perinatal Education* 16(1) (2007) (Suppl.): 20S–22S.

19. United States, the Health Insurance Portability and Accountability Act, http://www.opm.gov/insure/health/cbrr.htm#chpt4 (last accessed May 17, 2008).

20. E. R. Declercq, C. Sakala, M. P. Corry, and S. Applebaum, Listening to Mothers II. Report of the Second National U.S. Survey of Women's Childbearing Experiences, New York: Childbirth Connection, October 2006.

21. American College of Surgeons (ACS), When You Need an Operation. About Cesarean Childbirth, American College of Surgeons, http://www.facs.org/public_info/operation/aboutbroch.html (last accessed July 8, 2008).

22. American College of Obstetricians and Gynecologists, Cesarean Birth. Patient Education, ACOG, http://www.acog.org/publications/patient_education/bp006.cfm (last accessed July 8, 2008).

23. H. Goer, M. Sagady Leslie, and M. Romano, Coalition for Improving Maternity Services, Evidence Basis for the Ten Steps of Mother-Friendly Care. Step 6. Does Not Routinely Employ Practices, Procedures Unsupported by Scientific Evidence, *Journal of Perinatal Education* 16(1) (Suppl.) (2007): 32S–64S.

24. *Journal of the American Medical Association*, Patient Page, Cesarean Delivery, http://medem.com/search/article_display.cfm?path=\\TANQUERAY\M_ContentItem&mstr=/M_ContentItem/ZZZEO7LAB1D.html&soc=JAMA/Archives&srch_typ=NAV_SERCH) (last accessed on January 21, 2006).

25. National Library of Medicine, MedlinePlus, X-Plain.com, Patient Education Institute, C-Section Interactive Tutorial, http://www.nlm.nih.gov/medlineplus/tutorials/csection/htm/index.htm (last accessed on July 9, 2008).

26. National Library of Medicine, MedlinePlus, X-Plain Vaginal Birth, Interactive Tutorial, X-Plain Program, http://www.nlm.nih.gov/medlineplus/tutorials/vaginalbirth/htm/index.htm (last accessed on July 9, 2008).

27. Childbirth Connection Preventing Pelvic Floor Dysfunction. http://www.childbirthconnection.com/article.asp?ck=10206 (last accessed on July 25, 2008).

28. M. Kroeger and L. Smith, *Impact of Birthing Practices on Breastfeeding* (Boston: Jones and Bartlett, 2004).

29. Healthy Pregnancy, Childbirth and Beyond, http://www.4women.gov/pregnancy/childbirthandbeyond/laborandbirth.cfm#cesarean (last accessed on July 9, 2008).

30. University of Michigan Health Systems, Vaginal Birth after a Previous Cesarean Delivery, http://www.med.umich.edu/1libr/wha/wha_vbac_crs.htm (last accessed on July 9, 2008).

31. Patient Education Institute, Vaginal Birth, http://www.nlm.nih.gov/medlineplus/tutorials/vaginalbirth/htm/index.htm (last accessed on July 9, 2008).

32. American Society of Anesthesiologist, Anesthesia and You. Planning Your Childbirth: Pain Relief during Labor and Delivery, http://www.asahq.org/patientEducation/labordelivery.pdf (last accessed on July 9, 2008).

33. Painfree Birthing, http://www.painfreebirthing.com/english/welcome.html (last accessed on July 9, 2008).

34. Street Drugs, http://www.streetdrugs.org/fentanyl.htm (last accessed on July 9, 2008).

35. National Institutes of Health, National Institute on Drug Abuse, http://www.drugabuse.gov/drugpages/fentanyl.html (last accessed May 25, 2008).

36. S. Jordan et al., The Impact of Intrapartum Analgesia on Infant Feeding, *BJOG: An International Journal of Obstetrics and Gynecology* 112(7) (2005): 927–934, doi:10.1111/j.1471-0528.2005.00548.x, Abstract (last accessed May 25, 2008).

37. S. Jordan, Infant Feeding and Analgesia in Labour: The Evidence Is Accumulating. Commentary, *International Breastfeeding Journal,* Biomed Central, http://www.internationalbreastfeedingjournal.com/content/1/125 (last accessed May 25, 2008).

38. A. Montgomery, T. W. Hale, and the Academy of Breastfeeding Medicine Protocol Committee, ABM Clinical Protocol # 15, Analgesia and Anesthesia for the Breastfeeding Mother, *Breastfeeding Medicine* 1(4) (2006): 271–277.

39. M. Anim-Somuah,R. Smyth, and C. Howell, Epidural versus Non-Epidural or No Analgesia in Labour, *Cochrane Database of Systematic Reviews 1998*, Issue 1, Art. No.: CD000331. DOI: 10.1002/14651858.CD000331.pub2, Abstract (last accessed on May 25, 2008).

40. U.S. Department of Health and Human Services, Women's Health.gov, http://www.4woman.gov/pregnancy/childbirthandbeyond/laborandbirth.cfm#where (last accessed on July 25, 2008).

41. M. Sagady Leslie and M. Romano, Coalition for Improving Maternity Services, Evidence Basis for the Ten Steps of Mother-Friendly Care. Appendix: Birth Can Safely Take Place at Home and in Birthing Centers. *Journal of Perinatal Education* 16(1) (Suppl.) (2007): 381S–388S.

42. H. Goer, M. Sagady Leslie, and M. Romano, Coalition for Improving Maternity Services, Evidence Basis for the Ten Steps of Mother-Friendly Care. Step 6. Does Not

Routinely Employ Practices, Procedures Unsupported By Scientific Evidence, *Journal of Perinatal Education* 16(1) (Suppl.) (2007): 32S–364S.

43. Public Advocate for the City of New York, A Mother's Right to Know: New York City Hospitals Fail to Provide Legally Mandated Maternity Information, July 2005, http://www.pubadvocate.nyc.gov (last accessed on May 25, 2008).

44. Public Advocate for the City of New York Betsy Gotbaum, Giving Birth in the Dark, December 2006, http://www.pubadvocate.nyc.gov/policy/documents/GivingBirthInTheDark12.06.pdf (last accessed on May 25, 2008).

45. MIDIRS. Caesarean Section and Subsequent Births, http://www.infochoice.org/ (last accessed on May 25, 2008).

46. National Institute for Clinical Excellence (NICE), Caesarean Section. Information for the Public, April 2004, http://www.nice.org.uk/nicemedia/pdf/CG013publicinfoenglish.pdf (last accessed on May 25, 2008).

47. NICE, Caesarean Section Clinical Guidelines, April 2004, http://www.nice.org.uk/nicemedia/pdf/CG013fullguideline.pdf (last accessed May 25, 2008).

48. MIDIRS, Informed Choice. Non-Epidural Pain Relief, http://www.Infochoice.org (last accessed on May 25, 2008).

49. Ministry of Health, Government of New Zealand, http://www.moh.govt.nz/cochranelibrary (last accessed on May 25, 2008).

50. Institute of Medicine, To Err Is Human: Building a Safer Health System, Report Brief, http://www.iom.edu/CMS/8089/5575/4117.aspx (last accessed on May 25, 2008).

51. G. J. Annas, *The Rights of Patients. The Authoritative ACLU Guide to Patient Rights*, third edition (Carbondale, IL: Southern Illinois University Press, 2004).

52. Childbirth Connection, The Rights of Childbearing Women, http://childbirthconnection.com/article.asp?ck=10084 (last accessed on April 20, 2008).

53. G. J. Annas, *The Rights of Patients. The Authoritative ACLU Guide to Patient Rights*, third edition (Carbondale, IL: Southern Illinois University Press, 2004), 64.

CHAPTER 3

1. H. L. Minkoff, MD in Jennifer Block, *Pushed* (Cambridge, MA: Da Capo Press, Perseus Books), 125–126.

2. National Institutes of Health, State-of-the-Science Conference, Cesarean Delivery on Maternal Request, March 27–29, 2006, National Institutes of Health, Natcher Conference Center, Bethesda, MD.

3. S. Donati et al., Do Italian Mothers Prefer Cesarean Delivery? *Birth: Issues in Perinatal Care* 30(2) (June 2003): 89–93.

4. J. A. Gamble and D. K. Creedy, Women's Request for Cesarean Section: A Critique of the Literature, *Birth: Issues in Perinatal Care* 27(4) (December 2000): 256–263.

5. K. Hopkins, Are Brazilian Women Really Choosing to Deliver by Cesarean? *Social Science and Medicine* 51(5) (September 2000): 725–740.

6. J. J. Weaver, H. Statham, and M. Richards, Are There "Unnecessary" Cesarean Sections? Perceptions of Women and Obstetricians about Cesarean Sections for Non-clinical Indications, *Birth* 34(1) (March 2007): 32–41.

7. C. McCourt, J. Weaver, H. Statham et al., Elective Cesarean Section and Decision Making: A Critical Review of the Literature, *Birth* 34(1) (March 2007): 65–79.

8. D. Béhague, C. G. Victoria, and F. C. Barros, Consumer Demand for Caesarean Sections in Brazil: Informed Decision Making, Patient Choice, or Social Inequality? A Population-Based Birth Cohort Study Linking Ethnographic and Epidemiological Methods, *British Medical Journal* 321 (April 20, 2002), http://www.bmj.com.

9. S. Pakenham, S. M. Chamberlain, and G. N. Smith, Women's Views on Elective Primary Caesarean Section, *Journal of Obstetrics and Gynecology of Canada* (December 2006): 1089–1094.

10. Hilde Nerum, B.Sc. (Midwifery), Lotta Halvorsen, B.Sc. (Midwifery), Tore Sørlie M.D., Ph.D., Pål Øian, M.D., Ph.D. Maternal Request for Cesarean Section Due to Fear of Birth: Can It Be Changed through Crisis-Oriented Counseling? *Birth* 33(3) 2006, 221–228.

11. B. Sjögren, Reasons for auxiety about childbirth, J. Psychosom Obstet gynecol 18 (1997): 820–826.

12. K. Hopkins, Are Brazilian Women Really Choosing to Deliver by Cesarean ? *Social Science and Medicine*, May 23, 2000, Abstract doi:10.1016/S0277-9536(99)00480-3.

13. J. E. Potter, E. Berquó, I. H. Perpétuo, O. F. Leal, K. Hopkins, M. R. Souza, and M. C. Formiga, Unwanted Caesarean Sections among Public and Private Patients in Brazil: Prospective Study 1, *BMJ* 323(7322) (November 17, 2001): 1155–1158, http://www.ncbi.nlm.nih.gov/sites/entrez?orig_db=PubMed&db=pubmed&cmd=Search&term=British%20Medical%20Journal%20%5BJour%5D%20AND%202001%5Bpdat%5D%20AND%20Potter%20J%20E%5Bauthor%5D.

14. http://www.partodoprincipio.com.br/, private communication, Federal Public Prosecutor Supports Parto do Principio and Sponsors Hearing on C-Section Abuse, CIMSInternational@yahoogroups.com.

15. E. R. Declercq, C. Sakala, M. P. Corry, and S. Applebaum, Listening to Mothers II. Report of the Second National U.S. Survey of Women's Childbearing Experiences, New York: Childbirth Connection, October 2006.

16. M. F. MacDorman, F. Menacker, and E. Declercq, Cesarean Birth in the United States: Epidemiology, Trends, and Outcomes, *Clinics in Perinatology* 35 (2008): 293–307.

17. F. Menacker, E. Declercq, and M. F. MacDorman, Cesarean Delivery: Background, Trends, and Epidemiology, *Seminars in Perinatology*, 30(5) (October 2006): 235–241, Abstract, Doi:10.1053/j.semperi.2006.07.002.

18. L. Pevzner, D. Goffman, M.Comerford Freda, and A. K. Dayal, Patients' Attitudes Associated with Cesarean Delivery on Maternal Request in an Urban Population, *American Journal of Obstetrics and Gynecology* 198(5) (May 2008): e35–e37.

19. Diony Young, Confrontation in Kansas City: Elective Cesareans and Maternal Choice, Editorial, *Birth* 27(3) (September 2000): 153–155.

20. Health Grades, Health Grades Quality Study, First-Time Preplanned and "Patient Choice" Cesarean Section Rates In the United States, July 2003, Health Grades, http://www.healthgrades.com/pressroom/index.cfm?fuseaction=modNBG&modtype=b2b&modact=HGNews&section=1 (last accessed on May 17, 2008).

21. Health Grades, Health Grades Quality Study, First-Time Preplanned and "Patient Choice" Cesarean Section Rates In the United States, July 2003, Health Grades, http://www.healthgrades.com/pressroom/index.cfm?fuseaction=modNBG&modtype=b2b&modact=HGNews&section=1 (last accessed on May 17, 2008.

22. ACOG, New ACOG Opinion Addresses Elective Cesarean Controversy, October 31, 2003, http://acog.com/from_home/publications/press_releases/nr10-31-03-1.cfm (last accessed on May 17, 2008).

23. American College of Nurse Midwives (last accessed on July 9, 2008).

24. Society of Obstetricians and Gynecologists of Canada, Advisory. C-Sections on Demand—SOGC's Position, March 10, 2004, http://www.sogc.org (last accessed on July 9, 2008).

25. Canadian Association of Midwives-Association, Canadienne des Sages-Femmes, Position Statement on Elective Cesarean Section, http://www.canadianmidwives.org (last accessed on July 9, 2008).

26. RCOG, Caesarean Section, April 2004, http://www.nice.org.uk/nicemedia/pdf/CG013fullguideline.pdf (last accessed on May 17, 2008).

27. Royal College of Midwives, Maternal Choice and Caesarean Section, September 2001, http://www.rcm.org.uk (last accessed on September 9, 2003).

28. FIGO, FIGO Statement on Caesarean Section, January 2007, http://www.figo.org/Caesarean.asp (last accessed on September 7, 2007).

29. Health Grades, Number of "Patient Choice" C-Sections Rises by 25 Percent Healthgrades Study Finds, June 29, 2004, http://www.healthgrades.com/pressroom/?tv_lid=lnk_press_bottom (last accessed on May 17, 2008).

30. Health Grades, June 29, 2004, Press Release (last accessed on May 17, 2008).

31. Childbirth Connection, Preventing Pelvic Floor Dysfunction, http://www.childbirthconnection.org.

32. Health Grades, Health Grades Third Annual Report on "Patient-Choice" Cesarean Section Rates in the United States, September 2005, http://www.healthgrades.com (last accessed on July 9, 2008).

33. Healthgrades.com, Healthgrades in the News, 2005, http://www.healthgrades.com/pressroom/index.cfm?fuseaction=modNBG&modtype=b2b&modact=HGNews&section=1, http://www.healthywomen.org/resources/womenshealthinthenews/dbhealthnews/morefirsttimemomsoptingforcsections (last accessed on May 25, 2008).

34. HealthGrades, The HealthGrades Maternity Care Report, June 2007, http://www.healthgrades.com (last accessed on May 26, 2008).

35. NIH State-of-the-Science Conference Statement on Cesarean Delivery on Maternal Request, NIH Consensus Science Statements, 23(1) (March 27–29, 2006): 1–29, Booklet, http://consensus.nih.gov.

36. Childbirth Connection, National Institutes of Health State-of-the-Science Conference, Cesarean Delivery on Maternal Request, Proposed Criteria for Assessing Adequacy of Response to Key Questions, March 2006, http://www.childbirthconnection.org/pdfs/NIH_cesarean_questions.pdf.

37. Childbirth Connection, Alert: NIH Cesarean Conference: Interpreting Meeting and Media Reports, updated October 2006 (last accessed on September 4, 2007).

38. Maternity Center Association, What Every Woman Needs to Know about Cesarean Section, Childbirth Connection, New York, http://childbirthconnection.org/article.asp?ck=10164.

39. J. Villar, E. Valladares, D. Wojdyla et al., World Health Organization, 2005, Global Survey on Maternal and Perinatal Health Research Group, Cesarean Delivery Rates and Pregnancy Outcomes: The 2005 WHO Survey on Maternal and Perinatal Health in Latin America, *Lancet*, May 23, 2006, DOI:10.1o16/S0140-6736(06)68744-7.

40. Childbirth Connection, National Institute of Health State-of-the-Science Conference, Cesarean Delivery on Maternal Request, Proposed Criteria for Assessing Adequacy of Response to Key Questions, Childbirth Connection, March 2006, http://www.childbirthconnection.org/pdfs/NIH_csaran_questions.pdf.

41. Childbirth Connection, Alert: NIH Cesarean Conference: Interpreting Meeting and Media Reports, updated October 2006, http://childbirthconnection.org/article. asp?ck=10375 (last accessed on September 9, 2007).

42. Diony Young, "Cesarean Delivery on Maternal Request": Was the NIH Conference Based on a Faulty Premise? *Birth* 33 (3) (2006): 171–174, doi:10.1111/j.1523-536X.2006.00101.x (last accessed on December 28, 2007).

43. Rob Stein, NIH Panel Finds No Extra Risk in Caesarean Section, *Washington Post*, March 30, 2006.

44. Lauran Neergaared, No Clear Advice on Elective C-Sections, March 29, 2006 7:29 PM (ET), Yahoo! News.

45. Rita Rubin, Panel Asks Women to Weigh Pros and Cons of C-Sections, *USA Today* March 29, 2006, http://www.usatoday.com/news/health/2006-03-29-csection-panel_x.htm.

46. Allison Aubrey, Section Births Gaining Popularity, March 30, 2006, http://www.npr.org/templates/story/story.php?storyId=5311258 (last accessed on January 5, 2008).

47. ACNM Press Release, March 30, 2006, American College of Nurse-Midwives Calls for Accurate Reporting on New NIH Findings about Cesarean Delivery (last accessed on April 5, 2006).

48. L. M. Leeman, Planted, L.A. Patient-Choice Vaginal Delivery? *Annals of Family Medicine* 4(3) (May/June 2006), http://annfammed.org/cgi/contnet/full/4/3/265.

49. ACOG, Cesarean Delivery Associated with Increased Risk of Maternal Death from Blood Clots, Infection, Anesthesia, Press Release, August 31, 2006, http://acog.com/from_home/publications/press_releases/nr08-31-06-2.cfm (last accessed on December 28, 2007).

50. A. F. MacDorman, E. Declercq, F. Menacker, and M. H. Malloy, Infant and Neonatal Mortality for Primary Cesarean and Vaginal Births to Women with "No Indicated Risks," United States, 1998–2001, Birth Cohorts, *Birth* 33(3) (September 2006).

51. Lamaze International, Elective Cesarean Surgery versus Planned Vaginal Birth. What Are the Consequences?, http://www.lamaze.org.

CHAPTER 4

1. M. Enkin, M. J. N. C. Keirse, J. Neilson et al., *A Guide to Effective Care in Pregnancy and Childbirth* (Oxford: Oxford University Press, 2000).

2. Ibid., 406.

3. Edgardo Abalos, Alternative Techniques and Materials for Caesarean Section: RHL Commentary (last revised December 3, 2004). The WHO Reproductive Health Library, No. 9, Update Software Ltd, Oxford, 2006; WHO Reproductive Library, http://www.rhlibrary.com/Commentaries/htm-print/eacom3.htm (last accessed on April 11, 2007).

4. D. Jacobs-Jokhan and G. J. Hofmeyr, Extra-Abdominal versus Intra-Abdominal Repair of the Uterine Incision at Caesarean Section (Cochrane Review), Abstract, *The Reproductive Health Library*, 10, 2007, Oxford, Update Software Ltd, WHO Reproductive Health Library, http://www.rhlibrary.com (last accessed on April 17, 2007).

5. A. A. Bamigboye and G. J. Hofmeyr, Closure versus Non-Closure of the Peritoneum at Caesarean Section (Cochrane Review), Abstract, The Reproductive Health

Library, 10, 2007, Oxford, Update Software Ltd, WHO Reproductive Health Library, http://www.rhlibrary.com (last accessed on May 10, 2007).

6. E. R. Anderson and S. Gates, Techniques and Materials for Closure of the Abdominal Wall in Caesarean Section (Cochrane Review), Abstract, The Reproductive Health Library, 10, 2007, Oxford, Update Software Ltd., WHO Reproductive Health Library, http://www.rhlibrary.com (last accessed on April 17, 2007).

7. J. G. Cecatti, Antibiotic Prophylaxis for Cesarean Section: RHL Commentary (last revised January 18, 2005). The WHO Reproductive Health Library, No. 9, Update Software Ltd, Oxford, 2006, WHO Reproductive Health Library, http://www.rhlibrary.com (last accessed on April 17, 2007).

8. M. F. MacDorman, E. Declerq, F. Menacker, and M. H. Malloy, Infant and Neonatal Mortality for Primary Cesarean and Vaginal Births to Women with "No Indicated Risk," United States, 1998–2001 Birth Cohorts, *Birth* 33(3) (2006): 175–182.

9. C. Deneux-Tharaux, E. Caromona, M. H. Bouvier-Colle, and G. Bréart, Postpartum Maternal Mortality and Cesarean Delivery, *Obstetrics & Gynecology* 108(3) (2006): 541–548.

10. National Institute for Clinical Guidance, Clinical Guideline, Caesarean Section, April 2004, http://www.nice.org (last accessed on March 10, 2007).

11. E. Declercq, F. Menacker, and M. MacDorman, Rise in "No Indicated Risk" Primary Caesareans in the United States, 1991–2001: Cross Sectional Analysis, *British Medical Journal* 330(7482) (January 8, 2005): 71–72.

12. J. G. Cecatti, Antibiotic Prophylaxis for Cesarean Section: RHL Commentary (last revised January 18, 2005), The WHO Reproductive Health Library, No. 9, Update Software Ltd, Oxford, 2006, WHO Reproductive Health Library, http://www.rhlibrary.com (last accessed on April 17, 2007).

13. American Society of Anesthesiologists, Anesthesia and You, http://www.asahq.org/patientEducation.htm (last accessed on March 17, 2007).

14. W. Camann and K. J. Alexander, Easy Labor: Every Woman's Guide to Choosing Less Pain and More Joy during Childbirth (New York: Ballantine Books, 2006), 77–79.

15. PainFreeBirthing, http://www.painfreebirthing.com/english/welcome.htm (last accessed on April 23, 2007).

16. K. Ng, J. Parsons, A. M. Cyna, and P. Middleton, Spinal versus Epidural Anesthesia for Caesarean Section (Cochrane Review), Abstract, The Reproductive Health Library, 9, 2006, Oxford, Update Software Ltd, WHO Reproductive Health Library, http://www.rhlibrary.com (last accessed on April 23, 2007).

17. M. Enkin et al., *A Guide to Effective Care in Pregnancy and Childbirth*, 405–406.

18. Painfreebirthing, http://www.painfreebirthing.com/english/welcome.htm (last accessed on May 15, 2008).

CHAPTER 5

1. National Institute for Clinical Excellence (NICE), Cesarean Section, April 2004, http://www.nice.org.uk/guidance/index.jsp?action=byID&o=10940 (last accessed on May 17, 2008).

2. U.S. Department of Health and Human Services, Cesarean Childbirth, NIH Publication No. 82–2067, 1981.

3. C. Deneux-Tharaux E. Carmona, M. H. Bouvier-Colle et al., Postpartum Maternal Mortality and Cesarean Delivery, *Obstetrics & Gynecology*, Part 1, 108(3): (September 2006): 541–548.

4. J. Vilar, E. Valladares, D. Wojdyla et al., Caesarean Delivery Rates and Pregnancy Outcomes: The 2005 WHO Global Survey on Maternal and Perinatal Health in Latin America, *The Lancet*.com, May 23, 2006, DOI:10.1016/S0140-6736(06)68704-7, http://www.thelancet.com.

5. S. Liu, M. Heaman, K. S. Joseph et al., Maternal Mortality and Severe Morbidity Associated with Low-Risk Planned Cesarean Delivery versus Planned Vaginal Delivery at Term, *Canadian Medical Association Journal*, 176(4) (February 13, 2007), Doi.10.1503/cmaj.olo870 (last accessed on May 20, 2008).

6. H. Goer, M. Sagady Leslie, and A. Romano, CIMS Evidence Basis for the Ten Steps of Mother-Friendly Care, *Journal of Perinatal Education* (Suppl.) (2007): S48–S56.

7. Childbirth Connection, What Every Pregnant Woman Needs to Know about Cesarean Section, 2006, http://www.childbirthconnection.org/article.asp?ck=10164, February 10, 2008.

8. M. Boukerro et al., A History of Cesareans Is a Risk Factor in Vaginal Hysterectomies, *Acta Obstetricia et Gynecologica Scandinavica*, 82(12) (2003): 1135–1139, Abstract, http://www.blackwell-synergy.com/doi/abs/.

9. American College of Obstetricians and Gynecologists, Evaluation of Cesarean Delivery, Author, 2000, 5.

10. F. Smaill and G. J. Hofmeyr, Antibiotic Prophylaxis for Cesarean Section, *Cochrane Database of Systematic Reviews*, Issue 3, 2002, Art. No. CD000933. DOI: 10.1002/14651858.CD000933, Abstract, Cochrane Collaboration, Cochrane Reviews, http://www.cochrane.org/reviews/en/ab000933.html (last accessed on May 17, 2008).

11. J. Griffitsh et al., Surgical Site Infection Following Elective Caesarean Section: A Case-Control Study of Postdischarge Surveillance, *Journal of Obstetrics and Gynecology of Canada* (JOGC), 27(4) (2005): 340–344, Abstract.

12. L. Bren, Battle of the Bugs: Fighting Antibiotic Resistance, U.S. Federal Drug Administration, http://www.fda.gov/fdac/special/testtubetopatient/antibiotics.html (last accessed on January 4, 2007).

13. Agency for Healthcare Research and Quality (AHRQ), personal communication, January 8, 2007.

14. NICE, Cesarean Section, April 2004.

15. MayoClinic.com, Sheehan's Syndrome, http://www.mayoclinic.com/health/sheehans-syndrome/DS00889 (last accessed on May 17, 2008).

16. M. Enkin et al., *A Guide to Effective Care in Pregnancy and Childbirth* (Oxford: Oxford University Press, 2000), 324.

17. NICE, Cesarean Section, April 2004.

18. E. Declerq, C. Sakala, M. P. Corry, and S. Applebaum, Listening to Mothers II. Report of the Second National U.S. Survey of Women's Childbearing Experiences, New York, Childbirth Connection, 2006.

19. Women's Health Resource Center. Pelvic Adhesions: Fast Facts, http://www.healthywomen.org/resources/nwhrcpublications/dbpubs/fastfactspelvicadhesions (last accessed on April 10, 2008).

20. Maternity Center Association, What Every Pregnant Woman Needs to Know About Cesarean Section, New York, MCA, July 2004.

21. Brady E. Hamilton, Ph.D., Joyce A. Martin, M.P.H., and Stephanie J. Ventura, M.A., Division of Vital Statistics. Births Preliminary Data for 2005, National Center for Health Statistics, Centers for Disease Control, http://www.cdc.gov/nchs/products/pubs/pubd/hestats/prelimbirths05/prelimbirths05.htm#fig4 (last accessed on May 17, 2008).

22. J. Kleinbart et al., *Prevention of Thromboembolism*, chapter 31, pp. 333–348, in Agency for Healthcare Quality and Research Evidence Report/Technology Assessment No. 43, Making Health Care Safer: A Critical Analysis of Patient Safety Practices, AHRQ Publication 01-E058, July 20, 2001, http://www.ahrq.gov/clinic/ptsafety/pdf/ptsafety.pdf (last accessed on May 17, 2008).

23. Maternity Center Association, What Every Pregnant Woman Needs to Know about Cesarean Section, Evidence tables, http://www.childbirthconnection.org/pdfs/tablesA-C.pdf (last accessed on May 18, 2008).

24. ACOG, Evaluation of Cesarean Delivery, Author, 2000.

25. Maternity Center Association, What Every Pregnant Woman Needs to Know about Cesarean Section, 21–22.

26. NICE, Clinical Guideline, 13, Cesarean Section.

27. Maternity Center Association, What Every Pregnant Woman Needs to Know about Cesarean Section, April 14, 2004, Evidence Tables, http://www.childbirthconnection.org/pdfs/tablesA-C.pdf (last accessed on May 18, 2008).

28. S. Liu, M. Heaman, K. S. Joseph et al., Risk of Maternal Postpartum Readmission Associated with Mode of Delivery, *Obstetrics & Gynecology* 195(4) (2005): 836–842.

29. E. Declercq et al., 2006, Listening to Mothers.

30. Coalition for Improving Maternity Services, The Risks of Cesarean Delivery to Mother and Baby, http://www.motherfriendly.org (last accessed on March 15, 2008).

31. P. T. Simkin, Just Another Day in a Woman's Life? Women's Long-Term Perceptions of Their First Birth Experience, Part I, *Birth* 18(4) (1991): 203–210.

32. P. T. Simkin, Just Another Day in a Woman's Life? Part II: Nature and Consistency of Women's Long-Term Memories of Their First Birth Experiences, *Birth* 19 (2)(1992): 64–81.

33. M. Porter et al., Satisfaction with Cesarean Section: Qualitative Analysis of Open-Ended Questions in a Large Postal Survey, *Birth: Issues in Perinatal Care* 34(2) (June 2007): 148–154.

34. C. Deneux-Tharaux, E. Carmona, M. H, Bouvier-Colle et al., Postpartum Maternal Mortality and Cesarean Delivery, *Obstetrics and Gynecology* (108, Part 1) (September 2006): 541–548.

35. J. Villar et al., Cesarean Delivery Rates and Pregnancy Outcomes, WHO Global Survey on Maternal and Perinatal Health in Latin America (2005), *The Lancet* May 23, 2006, DOI:10.1016/S0140-6736(06)68704-7, http://www.thelancet.com.

36. National Institute for Clinical Excellence, CG46 Venous Thrombus Embolism: Understanding NICE Guidance, April 23, 2007, http://www.nice.org.uk/guidance/index.jsp?action=download&o=30471 (last accessed on May 18, 2008).

CHAPTER 6

1. Coalition for Improving Maternity Services, The Mother-Friendly Childbirth Initiative, http://www.motherfriendly.org.

2. P. T. Simkin, Just Another Day in a Woman's Life? Women's Long-Term Perceptions of Their First Birth Experience, Part I, *Birth* 18(4) (1991): 203–210.

3. P. T. Simkin, Just Another Day in a Woman's Life? Part II: Nature and Consistency of Women's Long-Term Memories of Their First Birth Experiences, *Birth* 19(2) (1992): 64–81.

4. E. R. Declercq, C. Sakala, M. P. Corry, and S. Applebaum, Listening to Mothers II: Report of the Second National U.S. Survey of Women's Childbearing Experiences, New York, Childbirth Connection, 2006.

5. U.S. Department of Health and Human Services Health Resources & Services Administration, http://www.mchb.hrsa.gov/pregnancyandbeyond/depression (last accessed on April 14, 2008).

6. S. Ayers and A. D. Pickering, Do Women Get Posttraumatic Stress Disorder as a Result of Childbirth? A Prospective Study of Incidence, *Birth* 28(2) (June 2001): 111–118.

7. D. K. Creedy, I. M. Shochet, and J. Horsfall, Childbirth and the Development of Acute Trauma Symptoms: Incidence and Contributing Factors, *Birth* 27 (June 2, 2000): 104–111.

8. J. L. Reynolds, Post-Traumatic Stress Disorder after Childbirth: The Phenomenon of Traumatic Birth, *Canadian Medical Association Journal* 156(6) (1997): 831–835.

9. C. T. Beck, Birth Trauma: In the Eye of the Beholder, *Nursing Research* 53(1) (2004): 28–35.

10. D. K. Creedy, I. M. Shochet, and J. Horsfall, Childbirth and the Development of Acute Trauma Symptoms: Incidence and Contributing Factors, *Birth* 27(2) (2000): 104–111.

11. D. Bailham and S. Joseph, Post-Traumatic Stress Following Childbirth: A Review of the Emerging Literature and Directions for Research and Practice, *Psychology, Health & Medicine* 8(2) (2003): 159–168.

12. H. J. Czarnocka and P. Slade, Prevalence and Predictors of Post-Traumatic Stress Symptoms Following Childbirth, *British Journal of Clinical Psychology* 39(1) (March 2000): 35–51.

13. U. Waldenström, I. Hildingsson, C. Rubertsson, and I. Rådestad, Negative Birth Experience: Prevalence and Risk Factors in a National Sample, *Birth* 31(1) (2004): 17–27.

14. P. Simkin and P. Klaus, *When Survivors Give Birth* (Seattle, WA: Classic Day Publishing, 2004).

15. T. Stojadinovic, For the First Time Somebody Wants to Hear. The Effects of Childhood Sexual Abuse on Women's Experiences of Pregnancy, Birth, and Mothering, June 2003, Women's Health Service, Government of South Australia, http://www.whs.sa.gov.au (last accessed on July 7, 2008).

16. J. E. Soet, G. A. Brack, and C. Diorio, Prevalence and Predictors of Women's Experience of Psychological Trauma during Childbirth, *Birth* 30(1) (2003): 36–46.

17. D. Swalm, Childbirth and Emotional Trauma: Why It's Important to Talk, Talk, Talk, Trauma and Birth Stress, http://www.TABShttp://www.tabs.org.nz/articles.htm (last accessed on June 21, 2008).

18. M. S. Cranley, K. J. Hedal, and S. H. Pegg, Perceptions of Vaginal and Cesarean Deliveries, *Nursing Research* 32(1) (1983): 10–15.

19. L. H. Cummings, C. M. Scrimshaw, and P. L. Engle, Views of Cesarean Birth among Primiparous Women of Mexican Origin in Los Angeles, *Birth* 15(3) (1988): 164–170.

20. J. Marut and R. Mercer, Comparison of Primiparas' Perceptions of Vaginal and Cesarean Births, *Nursing Research* 28 (1979): 260–266.

21. C. Sheppard-McLain, Why Women Choose Trial of Labor or Repeat Cesarean Section, *The Journal of Family Practice* 21(3) (1985): 210–216.

22. J. G. Lipson and V. P. Tilden, Psychological Integration of the Cesarean Birth Experience, *American Journal of Orthopsychiatry* 50(4) (1980): 598–609.

23. L. Baptisti-Richards, Healing the Couple, *Midwifery Today* (7) (1981): 22–25.

24. G. Peterson and L. Mehl, *Cesarean Birth Risk and Culture* (Berkeley, CA: Mind-body Press, 1985).

25. N. Wainer-Cohen and L. Estner, *Silent Knife* (Westport, CT: Bergin & Garvey, 1983).

26. C. S. Mutryn, Psychosocial Impact of Cesarean Section on the Family: A Literature Review, *Social Science and Medicine* 37(10) (1993):1271–1281.

27. L. Madsen, Rebounding from Childbirth: Toward Emotional Recovery (Westport, CT: Bergin & Garvey, 1994).

28. J. R. W. Fisher, R. O. Stanley, and G. D. Burros (1990), Psychological Adjustment to Cesarean Delivery: A Review of the Evidence, *Journal of Psychosomatic Obstetrics and Gynecology* 11(2): 91–206.

29. P. M. Boyce and A. L. Todd, Increased Risk of Postnatal Depression after Emergency Cesarean Section, *Medical Journal of Australia* 157(3) (1992): 172–174.

30. J. Jolly, J. Walker, and K. Bhabra, Subsequent Obstetric Performance Related to Primary Mode of Delivery. *British Journal of Obstetrics and Gynecology* 106 (3) (1999): 227–232.

31. T. Saisto, O. Ylikorkala, and E. Halmesmaki, Factors Associated with Fear of Delivery in Second Pregnancies, *Obstetrics & Gynecology* 94(5) (1999): 679–682.

32. D. Bailham and S. Joseph, Post-Traumatic Stress Following Childbirth; A Review of the Emerging Literature and Directions for Research And Practice, *Psychology, Health & Medicine* 8(2) (2003): 159–168.

33. E. L. Ryding, et al., Psychological Impact of Emergency Cesarean Section in Comparison with Elective Cesarean Section, Instrumental and Normal Vaginal Delivery, *Journal of Psychosomatic Obstetrics and Gynecology* 19(3) (1998): 135–144.

34. E. L. Ryding, K. Wijma, and B. Wijma, Experiences of Emergency Cesarean Section: A Phenomenological Study of 53 Women, *Birth* 25(4) (1999): 246–251.

35. S. Ayers and A. D. Pickering, Do Women Get Posttraumatic Stress Disorder As a Result of Childbirth? A Prospective Study of Incidence, *Birth* 28(2) (2001): 11–118.

36. D. K. Creedy, I. M. Shochet, and J. Horsfall, Childbirth and the Development of Acute Trauma Symptoms: Incidence and Contributing Factors, *Birth* 27(2) (2000): 104–111.

37. P. Simkin and P. Klaus, When Survivors Give Birth: Understanding and Healing the Effects of Early Sexual Abuse on Childbearing Women, Conference Proceedings, San Jose, CA: October 6, 2007.

38. International Cesarean Awareness Network, Cesarean Voices, Redondo Beach, CA: International Cesarean Awareness Network, 2007.

39. C. Beck, Post-Traumatic Stress Disorder Due to Childbirth: The Aftermath, *Nursing Research* 53(4) (2004): 216–224.

40. J. N. Mozingo, M. W. Davis, S. P. Thomas, et al. I Felt Violated: Women's Experience of Childbirth-Associated Anger, *American Journal of Maternal Child Nursing* 27(6) (2002): 342–348, Abstract.

41. D. Bailham and S. Joseph, Post-Traumatic Stress Following Childbirth: A Review of the Emerging Literature and Directions for Research and Practice, *Psychology, Health & Medicine* 8 (2003): 159–168.

42. American Psychiatric Association, *DSM-IV*, Author, Washington, DC, 2000.

43. D. Bailham and S. Joseph, Post-Traumatic Stress Following Childbirth.

44. Birthrites: Healing After Cesarean, *Newsletter*, June 1999.

45. Ibid.

46. VBAC/AVAC Canada, *Newsletter*, Fall 1999.

47. Cesarean Prevention Movement, *The Clarion*, April 1990.

48. Cesarean Voices, K. C. Scott, L. Hudson, J. MacCorkle, and P. Udy, eds., International Cesarean Awareness Network, Redondo Beach, CA: Laurie, 4.

49. Birthrites: Healing after Caesarean, Healing after Your Caeserean, http://www.birthrites.org (last accessed on July 8, 2008).

50. Cesarean Voices, Erica, 19.

51. Birthcut, http://www.birthcut.com (last accessed July 7, 2008).

52. Cesarean Voices, Kim, 52.

53. T. Lavender and S. A. Walkinshaw, Can Midwives Reduce Postpartum Psychological Morbidity? A Randomized Trial, *Birth* 25(4) (1998): 215–219.

54. Trauma and Birth Stress, http://www.tabs.org.nz (last accessed July 7, 2008).

55. Penny Simkin with Phyllis Klaus, Processing the Birth Experience with the Woman. When Survivors Give Birth: Understanding and Healing the Effects of Early Sexual Abuse on Childbearing Women, Conference Proceedings, San Jose, CA: October 6, 2007.

56. C/SEC, Cesarean/Support Education and Concern, Farmingham, MA, formed in 1973.

57. Sharon Storton, Why We Need an Organization Like SOLACE, Solace for Mothers, http://www.solaceformothers.org (last accessed on July 10, 2008).

58. American College of Obstetrics and Gynecology, Vaginal Birth after Previous Cesarean, Practice Bulletin, No. 5, July 1999.

CHAPTER 7

1. M. Kroeger and L. Smith, *Impact of Birth Practices on Breastfeeding* (Boston: Jones and Bartlett, 2004).

2. H. Goer, M. Sagady Leslie, and A. Romano, Coalition for Improving Maternity Services: Evidence Basis for the Ten Steps of Mother-Friendly Care, *Journal of Perinatal Education* 16(1) (Suppl.) (2007): 32S–64S.

3. J. R. Loftus, H. Hill, and S. E. Cohen, Placental Transfer and Neonatal Effects of Epidural Sufentanil and Fentanyl Administered with Bupivacaine during Labor, *Anesthesiology* 83(2) (August 1995): 300–308.

4. American Academy of Pediatrics, Breastfeeding and the Use of Human Milk, Revised, *Pediatrics* 115 (2005): 496–506, http://aappolicy.aappublications.org/cgi/content/full/pediatrics;115/2/496 (last accessed on May 18, 2008).

5. Cesarean Sections May Be Contributing to the Rise in Late Preterm Births, March of Dimes Press Release, March 29, 2006, March of Dimes, http://search.marchofdimes.com (last accessed on May 18, 2008).

6. National Institutes of Health, Report Shows Gains, Setbacks for Nation's Children (NIH WebWire), Webwire, http://www.webwire.com/ViewPressRel.asp?aId=42234 (last accessed on May 18, 2008).

7. K. Levit, K. Ryan, A. Elixhauser, E. Stranges, et al., HCUP Facts and Figures: Statistics on Hospital-Based Care in the United States in 2005, Rockville, MD, Agency for Healthcare Research and Quality, 2007, Healthcare Cost and Utilization Project,

http://www.hcup-us.ahrq.gov/reports/factsandfigures/HAR_2005.pdf (last accessed on May 18, 2008).

8. T. N. K. Raju, R. Higgins, A. R. Stark et al., Optimizing Care and Outcome for Late-Preterm (Near-Term) Infants: A Summary of the Workshop Sponsored by the National Institute of Child Health and Human Development, *Pediatrics* 118(3) (September 2006): 1207–1214.

9. W. A. Engle, K. M. Tomashek, C. Wallman, and the Committee on Fetus and Newborn, "Late-Preterm" Infants: A Population at Risk, *Pediatrics* 120(6) (December 2007): 1390–1399.

10. W. A. Engle and M. A. Kormniarek, Late Preterm Infants, Early Term Infants, and Timing of Elective Deliveries, *Clinics in Perinatology* 35(2008): 325–241.

11. March of Dimes Foundation, Understanding Late Preterm Birth, Background Information for March of Dimes Staff and Volunteers Using the Late Preterm Birth Brain Card, PowerPoint Presentation, Personal.

12. M. F. MacDorman, E. Declercq, F. Menacker, and M. H. Malloy, Infant and Neonatal Mortality for Primary Cesarean and Vaginal Births to Women with "No Indicated Risk," United States, 1998–2001 Birth Cohorts, *Birth* 33(3) (2006): 175–181.

13. K. Levit, K. Ryan, A. Elixhauser, E. Stranges et al., HCUP Facts and Figures: Statistics on Hospital-Based Care in the United States in 2005.

14. P. Simkin, Stress, Pain and Catecholamines in Labor: Part I. A Review, *Birth* 13(4) (1986): 227–233.

15. Coalition for Improving Maternity Services, the Risks of Cesarean Delivery to Mother and Baby Fact Sheet, http://www.motherfriendly.org (last accessed on May 18, 2007).

16. S. Storton, Coalition for Improving Maternity Services: Evidence Basis for the Ten Steps for Mother-Friendly Care. Step 8. Encourages All Mothers, Families, to Touch, Hold, Breastfeed, Care for Their Babies, *Journal of Perinatal Education* 16(1) (Suppl.) (2007): 74S–76S.

17. UNICEF/WHO Breastfeeding and Support in a Baby-Friendly Hospital Initiative, *American Academy of Pediatrics. Breastfeeding and the Use of Human Milk*, 2005.

18. Lamaze International, The Six Care Practice That Support Normal Birth, Care Practice # 6: No Separation of Mother and Baby after Birth with Unlimited Opportunity for Breastfeeding, Lamaze, http://www.lamaze.org/ChildbirthEducators/ResourcesforEducators/CarePracticePapers/NoSeparation/tabid/488/Default.aspx (last accessed on May 18, 2008).

19. E. Declercq, C. Sakala, M. P. Corry, and S. Applebaum, Listening to Mothers II. Report of the Second National U.S. Survey of Women's Childbearing Experiences, New York, Childbirth Connection, 2006.

20. National Institute for Clinical Excellence, Cesarean Section, April 2004.

21. G. C. Anderson, E. Moore, J. Hepworth, and N. Bergman, Early Skin-to-Skin Contact for Mothers and Their Healthy Newborn Infants, Cochrane Database of Systematic Reviews, Abstract, 2003, Issue 2, Art. No. CD003519, DOI: 10.1002/14651858.CD003519.

22. K. Erlandsson, A. Dsilna, and I. Fagerberg, Skin-to-Skin Care with the Father after Cesarean Birth and Its Effect on Newborn Crying and Prefeeding Behavior, *Birth* 34(2) (2007), 105–114.

23. Office of Disease Prevention and Health Promotion, U.S. Department of Health and Human Services, Healthy People 2010, Maternal, Infant, and Child Health, 16–30.

Washington, DC, http://www.healthypeople.gov/document/word/Volume2/16MICH. doc (last accessed on May 18, 2008).

24. U.S. Centers for Disease Control, Breastfeeding Report Card, United States, 2007: P, Outcome Indicators, http://www.cdc.gov/breastfeeding/data/report_card2. htm (last accessed on May 18, 2008).

25. K. Shealy, L. Ruowei, S. Benton-Davis, and L. M. Grummer-Strawn, The CDC Guide to Breastfeeding Interventions, Atlanta: U.S. Department of Health and Human Services, Centers for Disease Control and Prevention, 2005, http://www.cdc. gov/breastfeeding/pdf/BF_guide_1.pdf (last accessed on May 18, 2008).

26. U.S. Agency for Healthcare Research and Quality. Breastfeeding and Maternal and Infant Outcomes in Developed Countries, http//www.ahrq.gov/clinic/tp/brfouttp. htm (last accessed on May 18, 2008).

27. U.S. Agency for Health Research and Quality, Breastfeeding and Maternal and Infant Outcomes.

28. U.S. Breastfeeding Committee, Economic Benefits of Breastfeeding, http:// usbreastfeeding.org/Issue-Papers/Economics.pdf (last accessed on May 18, 2008).

29. Baby-Friendly U.S.A., http//www.bbyfriendlyusa.org (last accessed on May 18, 2008).

CHAPTER 8

1. Childbirth Connection.org, Cesarean Section-Best Evidence, http://childbirth-connection.com/article.asp?ck=10166&ClickedLink=274&area=27#future (last accessed on July 6, 2008).

2. Childbirth Connection, What Every Pregnant Woman Needs to Know About Cesarean Section, revised edition, 2006, http://childbirthconnection.org/article.asp? ck=10164 (last accessed on July 10, 2008).

3. NICE, Cesarean Section, April 2004.

4. Childbirth Connection, What Every Pregnant Woman Needs to Know about Cesarean Section, 2006.

5. Coalition for Improving Maternity Services. The Risks of Cesarean Delivery to Mother and Baby, http://www.motherfriendly.org (last accessed on March 10, 2007).

6. M. Wagner, Cytotec Induction and Off-Label Use, *Midwifery Today* (67) (Autumn 2003), http://www.midwiferytoday.com/articles/cytotec.asp (last accessed on February 5, 2008).

7. ACOG, Evaluation of Cesarean Delivery, 2000.

8. Royal College of Obstetricians and Gynecologists, Guideline No. 27, Placenta Praevia and Placenta Praevia Accreta: Diagnosis and Management, October 2005, http://www.rcog.org.uk/index.asp?PageID=527 (last accessed on July 10, 2008).

9. Childbirth Connection, 2006.

10. C. V. Ananth, J. C. Smulian, and A. M. Vintzileos, The Association of Placenta Previa with History of Cesarean Delivery and Abortion: A Meta Analysis, *American Journal of Obstetrics and Gynecology* 177(5) (1997): 1071–1078.

11. Childbirth Connection, 2006, Cesarean Section, Best Evidence: C-Section, http://www.childbirthconnection.org/article.asp?ck=10166#future (last accessed on July 6, 2008).

12. Coalition for Improving Maternity Services, Cesarean Fact Sheet.

13. ACOG, Evaluation of Cesarean Delivery, 2000.

14. Ibid.

15. D. W. Skupski, I. P. Lowenwirt, F.I. Weinbaum et al., Improving Hospital Systems for the Care of Women with Major Obstetric Hemorrhage, *Obstetrics & Gynecology* 107 (2006): 977–983.

16. March of Dimes, Preterm Birth, Quick Reference: Fact Sheets, Preterm Birth http://www.marchofdimes.com (last accessed on July 10, 2008).

17. March of Dimes, Costs of Maternity and Infant Care, Thompson Healthcare Report, June 2007, http://www.marchofdimes.com/advocacy (last accessed on June 12, 2007).

18. G. C. Smith., J. P. Pell, and R. Dobbie, Caesarean Section and Risk of Unexplained Still Birth in Subsequent Pregnancy, *Lancet* 362(9398) (November 29, 2003): 1779–1784.

19. R. M. Silver, M. B. Landon, and D. J. Rouse, Maternal Morbidity Associated with Multiple Repeat Cesarean Deliveries, *Obstetrics & Gynecology* 107 (2006): 1226–1232.

20. V. Nisenblat, S. Barak, O. Barnett Griness et al., Maternal Complications Associated with Multiple Cesarean Deliveries, *Obstetrics & Gynecology* 108 (2006): 21–26, Abstract.

CHAPTER 9

1. M. Enkin et al., *Effective Care for Pregnancy and Childbirth* (Oxford: Oxford University Press, 2000), 249.

2. M. Sagady Leslie and A. Romano, Coalition for Improving Maternity Services: Evidence Basis for the Ten Steps of Mother-Friendly Care. Appendix: Birth Can Safely Take Place at Home and in Birthing Centers, *Journal of Perinatal Education* (Suppl.) (Winter 2007): 81S–88S.

3. Medical Leadership Council, Coming to Term, Innovations in Safely Reducing Cesarean Rates, The Advisory Board Company, 1996, 87–106

4. E. A. Friedman, Dystocia and "Failure to Progress" in Labor, *Cesarean Section: Guidelines for Appropriate Utilization*, B. L. Flamm and E. J. Quilligan, eds. (New York: Springer-Verlag, 1995).

5. P. Simkin and R. Ancheta, *The Labor Progress Handbook*, second edition (Oxford: Blackwell Publishing, 2005), 15.

6. National Institutes of Health, Cesarean Childbirth, 1981, 331–349.

7. L. Silver and S. M. Wolfe, *Unnecessary Cesarean Sections: How to Cure a National Epidemic* (Washington, DC: Public Citizen Health Research Group 1989).

8. Medical Leadership Council, Coming to Term: Innovations in Safely Reducing Cesarean Rates, Author, 1996, 87–106.

9. Institute for Healthcare Improvement (IHI), Breakthrough Series Guides, Reducing Cesarean Section Rates While Maintaining Maternal and Infant Outcomes (Boston: IHI, 1997).

10. D. S. Gifford, S. C. Morton, M. Fiske et al., Lack of Progress in Labor as a Reason for Cesarean, *Obstetrics & Gynecology* 95 (2000): 589–595.

11. E. A. Friedman, Dystocia and "Failure to Progress" in Labor, in Bruce L. Flamm and Edward J. Quilligan, *Cesarean Section: Guidelines for Appropriate Utilization* (New York: Springer-Verlag, 1995), 23–41.

12. L. L. Albers, M. Schiff, and J. G. Gorwoda, The Length of Active Labor in Normal Pregnancies, *Obstetrics & Gynecology* 87(3) (1996): 355–359.

13. M. Jones and E. Larson, Length of Labor in Women of Hispanic Origin, *Journal of Midwifery & Women's Health* 48(1) (2003): 2–9.

14. World Health Organization, Managing Complications in Pregnancy and Childbirth: A Guide for Midwives and Doctors, Department of Reproductive Health and Research Family and Community Health, WHO, Geneva, 2003.

15. J. Zhang, J. F. Troendle, and M. K. Yancey, Reassessing the Labor Curve in Nulliparous Women, Transactions of the Twenty–Second Annual Meeting of the Society for Maternal-Fetal Medicine, *American Journal of Obstetrics and Gynecology* 187(824) (2002): 8.

16. E. K. Diegmann, C. M. Andrews, and C. A. Niemezura, The Length of the Second Stage of Labor in Uncomplicated, Nulliparous African American and Puerto Rican Women, *Journal of Midwifery & Women's Health* 45(1) (2000): 67–71.

17. Kathleen Rice Simpson, When and How to Push: Providing the Most Current Information about Second-Stage Labor to Women during Childbirth Education, *Journal of Perinatal Education* 15(4) (2006): 6–9.

18. World Health Organization, Managing Complications in Pregnancy and Childbirth: A Guide for Midwives and Doctors, Department of Reproductive Health and Research Family and Community Health, Geneva, WHO, 2003.

19. E. R. Declerq, C. Sakala, M. P. Corry, and S. Applebaum, Listening to Mothers II. Report of the Second National U.S. Survey of Women's Childbearing Experiences, New York, Childbirth Connection, October 2006.

20. MIDIRS, Positions in Labour and Delivery, an Informed Choice, Pamphlet, http://www.infochoice.org, May 18, 2008.

21. L. Fenwick and P. Simkin, Maternal Positioning to Prevent or Alleviate Dystocia in Labor, *Clinical Obstetrics and Gynecology* 30(1) (1987), 83–89.

22. P. Simkin and R. Ancheta, *The Labor Progress Handbook*, second edition (Oxford: Blackwell Publishing, 2005), 16–20, 134–145.

23. P. Simkin and P. Klaus, *When Survivors Give Birth: Understanding and Healing the Effects of Early Sexual Abuse on Childbearing Women* (Seattle, WA: Classic Day Publishing, 2004.)

24. J. A. Thorp, D. H. Hu, R. M. Albin et al., The Effect of Intrapartum Epidural Analgesia on Nulliparous Labor: A Randomized, Controlled, Prospective Trial, *American Journal of Obstetrics and Gynecology* 169 (1993): 851–858.

25. C. J. Howell, C. Kidd, W. Roberts et al., A Randomized Controlled Trial of Epidural Compared with Non-Epidural Analgesia in Labour, *British Journal of Obstetrics and Gynecology* 108 (2001): 27–33.

26. B. L. Leighton and S. H. Halpern, The Effects of Epidural Analgesia on Labor, Maternal, and Neonatal Outcomes: A Systematic Review, *American Journal of Obstetrics and Gynecology* 186 (Suppl.) (2002): S69–S77.

27. E. Lieberman, K. Davidson, A. Lee-Parritz et al., Changes in Fetal Position during Labor and Their Association with Epidural Analgesia, Obstetrics and Cynecology 105 (2005): 974–982.

28. R. M. Brancato, S. Church, and P. W. Stone, A Meta-Analysis of Passive Descent versus Immediate Pushing in Nulliparous Women with Epidural Analgesia in the Second Stage of Labor, *Journal of Obstetric, Gynecologic, and Neonatal Nursing* 37(1) (2008): 4–12.

29. P. Simkin and R. Ancheta, *The Labor Progress Handbook*, 158–160.

CHAPTER 10

1. Coalition for Improving Maternity Services (CIMS), Having a Baby? Ten Questions to Ask. Pamphlet, Author, 2000, http://www.motherfriendly.org (last accessed May 18, 2008).

2. P. Simkin and R. Ancheta, *Labor Progress Handbook* (London: Blackwell Publishing, 2005).

3. Common Knowledge Charitable Trust, *The Pink Kit: Essential Preparations for Your Birthing Body* (New Zealand: Anchor Press, 2001).

4. J. Sutton and P. Scott, *Understanding and Teaching Optimal Fetal Positioning*, second revised edition (New Zealand: Birth Concepts, 1996).

5. Association of Women's Health, Obstetric and Neonatal Nurses. *Second Stage Labor Management: Promotion of Evidence-Based Practice and a Collaborative Approach to Patient Care*, Author, 2002.

6. P. Simkin and P. Klaus, *When Survivors Give Birth*: Understanding and Healing the Effects of Early Sexual Abuse on Childbearing Women (Seattle, WA: Classic Day Publishing, 2004).

7. P. Simkin and R. Ancheta, *The Labor Progress Handbook*.

CHAPTER 11

1. E-mail sent to VBAC.com, September 15 and 17, 2002, with permission to post on Web site.

2. Maternal, Infant, and Child Health Goals 2010, http://healthypeople.gov/document/html/objectives/16-09.htm (last accessed May 20, 2008).

3. Centers for Disease Control and Prevention, Births: Final Data for 2005, in *National Vital Statistics Report*, vol. 56, no. 6 (December 5, 2007), www.cdc.gov/nchs/data/nvsr/nvsr56/nvsr56_06.pdf.

4. H. Goer, M. Sagady Leslie, and A. Romano, Coaliton for Imrproving Maternity Services: Evidence Basis for the Ten Steps of Mother-Friendly Care. Step 6: Does Not Routinely Employ Practices, Procedures Unsupported by Scientific Evidence, *The Journal of Perinatal Education* 16(1) (2007) (Suppl.): 32S–64S.

5. Childbirth Connection, Best Evidence VBAC or Repeat C-Section, http://childbirthconnection.org/article.asp?ck=10210 (last accessed May 20, 2008).

6. M. Enkin, M. J. N. C. Keirse, J. Nielson, C. Crowther, L. Duley, E. Hodnett, and J. Hofmeyr, *Effective Care in Pregnancy and Childbirth* (New York: Oxford University Press, 2000).

7. B. M. Mercer, S. Gilbert, B. Mark, M. B. Landon, et al., Labor Outcomes with Increasing Number of Prior Vaginal Births after Cesarean Delivery. *Obstetrics & Gynecology* 111 (2008): 285–291.

8. R. M. Silver, M. B. Landon, D. J. Rouse, et al., Maternal Morbidity Associated with Multiple Repeat Cesarean Deliveries, *Obstetrics & Gynecology* 107 (2006): 1226–1232.

9. U.S. Department of Health and Human Services, National Institutes of Health, *Cesarean Childbirth*, NIH Publication No. 82-2067, October 1981, 11–12.

10. ACOG, Guidelines for Vaginal Delivery after a Previous Cesarean Birth. Committee Statement, Committee on Obstetrics: Maternal and Fetal Medicine, 1984, author, Washington, DC.

11. ACOG, Guidelines for Vaginal Delivery after a Previous Cesarean Birth. Committee Opinion, # 64, October 1988, author, Washington, DC.

12. Institute for Healthcare Improvement (IHI), *Reducing Cesarean Section Rates While Maintaining Maternal and Infant Outcomes* (Boston: IHI, 1997).

13. B. Flamm and E. J. Quilligan, *Cesarean Section: Guidelines for Appropriate Utilization* (New York: Springer-Verlag, 1995).

14. B. L. Flamm, *Birth after Cesarean: The Medical Facts* (Upper Saddle River, NJ: Prentice Hall, 1990).

15. Institute for Healthcare Improvement, *Reducing Cesarean Section Rates While Maintaining Maternal and Infant Outcomes.*

16. Cambridge Health Resources, Safely Reducing Cesarean Rates, in *Conference Proceedings* (Fairmont Copley Plaza, Boston, MA, June 8–9, 1998).

17. C. Sufrin-Disler, Vaginal Birth After Cesarean, *International Childbirth Education Association Review* (ICEA, Minneapolis, MI, August 1990).

18. ACOG, Vaginal Delivery after a Previous Cesarean Birth. Committee Opinion. Committee on Obstetrics Practice, #143, 1994, author, Washington, DC.

19. ACOG, Vaginal Delivery after a Previous Cesarean Birth. Practice Patterns, #1, August 1995, Washington, DC.

20. B. Flamm, A. Kabcenell, D. M. Berwick, et al., *Safely Reducing Cesarean Section Rates While Maintaining Maternal and Infant Outcomes* (Boston: Institute for Healthcare Improvement, 1997).

21. Ibid., xv.

22. ACOG, Vaginal Delivery after a Previous Cesarean Delivery. ACOG Practice Bulletin Number 5, July 1999, Washington, DC.

23. B. W. Harer, Jr., Vaginal Birth after Cesarean Delivery, Current Status, *Journal of the American Medical Association* 287(20) (May 22, 2002): 2627–2630.

24. M. E. Schneider, Insurers Set Criteria for VBAC Coverage, *Ob.Gyn.News* 40(3) (February 1, 2005): 1–2.

25. D. Mecoy, State's Largest Malpractice Insurer Limits Birthing Choices for Some, *The Oklahoman*, 2005, http://newsok.com/home/theoklahoman (last accessed May 20, 2008).

26. G. Gochnour, S. Ratcliffe, and M. B. Stone, The Utah VBAC Study, *Maternal Child Health Journal* 9(2) (June 2005): 181–188.

27. E. D. Bell, D. H. Penning, E. F. Cousineau, et al., How Much Labor Is in a Labor Epidural? Manpower Cost and Reimbursement for an Obstetric Analgesia Service in a Teaching Institution, *Anesthesiology* 92 (2000): 851–858.

28. International Cesarean Awareness Network, Hospital VBAC Bans Push Record-High Cesarean Rates, Press Release, November 23, 2004.

29. Tonya Jamois, ICAN president, personal communication with the author, October 9, 2003.

30. Northern New England Perinatal Quality Improvement Project, http://www.nnepqin.org/ViewPage?id=3 (last accessed June 6, 2008).

31. Michelle Lauria, M.D., personal conversation with the author, September 10, 2007, and January 22, 2007.

32. Northern New England Perinatal Quality Improvement Project, http://www.nnepqin.org/ViewPage?id=3 (last accessed July 6, 2008).

33. J. A. Martin, B. E. Hamilton, P. D. Sutton, et al., Birth: Final Data for 2005, in *National Vital Statistics Reports*, vol. 56, no. 6 (Hyattsville, MD: National Center for Health Statistics, December 5, 2007).

34. J. Zweifler, A. Garsa, S. Hughes, et al., Vaginal Birth after Cesarean in California: Before and after a Change in Guidelines, *Annals of Family Medicine* 4(3) (2006): 228–234.

35. American Academy of Family Physicians, Trial of Labor after Cesarean (TOLAC). Policy action. March 2005, http://www.aafp.org/online/en/home/clinical/clinicalrecs/tolac.html (last accessed May 20, 2008).

36. Society of Obstetricians and Gynaecologists of Canada, Clinical Practice Guidelines# 155: Guidelines for Vaginal Birth after Prior Caeserean Birth, July 2004, http://www.sogc.org/guidelines/index_e.asp#Obstetrics (last accessed May 20, 2008).

37. Royal College of Obstetricians and Gynaecologists, Birth after Previous Cesarean. Green-Top Guidelines (45), http://www.rcog.org.uk/index.asp?PageID=1913 (last accessed May 20, 2008).

38. ACOG, Vaginal Birth after Previous Cesarean Delivery. Practice Bulletin Number 5, July 1999, Washington, DC.

39. E. Lieberman, E. K. Ernst, J. P. Rooks, et al., Results of the National Study of Vaginal Birth after Cesarean in Birth Centers, Obstetrics & Gynecology 104 (2004): 933–942.

CHAPTER 12

1. H. D. Banta and S. B.Thacker, Policies toward Medical Technology: The Case of Electronic Fetal Monitoring, *American Journal of Public Health*, 69(9) (1979): 931–935, http://www.ajph.org/cgi/reprint/69/9/931 (last accessed May 21, 2008).

2. M. Wagner, Pursuing the Birth Machine: The Search for Appropriate Birth Technology (Australia: Ace Graphics, 1994), 158–159.

3. U.S. Department of Health and Human Services, *Cesarean Childbirth: Report of a Consensus Development Conference* (Washington, DC: NIH Publication # 82-2067, 1981), 14–15.

4. M. Wagner, *Pursuing the Birth Machine*, 159.

5. St. Paul., Minnesota, Health Care Commission 1996, Executive Summary, in *Surgeon General Reports, SAMHSA TIPs, SAMHSA PEPs*, http://www.ncbi.nlm.nih.gov/books/bv.fcgi?rid=hstat6.section.666 (last accessed May 21, 2008).

6. H. Goer, M. Sagady Leslie, and A. Romano, Coalition for Improving Maternity Services: Evidence Basis for the Ten Steps of Mother-Friendly Care. Step 6: Does Not Routinely Employ Practices, Procedures Unsupported by Scientific Evidence, *The Journal of Perinatal Education* 16(1) (Suppl.) (2007): 32S–64S.

7. E. R. Declercq, C., Sakala, M. P. Corry, and S. Applebaum, *Listening to Mothers II: Report of the Second National U.S. Survey of Women's Childbearing Experiences* (New York: Childbirth Connection, 2006).

8. UCSF Medical Center UCSF Children's Hospital, Birth Asphyxia, http://www.ucsfhealth.org/childrens/medical_services/critical/asphyxia/index.html (last accessed May 21, 2008).

9. Z. Alfirevic, D. Devane, and G. M. L. Gyte, Continuous Cardiotocography (CTG) as a Form of Electronic Fetal Monitoring (EFM) for Fetal Assessment during Labour: Abstract, *Cochrane Database of Systematic Reviews* (3) (2006), Art. No. CD006066, DOI: 10.1002/14651858.CD006066.

CHAPTER 13

1. MIDIRS, Breech Presentation: Options for Care—The Informed Choice Initiative for Professionals, http://infochoice.org/ic/ic.nsf/TheLeaflets?openform (last accessed May 21, 2008).

2. Ibid.

3. J. A. Martin and F. Menacker, Expanded Health Data from the New Birth Certificate, 2004, *National Vital Statistics Reports* 55(12) (April 19, 2007), www.cdc.gov/nchs/data/nvsr/nvsr55/nvsr55_12.pdf (last accessed May 21, 2008).

4. A. Jenis, Pregnancy, Breech Delivery, May 10, 2006, http://www.emedicine.com/emerg/TOPIC868.HTM (last accessed May 21, 2008).

5. US. Health and Human Services, *Cesarean Childbirth*, NIH Publication No. 82-2067 (Bethesda, MD: National Institutes of Health, 1981).

6. L. A. Cibils, Breech Presentation, in *Cesarean Section: Guidelines for Appropriate Utilization*, edited by B. L. Flamm and E. J. Quilligan (New York: Springer-Verlag, 1995), 65–93.

7. M. Enkin, M. J. N. C. Kerise, J. Neilson, et al., *A Guide to Effective Care in Pregnancy and Chidlbirth* (New York: Oxford University Press, 2000), 188.

8. New Zealand Guidelines Group, Care of Women with Breech Presentation or Previous Caesarean Birth. Evidence-based Best Practice Guideline, March 2004, http://www.nzgg.org.nz/index.cfm?fuseaction=download&fusesubaction=template&libraryID=190 (last accessed May 21, 2008).

9. Royal College of Obstetricians and Gynaecologists, Management of Breech, Guideline No. 20b, December 2006. http://www.rcog.org.uk/resources/public/pdf/green_top20b_breech.pdf (last accessed May 21, 2008).

10. G. J. Hofmeyr and M. E. Hannah, Planned Caesarean Section for Term Breech Delivery: Abstract, *Cochrane Database of Systematic Reviews* 2 (2003), Art. No. CD000166, DOI: 10.1002/14651858.CD000166, http://www.cochrane.org/reviews/en/ab000166.html (last accessed May 21, 2008).

11. L. A. Cibils, Breech Presentation, 65–94.

12. Royal College of Obstetricians and Gynaecologists, The Management of Breech Presentation Guideline No. 20b, December 2006, http://www.rcog.org.uk/resources/public/pdf/green_top20b_breech.pdf (last accessed May 21, 2008).

13. G. J. Hofmeyer and R. Kulier, External Cephalic Version for Breech at Term: Abstract, *Cochrane Data Base of Systematic Reviews* 2 (2006), http://www.cochrane.org/reviews/en/ab000083.html (last accessed June 21, 2006).

14. Royal of College of Obstetricians and Gynaecologists, External Cephalic Version and Reducing the Incidence of Breech Presentation. Guideline No. 20a, December 2006, http://www.rcog.org.uk/index.asp?PageID=1811 (last accessed January 20, 2007).

15. A. S. Coco and S. D. Silverman, External Cephalic Version, *American Family Physician* 58(3) (1998): 731–738, http://www.aafp.org/afp/980901ap/coco.html (last accessed May 21, 2008).

16. Royal College of Obstetricians and Gynaecologists, External Cepahlic Version.

17. E. K. Hutton and G. J. Hofmeyr, External Cephalic Version for Breech Presentation before Term, in *The Reproductive Health Library*, Issue 9 (Oxford: Update Software Ltd., 2006), available from http://www.rhlibrary.com.

18. G. J. Hofmeyer and R. Kulier, External Cephalic Version.

19. Royal College of Obstetricians and Gynaecologists, Guideline No. 20a.

20. MIDIRS, Infochoice, Breech Presentation.

21. Royal College of Obstetricians and Gynaecologists, Guideline No. 20a.

22. New Zealand Guidelines Group, Care of Women with Breech Presentation or Previous Caesarean Birth.

23. Royal College of Obstetricians and Gynaecologists, Guideline No. 20a; A. S. Coco and S. D. Silverman, External Cephalic Version, 731–738.

24. Royal College of Obstetricians and Gynaecologists, Guideline No. 20a.

25. G. J. Hofmeyr and R. Kulier, Cephalic Version by Postural Management for Breech Presentation, in *The Reproductive Health Library*, Issue 9 (Oxford: Update Software Ltd., 2006), available from http://www.rhlibrary.com.

26. Healthline, Moxibustion, http://healthline.com/galecontent/moxibustion (last accessed May 21, 2008).

27. M. E.Coyle, C. A. Smith, and B. Peat, Cephalic Version by Moxibustion for Breech Presentation: Abstract, *Cochrane Database of Systematic Reviews* 2 (2005), Art. No. CD003928, DOI 10.1002/14651858.CD003928.pub2 (last accessed May 21, 2008).

28. M. E. Hannah, W. J. Hannah, S. A. Hewson, E. D. Hodnett, S. Saigal, and A. R. Willan, Planned Caesarean Section versus Planned Vaginal Birth for Breech Presentation at Term: A Randomised Multicentre Trial, *The Lancet*, 356(9239) (2000): 1375–1383.

29. H. Goer, When Research Is Flawed: Planned Vaginal Birth versus Elective Cesarean for Breech Presentation, http://www.lamaze.org/Research/WhenResearchisFlawed/VaginalBreechBirth/tabid/167/Default.aspx (last accessed January 23, 2007).

30. F. Goffinet, M. Carayol, J. M. Doidart, et al., Is Planned Vaginal Breech Presentation at Term Still an Option? Results of an Observational Prospective Survey in France and Belgium, *American Journal of Obstetrics and Gynecology* 194(4) (April 2006): 1001–19011.

31. A. Kotaska, Inappropriate Use of Randomized Trials to Evaluate the Complex Phenomena: A Case Study of Vaginal Breech Delivery, *British Medical Journal* 329 (2004): 1039–1042, http://bmj.com/cgi/content/full/329/7473/1039 (last accessed May 21, 2008).

32. Childbirth Connection, What Every Pregnant Woman Needs to Know about Cesarean Section, 2006, http://childbirthconnection.com/pdf.asp?PDFDownload=cesareanbooklet (last accessed May 21, 2008).

33. MIDIRS, Infochoice, Breech Presentation.

34. Richard E. Fisher, Emedicine Breech Presentation, July 10, 2006, http://emedicine.com/med/topic3272.htm (last accessed May 21, 2008).

35. L. Sanchez-Ramos, T. L. Wells, C. D. Adair, et al., Route of Breech Delivery and Maternal and Neonatal Outcomes, *International Journal of Gynaecology and Obstetrics* 73(1) (April 2001): 7–14.

36. F. Goffinet, M. Carayol, J. M. Doidart, et al., Is Planned Vaginal Breech Presentation at Term Still an Option?

37. Richard E. Fisher, Breech Presentation.

38. New Zealand Guidelines Group, Care of Women with Breech Presentation or Previous Caesarean Birth.

39. Royal College of Obstetrics and Gynaecologists, The Management of Breech Presentation. Guideline No. 20b.

40. World Health Organization Reproductive Health Library, Managing Complications in Pregnancy and Childbirth: A Guide for Midwives and Doctors. Breach Delivery, http://www.who.int/reproductive-health/impac/Procedures/Breech_delivery_P37_P42.html (last accessed May 21, 2008).

41. Royal College of Obstetricians and Gynaecologists, The Management of Breech Presentation. Guideline No. 20b.

42. P. Simkin, *The Birth Partner*, second edition (Boston: Harvard Common Press. 2001).

43. Acupunture Today, http://www.acupuncturetoday.com/abc/moxbustion.php, December 21, 2006.

44. A. S. Coco and S. D. Silverman, External Cephalic Version, 731–738.

CHAPTER 14

1. Marsden Wagner, *Born in the USA: How a Broken Maternity System Must Be Fixed to Put Mothers and Infants First* (Berkeley, CA: University of California Press), 85.

2. E. R. Declercq, C. Sakala, M. P. Corry, and S. Applebaum, *Listening to Mothers II: Report of the Second National U.S. Survey or Women's Childbearing Experiences* (New York: Childbirth Connection, 2006).

3. J. A. Martin, B. E. Hamilton, P. D. Sutton, et al., Births: Final Data for 2005, *National Vital Statistics Report* 56(6) (December 5, 2007).

4. J. C. Glantz, Labor Induction Rate Variation in Upstate New York: What Is the Difference? *Birth* 30(3) (2003): 168–174.

5. A. Romano, Risk of Cesarean Section Following Elective Induction Is Influenced by Choice of Physician, *Research Summaries for Normal Birth* 2(1) (January 2005), www.lamaze.org/institute/advancing/rsnb/January 2005.asp.

6. Coalition for Improving Maternity Services, Problems and Hazards of Induction of Labor, http://www.motherfriendly.org/Resources.

7. Society of Obstetricians and Gynecologists of Canada, Induction of Labour at Term. SOGC Clinical Practice Guideline, No. 107, August 2001, http://www.sogc.org/guidelines/public/107E-CPG-August2001.pdf.

8. H. Goer, M. Sagady Leslie, and M. Romano, Coalition for Improving Maternity Services: Evidence Basis for the Ten Steps of Mother-Friendly Care. Step 6: Does Not Routinely Employ Practices, Procedures, Unsupported by Scientific Evidence, *The Journal of Perinatal Education* 16(1) (Suppl.) (2007): 42S–45S.

9. Royal College of Obstetricians and Gynaecologists, Green-Top Guideline No. 29. The Management of Third- and Fourth-Degreee Perineal Tears, http://www.rcog.org.uk/index.asp?PageID=532.

10. Society of Obstetricians and Gynaecologists of Canada, Induction of Labor at Term.

11. M. S. Kraemer et al., Amniotic-Fluid Embolism and Medical Induction of Labour: A Retrospective, Population-Based Cohort Study, *The Lancet* 368 (October 21, 2006): 1444–1448.

12. H. Goer, M. Sagady Leslie, and M. Romano, Coalition for Improving Maternity Services: Evidence Basis for the Ten Steps of Mother-Friendly Care. Step 6, 42S–45S.

13. March of Dimes, Induction by Request, http://www.modimes.com.

14. M. F. MacDorman, W. M. Callaghan, T. J. Mathews, et al., Trends in Preterm-Related Infant Mortality by Race and Ethnicity: United States, 1999–2004, *National Center for Health Statistics Health E-Stats*, http://www.cdc.gov/nchs/products/pubs/pubd/hestats/infantmort99-04/infantmort99-04.htm.

15. Intermountain Healthcare, Management of Elective Labor Induction. 2006 Update, http://intermountainhealthcare.org/xp/public/.

16. O. Irion and M. Boulvain, Induction of Labour for Suspected Fetal Macrosomia, Art. No. CD000938, DOI 10.1002/14651858.CD000938.

17. Lamaze International, Care Practice #1: Labor Begins on Its Own, http://www.lamaze.org/ChildbirthEducators/ResourcesforEducators/CarePracticePapers/LaborBeginsOnItsOwn/tabid/487/Default.aspx.

18. Royal College of Obstetricians and Gynaecologists, Induction of Labour, Full Guidelines. June 2001, http://guidance.nice.org.uk/CGD/guidance/pdf/English.

19. Royal College of Obstetricians and Gynaecologists, Induction of Labour, Full Guidelines.

20. NICE, Induction of Labour. Inherited Clinical Guidelines, June 2001, http://guidance.nice.org.uk/cgd/publicinfo/pdf/English.

21. H. Goer, M. Sagady Leslie, and M. Romano, Coalition for Improving Maternity Services: Evidence Basis for the Ten Steps of Mother-Friendly Care. Step 6, 38S–39S.

22. Society of Obstetricians and Gynaecologists of Canada, Induction of labour at Term.

23. Lamaze International, Care Practice #1.

24. Harman, Jr., and A. Kim, Current Trends in Cervical Ripening and Labor Induction, *American Family Physician* 60(2) (August 1999), http://www.aafp.org/afp/990800ap/477.html.

25. Searle, Letter to Health Care Practitioner: Important Drug Warning Concerning Unapproved Use of Intravaginal or Oral Misoprostol in Pregnant Women for Induction of Labor or Abortion, August 23, 2000.

26. ACOG, Letter to the FDA: Citizen Petition, November 1, 2000.

27. FDA. Patient Information Sheet. Misoprostol (Marketed as Cytotec), http://www.fda.gov/cder/drug/InfoSheets/patient/MisoprostolPIS.pdf.

28. H. Goer, Elective Induction of Labor, http://hencigoer.com/articles/elective_induction (last accessed May 22, 2008); Cytotec: Safe for Inducing Labor?, http://parenting.ivillage.com/pregnancy/plabor/0,,6xr4,00.html (last accessed May 22, 2008).

29. Marsden Wagner, Cytotec Induction and Off-Label Use, *Midwifery Today* 67 (Fall 2003), http://www.midwiferytoday.com/articles/cytotec.asp (last accessed May 22, 2008).

30. Tatia Oden French Memorial Foundation, http://tatia.org (last accessed May 22, 2008).

31. M. Boulvain, A. Kelly, C. Lohse, C. Stan, O. Irioin, Mechanical Methods for Induction of Labour: Abstract, *Cochrane Database of Systematic Reviews* 4 (2001), Art. No. CD001233, DOI 10.1002/14651858.CD001233, http://www.cochrane.org/reviews/en/ab001233.html (last accessed May 22, 2008).

32. Royal College of Obstetricians and Gynaecologists, Induction of Labour, Full Guidelines, June 2001, http://www.rcog.org.uk/index.asp?PageID=697 (last accessed May 22, 2008).

33. J. Kavanagh A. J. Kelly, and J. Thomas, Breast Stimulation for Cervical Ripening and Induction of Labour, Cochrane Database of Systematic Reviews 4, Abstract (2001), Art. No. CD003392, DOI 10.1002/14651858.CD003392.pub2, http://www.cochrane.org/reviews/en/ab003392.html (last accessed May 22, 2008).

34. Lamaze International, Care Practice #1.

35. NICE, Induction of Labor, Information for pregnant women, their partner, and their families., http://www.nice.org.uk/guidance/index.jsp?action=download&o= 28989 (last accessed May 22, 2008).

CHAPTER 16

1. Douglas Brooks, M.D., personal communication with the author, August 28, 2007.

2. O. Olson and O. Jewell, Home versus Hospital Birth: Abstract, *Cochrane Database of Systematic Reviews* 3 (1998), Art. No. CD000352, DOI 10.1002/14651858. CD000352, http://www.cochrane.org/reviews/en/ab000352.html.

3. E. D. Hodnett, S. Gates, G. J. Hofmeyr, and C. Sakala, Continuous Support for Women during Childbirth: Abstract, *The Cochrane Database of Systematic Reviews* 3 (2003), Art. No. CD003766, DOI 10.1002/14651858.CD003766; Childbirth Connection, Labor Support, http://childbirthconnection.org/printerfriendly.asp?ck=10178 (last accessed May 22, 2008).

4. E. D. Hodnett, S. Gates, G. J. Hofmyer, and C. Sakala, Continuous Support for Women during Childbirth.

5. Ibid.

6. M. H. Klaus, J. H. Kennel, and P. H. Klaus, *The Doula Book*, second edition (Cambridge, MA: Perseus, 2002), 191–192.

7. M. Sagady Leslie and S. Storton, Coalition for Improving Maternity Services: Evidence Basis for the Ten Steps of Mother-Friendly Care, *The Journal of Perinatal Education* 16(1) (Suppl.) (2007): 10S–19S.

8. DONA International, Position Paper: The Birth Doula's Contribution to Maternity Care, Table 1, http://www.dona.org/publications/position_paper_birth_table1.php (last accessed May 22, 2008).

9. E. D. Hodnett, S. Gates, G. J. Hofmyer, and C. Sakala, Continuous Support for Women during Childbirth.

10. Ginger Breedlove, Ph.D., CNM, written for this book, forwarded by personal communication by Linda Herrick, October 16, 2007.

CHAPTER 17

1. J. Pence Rooks, *Midwifery and Childbirth in America* (Philadelphia: Temple University Press, 1997), 2.

2. Ibid., 128.

3. International Confederation of Midwives, Definition of the Midwife, The Hague, The Netherlands, 2005, http://www.internationalmidwives.org/pdf/ICM Definition of the Midwife 2005.pdf (last accessed May 22, 2008).

4. M. Sagady Leslie and S. Storton, The Coalition for Improving Maternity Services: Evidence Basis for the Ten Steps of Mother-Friendly Care, Step 1: Offers All Birthing Mothers Unrestricted Access to Birth Companions, Labor Support,

Professional Midwifery Care. *The Journal of Perinatal Education* 16(1) (Suppl.) (2007): 10S–19S, http://www.motherfriendly.org/downloads.htm (last accessed May 22, 2008).

5. Childbirth Connection, Preventing Pelvic Floor Dysfunction. Best Evidence: Pelvic Floor, http://www.childbirthconnection.org/article.asp?ck=10197#vacuum (last accessed May 22, 2008).

6. H. Varney, J. M. Kriebs, and C. L. Gegor, *Varney's Midwifery*, fourth edition (Boston: Jones and Bartlett, 2004), 705.

7. H. Goer, M. Sagady Leslie, and A. Romano, The Coalition for Improving Maternity Services: Evidence Basis for the Ten Steps of Mother-Friendly Care, Step 6: Does Not Routinely Employ Practices, Procedures, Unsupported by Scientific Evidence, *Journal of Perinatal Education* 16(1) (Suppl.) (2007): 32S–64S, http://www.motherfriendly.org/downloads.htm (last accessed May 22, 2008).

8. E. Declercq, C. Sakala, M. P. Corry and S. Applebaum, *Listening to Mothers II*, Report of the Second National U.S. Survey of Women's Childbearing Experiences (New York: Childbirth Connection, 2006).

9. Health Services, Technology Assessment Text (HSTAT): Fetal Heart Rate Assessment during Labor, available from the National Library of Medicine at http://www.ncbi.nlm.nih.gov/books/bv.fcgi?rid=hstat6.section.666 (last accessed May 22, 2008).

10. M. Sagady Leslie and S. Storton, Coalition for Improving Maternity Services, Evidence Basis for the Ten Steps of Mother-Friendly Care, Step 4. Provides the Birthing Woman With Freedom of Movement to Walk, Move, Assume Positions of Her Choice, *The Journal of Perinatal Education* 16(1) (Suppl.) (2007): 25S–27S.

11. H. Goer, M. Sagady Leslie, and A. Romano, Coalition for Improving Maternity Services: Evidence Basis for the Ten Steps of Mother-Friendly Care, Step 6, 36S.

12. Royal College of Midwives, Evidence Based Guidelines for Midwifery-Led Care in Labour, *Midwifery Practice Guideline* 1 (January 2005): 63–67, http://www.rcm.org.uk/professional/docs/guidelines_formatted_070105v2.doc (last accessed May 22, 2008).

13. M. Sagady Leslie, A. Romano, and D. Woolley, The Coalition for Improving Maternity Services: Evidence Basis for the Ten Steps of Mother-Friendly Care, Step 7. Educates Staff in Nondrug Methods of Pain Relief and Does Not Promote Use of Analgesics, Anesthetic Drugs, *The Journal of Perinatal Education* 16(1) (Suppl.) (2007): 69S–73S.

14. E. Lieberman, K. Davidson, A. Lee-Parritz, and E. Shearer, Changes in Fetal Position during Labor and Their Association with Epidural Analgesia, *Obstetrics and Gynecology* 105 (Pt. 5) (2005): 974–982, http://www.greenjournal.org/cgi/content/full/105/5/974 (last accessed May 22, 2008).

15. P. Simkin and M. A. O'Hara, Non-Pharmacological Relief of Pain during Labor: Systematic Reviews of Five Methods, *American Journal of Obstetrics & Gynecology* 186(5) (Suppl.) (2001): S131–S159.

16. H. Varney, J. M. Kriebs, and C. L. Gegor, *Varney's Midwifery*, 883–890.

17. K. Johnson, S. F. Posner, and J. Biermann, Morbidity and Mortality, *Weekly Report* (April 21, 2006), vol. 55, no. RR-6, In Recommendations to Improve Preconception Health and Health Care—United States, http://www.cdc.gov/mmwr/preview/mmwrhtml/rr5506a1.htm (last accessed May 22, 2008).

18. March of Dimes, Inducing Labor, http://search.marchofdimes.com/cgi-bin/MsmGo.exe?grab_id=2&page_id=15401472&query=induction&hiword=INDUCTED+INDUCTIONS+induction+ (last accessed May 22, 2008).

19. American Academy of Pediatrics, Breastfeeding and the Use of Human Milk, *Pediatrics* 115(2) (2005): 496–506, DOI 10.1542/peds.2004-2491, http://aapplolicy.aappublications.org/cgi/content/full/pediatrics;115/2/496 (last accessed May 22, 2008).

20. K. R. Shealy, R. Li, S. Benton-Davis, and L. M. Grummer-Strawn, *The CDC Guide to Breastfeeding Interventions* (Atlanta, GA: U.S. Department of Health and Human Services, Centers for Disease Control and Prevention, 2005).

21. M. Enkin, M. J. N. C. Keirse, J. Neilson, et al., *A Guide to Effective Care in Pregnancy and Childbirth* (New York: Oxford University Press, 2000), 221.

22. J. A. Martin, B. E. Hamilton, P. D. Sutton, et al., Births: Final Data for 2005, *National Vital Statistics Reports*, vol. 56, no.6 (Hyattsville, MD: National Center for Health Statistics, December 5, 2007).

23. North American Registry of Midwives, http://www.narm.org/certification.htm (last accessed May 22, 2008).

24. Midwives Alliance of North America, Midwives Model of Care, http://www.mana.org/definitions.html#MMOC (last accessed May 22, 2008).

25. R. Davis-Floyd and C. B. Johnson, *Mainstreaming Midwives: The Politics of Change* (New York: Routledge, 2006), 510–526.

26. M. Wagner, *Born in the U.S.A.* (Berkley, CA: University of California Press, 2006), 5.

27. L. L. Paine, C. D. Dower, and E. H. O'Neil, Midwifery in the 21st Century. Recommendations from the Pew Health Professions Commission/ UCSF Center for the Health Professions 1998 Taskforce on Midwifery, *Journal of Nurse-Midwifery* 44(4) (July–August 1999): 341–348.

28. J. Pence Rooks, *Midwifery and Childbirth in America*, 216–219.

29. American College of Nurse Midwives, Legislation and Health Policy, State Legislative and Regulatory Developments, http://www.midwife.org/state_legislation.cfm (last accessed May 22, 2008).

30. American College of Nurse Midwives, Legislation and Health Policy, http://www.midwife.org/ama.cfm (last accessed May 22, 2008).

31. R. Davis-Floyd and C. B. Johnson, *Mainstreaming Midwives*, 21.

32. S. M. Jenkins, J.D., The Myth of Vicarious Liability. Impact on Barriers to Nurse-Midwifery Practice, http://www.midwife.org/display.cfm?id=495 (last accessed May 22, 2008).

33. Friends of Missouri Midwives, Midwives Licensure Bill Passes Missouri Senate, Press Release, Friday, May 16, 2008, http://www.friendsofmomidwives.org/FoMMHome/tabid/36/Default.aspx (last accessed May 22, 2008).

34. R. Davis-Floyd and C. B. Johnson, *Mainstreaming Midwives*, 21.

CHAPTER 18

1. H. Varney, J. M. Kriebs, and C. L. Gegor (eds.), *Varney's Midwifery*, fourth edition, (Boston: Jones and Bartlett, 2004), 928.

2. M. Sagady Leslie and A. Romano, Birth Can Safely Take Place at Home and in Birthing Centers: Appendix in CIMS–Evidence Basis for the Ten Steps of Mother-Friendly Care, *The Journal of Perinatal Education* 6(1) (Suppl.) (2007): 81S–88S.

3. M. Enkin, M. J. N. C. Kierse, J. Neilson, et al., *A Guide to Effective Care in Pregnancy and Childbirth* (New York: Oxford University Press, 2000), 250–251.

4. M. Sagady Leslie and A. Romano, Birth Can Safely Take Place at Home and in Birthing Centers.

5. WHO, *Care in Normal Birth: A Practical Guide. Report of a Technical Working Group* (Geneva: World Health Organization, 1996).

6. Parenting in Holland, http://www.parentinginholland.com/pregnancy/pregnancy-and-birth/midwives (last accessed May 23, 2008).

7. Mary Zwart (professional Dutch midwife), personal communication with the author, May 5, 2007.

8. Welsh Government Assembly, Realizing the Potential. Briefing Paper 4, Delivering the Future in Wales: A Framework for Realizing the Potential of Midwives in Wales, June 2002, http://www.wales.nhs.uk/documents/briefing-4-e.pdf (last accessed May 23, 2008).

9. U.K. Department of Health, The Pregnancy Book: May 2007, http://www.dh.gov.uk/en/Publicationsandstatistics/Publications/PublicationsPolicyAndGuidance/DH_074920 (last accessed May 23, 2008).

10. New Zealand College of Midwives, http://www.midwife.org.nz (last accessed May 23, 2008).

11. New Zealand Health Information Services, http://www.nzhis.govt.nz/stats/maternitystats.html (last accessed May 23, 2008).

12. S. Buckley, M.D., personal communication with the author, January 21, 2007.

13. Canadian Association of Midwives, http://www.canadianmidwives.org (last accessed May 23, 2008).

14. J. A. Martin, B. E. Sutton, S. J. Ventura et al., Final Data for 2005. *National Vital Statistics Reports*, vol. 56, no. 6 (Hyattsville, MD: National Center for Health Statistics, December 5, 2007).

15. K. C. Johnson and B. A. Davis, Outcomes of Planned Homebirths with Certified Professional Midwives: Large Prospective Study in North America, *British Medical Journal* 330(7505) (2005): 1416.

16. O. Jewell, Home Versus Hospital Birth: Plain Language Summary; Abstract, *Cochrane Database of Systematic Reviews* 4 (2006), http://www.cochrane.org/reviews/en/ab000352.html (last accessed May 23, 2008).

17. W. Y. Pang et al., Outcomes of Planned Home Births in Washington State: 1989–1996, *Obstetrics & Gynecology* 100 (2002): 252–259.

18. H. Goer, When Research Is Flawed: The Safety of Home Birth, Commentary on W. Y. Pang Pang et al., Outcomes of Planned Home Births in Washington State: 1989–1996, http://www.lamaze.org/Research/WhenResearchisFlawed/homebirth/tabid/172/Default.aspx (last accessed May 23, 2008).

19. L. Sagady-Leslie and A. Romano, Birth Can Safely Take Place at Home and in Birthing Centers, appendix in the Coalition for Improving Maternity Services: Evidence Basis for the Ten Steps of Mother-Friendly Care, *The Journal of Perinatal Education* 16(1) (Suppl.) (Winter 2007): 81S–87S.

20. K. C. Johnson and B. A. Daviss, Outcomes of Planned Homebirths with Certified Professional Midwives.

21. M. Sagady Leslie and A. Romano, The Coalition for Improving Maternity Services: Evidence Basis for the Ten Steps of Mother-Friendly Care, *The Journal of Perinatal Education* 16(1) (2007): 81S–88S.

22. American Association of Birth Centers, Position Statement: Legal Definition of Childbearing Center, http://www.birthcenters.org/about-aabc/position-statements/legal-definition-of-bc.php (last accessed May 23, 2008).

23. J. A. Martin, B. E. Hamilton, P. D. Sutton, et al., Births: Final Data for 2005, *National Vital Statistics Reports*, vol. 56, no. 6 (Hyattsville, MD: National Center for Health Statistics, December 5, 2007).

24. M. Sagady Leslie and A. Romano, The Coalition for Improving Maternity Services.

25. J. P. Rooks, N. L. Weatherby, and E. K. Ernst, The National Birth Center Study. Part II. Intrapartum and Immediate Postpartum and Neonatal Care, *Journal of Nurse-Midwifery* 37(5) (September–October 1992): 301–330.

26. J. P. Rooks, The National Birth Center Study. Part III. Intrapartum and Immediate Postpartum and Neonatal Complications and Transfers, Postpartum and Neonatal Care, Outcomes, and Client Satisfaction, *Journal of Nurse-Midwifery* 37(6) (November–December 1992): 361–397.

27. M. Sagady Leslie and A. Romano, The Coalition for Improving Maternity Services.

28. ACOG, Out-of-Hospital Births in the United States. ACOG Statement of Policy As Issued by the ACOG Executive Board, October 2006, http://mana.org/ACOGStatement.html (last accessed May 23, 2008).

29. Katherine Camacho Carr, CNM, Ph.D., FACNM, president, American College of Nurse-Midwives, Letter Addressed to Dr. Douglas W. Laube, M.D., President of ACOG, November 20, 2006, http://www.mana.org/ACOGStatement.html (last accessed May 23, 2008).

30. Jill Alleman, MSN, CNM, president, American Association of Birth Centers, Letter to Douglas Laube, M.D., Med., President, American College of Obstetricians and Gynecologists, November 16, 2006, www.acnm.org/siteFiles/education/AABCACOG11162006.pdf (last accessed May 23, 2008).

31. Childbirth Connection, Letter to Douglas W. Laube, M.D., Med., President, American College of Obstetrics and Gynecology. December 22, 2006, http://www.childbirthconnection.org/pdf.asp?PDFDownload=ACOG-place-of-birth (last accessed May 23, 2008).

32. ACOG, Statement of Policy. Home Births in the United States. http://www.mana.org/ACOGStatement.html (last accessed May 4, 2007).

33. Childbirth Connection, ACOG Place of Birth Policies Limit Women's Choices Without Justification and Contrary to the Evidence, http://childbirthconnection.org/article.asp?ck=10465 (last accessed on July 10, 2008).

34. ACOG, ACOG Statement on Home Birth, Press Release, February 6, 2008. http://www.acog.org/from_home/publications/press_releases/nr02-06-08-2.cfm (last accessed May 23, 2008).

35. K. Salt, Coalition for Improving Maternity Services: Evidence Basis for the Ten Steps to Mother-Friendly Care Step 5: Has Clearly Defined Policies, Procedures for Collaboration, Consultation, and Links to Community Resources, *The Journal of Perinatal Education* 16(1) (Suppl.) (2007): 28S–30S.

CHAPTER 19

1. Coalition for Improving Maternity Services, The Mother-Friendly Childbirth Initiative, http://motherfriendly.org/downloads.htm.

2. M. Sagady-Leslie and S. Storton, Coalition for Improving Maternity Services: Evidence Basis for the Ten Steps of Mother-Friendly Care. Step 1: Offers All Birthing

Mothers Unrestricted Access to Birth Companions, Labor Support, Professional Midwifery Care, *The Journal of Perinatal Education* 16(1) (Suppl.) (2007): 10S–19S.

3. M. Sagady-Leslie and A. Romano, Coalition for Improving Maternity Services: Evidence Basis for the Ten Steps of Mother-Friendly Care. Appendix: Birth Can Safely Take Place at Home and in Birthing Centers, *The Journal of Perinatal Education* 16(1) (Suppl.) (2007): 81S–88S.

4. MIDIRS, Midwife Information and Research Service. Informed Choice, for Women. When Your Baby is Overdue. Bristol, England (2005); MIDIRS, Midwife Information and Research Service. The Informed Choice Initiative, for Professionals. Prolonged Pregnancy. Bristol, England (2005), http://infochoice.org/ic/ic.nsf/TheLeaflets?openform (last accessed May 23, 2008).

5. L. Bricker and J. P. Neilson, Routine Ultrasound in Late Pregnancy (after 24 Weeks' Gestation): Abstract, *Cochrane Database of Systematic Reviews* 1 (2000), Art. No. CD001451, DOI 10.1002/14651858.CD001451.pub2, http://www.cochrane.org/reviews/en/ab001451.html (last accessed May 23, 2008).

6. R. C. Pattinson and E. Farrell, Pelvimetry for Fetal Cephalic Presentations at or Near Term: Abstract, *Cochrane Database of Systematic Reviews* 2 (1997), Art. No. CD000161, DOI 10.1002/14651858.CD000161, http://www.cochrane.org/reviews/en/ab000161.html.

7. ACOG, Fetal Macrosomia. Practice Bulletin No. 22. November 2000, (NGC-3110), online from National Guideline Clearinghouse, AHRQ (withdrawn), http://www.guideline.gov/browse/gawithdrawn.aspx?st=A (last accessed May 23, 2008).

8. M. Enkin, M. J. N. C. Kierse, J. Neilson, et al., *A Guide to Effective Care in Pregnancy and Childbirth* (New York: Oxford University Press, 2000), 187.

9. Simkin and Ancheta, 188.

10. M. Enkin et al., *A Guide to Effective Care in Pregnancy and Childbirth.*

11. M. Sagady-Leslie and S. Storton, Coalition for Improving Maternity Services: Evidence Basis for the Ten Steps of Mother-Friendly Care. Step 1, 10S–19S.

12. NICE, Cesarean Section, April 2004. http://www.nice.org.uk/guidance/index.jsp?action=byID&o=10940 (last accessed May 23, 2008).

13. J. M. Dodd and C. A. Crowther, Elective Delivery of Women with a Twin Pregnancy from 37 Weeks' Gestation: Abstract, *Cochrane Database of Systematic Reviews* 1 (2003), Art. No. CD003582, DOI: 10.1002/14651858.CD003582, http://www.cochrane.org/reviews/en/ab003582.html (last accessed May 23, 2008).

14. A. Grant and C. M. A. Glazener, Elective Caesarean Section versus Expectant Management for Delivery of the Small Baby: Abstract, *Cochrane Database of Systematic Reviews* 4 (1995), Art. No. CD000078, DOI: 10.1002/14651858.CD000078, http://www.cochrane.org/reviews/en/ab000078.html (last accessed May 23, 2008).

15. Maternity Center Association, What Every Pregnant Woman Needs to Know About Cesarean Section, http://childbirthconnection.com/article.asp?ck=10164 (last accessed May 23, 2008).

16. J. M. Dodd, C. A. Crowther E. Huertas, J. M. Guise, and D. Horey, Planned Elective Repeat Caesarean Section versus Planned Vaginal Birth for Women with a Previous Caesarean Birth: Abstract, *Cochrane Database of Systematic Reviews* 4 (2004), Art. No. CD004224, DOI 10.1002/14651858.CD004224.pub2, http://www.cochrane.org/reviews/en/ab004224.html (last accessed May 23, 2008).

17. J. Z. Press, M. C. Klein, J. Kaczorowske, et al., Does Cesarean Section Reduce Postpartum Urinary Incontinence? *Birth* 34(3) (2007): 228–237.

18. Centers for Medicare & Medicaid Services (CMS), The Joint Commission, Pregnancy and Related Conditions: Percent of Patients Who Have Vaginal Deliveries with Third or Fourth Degree Perineal Laceration, in *Specification Manual for National Hospital Quality Measures*, version 2.3b, October 2007, http://www.qualitymeasures.ahrq.gov/summary/summary.aspx?doc_id=11646 (last accessed May 23, 2008).

19. R. L. Nelson, M. Westercamp, and S. E. Furner, A Systematic Review of the Efficacy of Cesarean Section in the Preservation of Anal Continence, *Diseases of the Colon & Rectum* 49(10) (2006): 1587–1595.

20. Childbirth Connection, Preventing Pelvic Floor Dysfunction. Best Evidence Pelvic Floor, http://childbirthconnection.com/article.asp?ck=1019 (last accessed May 23, 2008).

21. National Collaborating Center for Women's and Children's Health. Cesarean Section Clinical Guideline. http://www.nice.org.uk/guidance/index.jsp?action=byID&o=10940 (last accessed May 23, 2008).

22. P. G. McIntyre, K. Tosh K, and W. McGuire, Caesarean Section versus Vaginal Delivery for Preventing Mother to Infant Hepatitis C Virus Transmission: Abstract, *Cochrane Database of Systematic Reviews* 4 (2006), Art. No. CD005546, DOI 10.1002/14651858.CD005546.pub2, http://www.cochrane.org/reviews/en/ab005546.html (last accessed May 23, 2008).

23. National Collaborating Center for Women's and Children's Health, Cesarean Section Clinical Guideline, 2004, http://www.nice.org.uk/guidance/index.jsp?action=byID&o=10940 (last accessed May 23, 2008).

24. Ibid.

25. Royal College of Obstetricians and Gynaecologists, Green-top Guideline No. 30. Management of Genital Herpes in Pregnancy. September 2007, http://www.rcog.org.uk/index.asp?PageID=518 (last accessed May 23, 2008).

CHAPTER 20

1. Royal College of Obstetricians and Gynaecologist, U.K., Making Normal Birth a Reality, Normal Birth Consensus Statement, November 2007, http://www.rcog.org.uk/index.asp?PageID=2230 (last accessed May 23, 2008).

2. L. Lauzon and E. Hodnett, Labour Assessment Programs to Delay Admission to Labour Wards: Abstract, *Cochrane Database of Systematic Reviews* 3 (2001), Art. No. CD000936, DOI 10.1002/14651858.CD000936, http://www.cochrane.org/reviews/en/ab000936.html (last accessed May 23, 2008).

3. Z. Alfirevic, D. Devane, and G. M. L. Gyte, Continuous Cardiotocography (CTG) as a Form of Electronic Fetal Monitoring (EFM) for Fetal Assessment during Labour: Abstract, *Cochrane Database of Systematic Reviews* 3 (2006), Art. No. CD006066, DOI 10.1002/14651858.CD006066, http://www.cochrane.org/reviews/en/ab006066.html (last accessed May 23, 2008).

4. The Informed Choice Initiative, Fetal Heart Monitoring in Labour, for Professionals. September 2007, http://www.infochoice.org (last accessed April 14, 2008).

5. MIDIRS, Mode of Delivery and Events Around the Second Stage of Labour. Professional Pamphlet, http://www.midirs.org (last accessed April 14, 2008).

6. L. Bricker and M. Luckas, Amniotomy Alone for Induction of Labour: Abstract, Cochrane Database of Systematic Reviews 4 (2000), Art. No. CD002862, DOI

10.1002/14651858.CD002862, http://www.cochrane.org/reviews/en/ab002862. html (last accessed May 23, 2008).

7. H. Goer, M. Sagady Leslie, and M. Romano, Coaltion for Improving Maternity Services: Evidence Basis for the Ten Steps of Mother-Friendly Care. Step 6: Does not Routinely Employ Practices, Procedures, Unsupported by Scientific Evidence, *The Journal of Perinatal Education* 6(1) (Suppl.) (2007): 38S–39S.

8. World Health Organization, Care in Normal Birth: A Practical Guide, 1996, http://www.who.int/reproductive-health/publications/MSM_96_24/MSM_96_ 24_table_of_contents.en.html (last accessed May 23, 2008).

9. National Collaborating Center for Women's and Children's Health, Cesarean Section Clinical Guideline, April 2004, http://www.nice.org.uk/guidance/index.jsp? action=byID&o=10940 (last accessed May 23, 2008).

CHAPTER 21

1. Ami McKay, *The Birth House* (Toronto, Canada: Vintage, 2007), 132.

2. Royal College of Obstetrics and Gynaecology, Maternity Care Working Party. Making Normal Birth a Reality, a Consensus Statement, http://www.rcog.org.uk/ resources/public/pdf/normal_birth_consensus.pdf (last accessed on July 10, 2008).

3. Alliance Francophone pour L'Accouchement Respecte, http://afar.naissance.asso. fr (last accessed May 23, 2008).

4. R. Davis-Floyd, Changing Childbirth: The Latin American Example, *Midwifery Today* 84 (Winter 2007): 9.

CHAPTER 22

1. Lamaze International, Why Transparency in Maternity Care Matters: A Fact Sheet for BirthAdvocates, http://www.lamaze.org/Advocacy/BirthNetworks OrganizingYourCommunity/ToolsTipsandResources/WhyTransparencyMatters/tabid/ 530/Default.aspx.

2. The Coalition for Improving Maternity Services, Evidence-Basis for the Ten Steps of Mother-Friendly Care, *The Journal of Perinatal Education* 16(1) (Suppl.) (2007).

INDEX

About the Author

NICETTE JUKELEVICS is a Childbirth Educator certified by the International Childbirth Education Association and Co-Founder as well as Parent Educator at the Center for Family in Torrance, California. A childbirth educator and researcher for over 25 years, she is also an experienced doula. Jukelevics served as Chair and Co-Chair of the ICEA's Cesarean Options Committee and Co-Chair of the Coalition for Improving Maternity Services. Her articles have been featured in publications including *Mothering Magazine, Childbirth Instructor Magazine*, and the *International Journal of Childbirth Education*. Her VBAC Fact Sheet was included in the Institute for Healthcare Improvement's Reducing Cesarean Section Rates While Maintaining Maternal and Infant Outcomes, Breakthrough Series Guide.

About the Series Editor

JULIE SILVER, M.D., is assistant professor, Harvard Medical School, Department of Physical Medicine and Rehabilitation, and is on the medical staff at Brigham & Women's, Massachusetts General, and Spaulding Rehabilitation Hospitals in Boston, Massachusetts. Dr. Silver has authored, edited, or coedited more than a dozen books including medical textbooks and consumer health guides. She is also the chief editor of books at Harvard Health Publications. Dr. Silver has won many awards including the American Medical Writers Association Solimene Award for Excellence in Medical Writing and the prestigious Lane Adams Quality of Life Award from the American Cancer Society. She is active teaching health care providers how to write and publish, and she is the founder and director of an annual seminar facilitated by the Harvard Medical School Department of Continuing Education, "Publishing Books, Memoirs and Other Creative Nonfiction."